Antipsychotic Long-acting Injections

Antipsychotic Long-acting Injections

Edited by

Peter Haddad
Consultant Psychiatrist,
Greater Manchester West Mental Health
NHS Foundation Trust, UK

Honorary Senior Lecturer,
Neuroscience and Psychiatry Unit,
University of Manchester
Manchester, UK

Tim Lambert
Professor of Psychiatry,
University of Sydney

Head, Schizophrenia Treatments and
Outcomes Research Group,
Brain and Mind Research Institute,
Sydney, Australia

John Lauriello
Professor and Chairman,
University of Missouri Medical School,
Department of Psychiatry,
Columbia, Missouri, USA

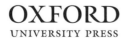
OXFORD
UNIVERSITY PRESS

OXFORD

UNIVERSITY PRESS

Great Clarendon Street, Oxford OX2 6DP

Oxford University Press is a department of the University of Oxford.
It furthers the University's objective of excellence in research, scholarship,
and education by publishing worldwide in

Oxford New York

Auckland Cape Town Dar es Salaam Hong Kong Karachi
Kuala Lumpur Madrid Melbourne Mexico City Nairobi
New Delhi Shanghai Taipei Toronto

With offices in

Argentina Austria Brazil Chile Czech Republic France Greece
Guatemala Hungary Italy Japan Poland Portugal Singapore
South Korea Switzerland Thailand Turkey Ukraine Vietnam

Oxford is a registered trade mark of Oxford University Press
in the UK and in certain other countries

Published in the United States
by Oxford University Press Inc., New York

© Oxford University Press, 2011

The moral rights of the author have been asserted
Database right Oxford University Press (maker)

First published 2011

British Library Cataloguing in Publication Data
Data available

Library of Congress Cataloging in Publication Data
Data available

Typeset in Minion by Glyph International Bangalore, India
Printed and bound by
CPI Group (UK) Ltd, Croydon, CR0 4YY

ISBN 978–0–19–958604–2

10 9 8 7 6 5 4

Preface

The first antipsychotic long-acting injection (LAI) was fluphenazine enantate that was introduced in 1966. Other LAIs soon followed, including fluphenazine decanoate and haloperidol decanoate. The LAIs were developed as a way of improving antipsychotic adherence and became widely used in many countries. However, interest and research in these compounds waned, particularly in the 1990s after the introduction of oral second-generation antipsychotics (SGAs) or 'atypicals'. Recently there has been a resurgence of interest in LAIs. The editors are unaware of any current books that bring together clinical and research findings regarding LAIs. This book was designed to fill this void.

It is worth considering why LAIs have attracted more interest recently. A major factor is the introduction of several SGA-LAIs starting with risperidone LAI, which was first licensed in Europe in 2002 and in the United States the following year. Recently two other SGA-LAIs, olanzapine pamoate and paliperidone palmitate, have been licensed in various countries, and other SGA-LAIs are in development. The introduction of these drugs has been accompanied by the completion of several large randomized controlled trials (RCTs) and observational studies that have assessed their efficacy and effectiveness. In contrast few studies of first-generation antipsychotic LAIs (FGA-LAIs) have been published in the last decade.

Second, several large randomized trials in schizophrenia, including the Clinical Antipsychotic Trials of Intervention Effectiveness (CATIE), have confirmed that although antipsychotics differ markedly in their side-effect profiles they are broadly similar in terms of efficacy in schizophrenia. The exception is clozapine, which is superior in treatment resistant schizophrenia. There is no sign of a major efficacy breakthrough in antipsychotic development. This means that ensuring the optimum benefit from current antipsychotics is important and for many patients this means improving adherence. LAIs provide one way, although not the only way, to improve adherence.

A third factor that may be responsible for the increased interest in LAIs is a re-appreciation of the extent and impact of poor medication adherence in schizophrenia. Although poor adherence has long been seen as a problem in schizophrenia, many thought it would lessen following the introduction of the oral SGAs in the 1990s. This did not happen. Indeed a key finding of the CATIE study was that even in the highly supported setting of a clinical trial, patient retention on a range of oral SGAs was disappointingly short. Recent studies show that poor adherence with oral antipsychotic medication occurs in at least 40% of patients with schizophrenia and is associated with a range of poor outcomes including relapse, rehospitalisation and self-harm.

The issue of terminology warrants some comments. We have used the term LAI (long-acting injection) rather than 'depot' throughout this book. This partly arises because of negative connotations that surround the term 'depot' in some quarters, and we believe any label used should always facilitate a sense of hope for recovery.

Notwithstanding this, the terms are interchangeable and which one is used is a matter of personal preference. 'Adherence' is used rather than 'compliance' to describe the extent to which medication taking matches a prescription. Compliance has been criticized for implying an unequal relationship between prescriber and patient with adherence been seen as a more neutral term. The terms first-generation antipsychotic (FGA) and second-generation antipsychotic (SGA) are used in preference to conventional and atypical antipsychotics although neither pair of terms is ideal. Both imply that antipsychotics can be neatly divided into two classes i.e. FGA and SGA, conventional and atypical. It is increasingly accepted that such divisions have little benefit and that it is preferable to consider a range of antipsychotic drugs that differ on various parameters with tolerability differences being more marked than efficacy differences. Many younger psychiatrists in developed countries will have had little or no experience of prescribing FGAs. For this reason, if no other, terms referring to these two 'classes' are likely to remain in use.

The main advantages of LAIs are that they eliminate covert non-adherence, can improve adherence rates, and can be a more convenient way of taking medication for some patients. Like any treatment LAIs have disadvantages and some patients in particular find it unacceptable to receive medication by injection. In addition adherence can be poor with an LAI just as it can with oral medication. The key difference is that non-adherence with an LAI is overt. Good adherence with an LAI, as with any drug, requires the prescribing decision to be the result of shared decision-making by the patient and prescriber. Prescribing an LAI in isolation will do little to overcome adherence problems. An LAI does not remove the need to ensure that other elements of treatment are provided. The best outcome in most major psychiatric disorders requires an optimized pharmacological treatment foundation to be put in place so that psychological and social treatments can be built around the patient's individual needs for their recovery. This book concentrates on the use of LAIs in schizophrenia as the literature on LAIs is heavily weighted to schizophrenia. In clinical practice LAIs are used in other psychiatric disorders where patients may benefit from maintenance antipsychotic treatment, in particular bipolar disorder. It is likely that in the coming years the evidence base for the use of LAIs in bipolar disorder will increase.

It is hoped that this book will be relevant to a range of health care professionals. We are fortunate that many experts agreed to contribute chapters. We have deliberately tried to give this book an international perspective by inviting experts from a range of countries. This is particularly helpful given the different patterns of LAI use across countries. As far as possible we have tried to avoid duplication in the different chapters although this is not always possible given that some chapters may be read in isolation. We hope that this book will stimulate interest in LAIs and contribute to these medications being used appropriately to help improve outcomes for patients.

Peter Haddad
Tim Lambert
John Lauriello

Contents

Contributors

Chris Abbott
Assistant Professor of Psychiatry,
Department of Psychiatry,
University of New Mexico,
Albuquerque, New Mexico, USA

Laila Asmal
Lecturer,
Department of Psychiatry,
University of Stellenbosch,
Cape Town, South Africa

Niels Beck
Professor and Vice Chair,
Department of Psychiatry,
University of Missouri Medical School,
Columbia, Missouri, USA

Bonga Chiliza
Senior Lecturer,
Department of Psychiatry,
University of Stellenbosch,
Cape Town, South Africa

Pierre Chue
Clinical Professor,
University of Alberta,
Edmonton, Canada

Mathias de Fleuriot
Research Psychiatrist,
Department of Psychiatry,
University of Stellenbosch,
Cape Town, South Africa

Robin Emsley
Professor and Executive Head,
Department of Psychiatry,
University of Stellenbosch,
Cape Town, South Africa

W. Wolfgang Fleischhacker
Professor of Psychiatry,
Biological Psychiatry Division,
Department of Psychiatry and
Psychotherapy,
Medical University,
Innsbruck, Austria

Peter Haddad
Consultant Psychiatrist,
Greater Manchester West Mental Health
NHS Foundation Trust, UK
Honorary Senior Lecturer,
Neuroscience and Psychiatry Unit,
University of Manchester,
Manchester, UK

Samuel J. Keith
Professor of Psychiatry and Psychology,
Chairman, Department of Psychiatry,
University of New Mexico,
Albuquerque, New Mexico, USA

Tim Lambert
Professor of Discipline of Psychiatry,
University of Sydney
Head, Schizophrenia Treatments
and Outcomes Research Group,
Brain and Mind Research Institute,
Sydney, Australia

John Lauriello
Professor and Chair,
Department of Psychiatry,
University of Missouri Medical School,
Columbia, Missouri, USA

Jennifer Nendick
Research Assistant
Academic Psychiatry,
Institute of Neuroscience,
Newcastle University,
Newcastle, UK

Maxine X. Patel
NIHR Clinician Scientist and
Consultant Psychiatrist,
Department of Psychosis Studies
Institute of Psychiatry
King's College London
London, UK

Jan Scott
Professor of Psychiatry,
Academic Psychiatry,
Institute of Neuroscience,
Newcastle University,
Newcastle, UK

Polash Shajahan
Consultant Psychiatrist,
NHS Lanarkshire,
Honorary Senior Clinical Lecturer,
University of Glasgow,
Glasgow, UK

Mary Jane Tacchi
Consultant Psychiatrist,
Northumberland, Tyne and
Wear NHS Trust, UK
Newcastle, UK

David Taylor
Professor of Psychopharmacology,
NHS Foundation Trust
Pharmacy Department,
Maudsley Hospital,
London, UK

Mark Taylor
Consultant Psychiatrist,
Honorary Senior Lecturer,
Intensive Home Treatment Team
Edinburgh, UK

Chapter 1

Antipsychotic treatment and adherence in schizophrenia

Chris Abbott and Sam Keith

Correspondence: cabbott@salud.unm.edu

Introduction

This chapter falls into two main sections. In the first section we provide an overview of schizophrenia and antipsychotic treatment. This includes the course of schizophrenia, the relationship between duration of untreated psychosis and relapse and disease progression, the role of antipsychotics in relapse prevention, and current treatment guidance for antipsychotic treatment in schizophrenia. Unfortunately the goals of antipsychotic treatment are frequently undermined by poor medication adherence. The second section of the chapter provides a comprehensive review of adherence with antipsychotic medication in schizophrenia. Many of the issues will apply to other disorders where long-term maintenance antipsychotic treatment is required such as bipolar disorder. We start by considering how adherence is defined and measured before considering its predictors, an area that is best understood by considering a health belief model. This is followed by a review of the extent and consequences of poor adherence in schizophrenia. We then consider interventions that can be employed to improve antipsychotic adherence, including psychosocial interventions, changes to the oral medication regimen, and a switch to a long-acting injection. The strategy or strategies that are adopted will depend on the individual patient and should be based on full discussion between the patient and doctor. The chapter ends with a brief summary of key points.

The course of schizophrenia

The course of schizophrenia can be divided into premorbid, prodromal, first-episode, and chronic phases. Patients in the premorbid phase often have subtle deficits in cognitive, motor, and social functioning (Fuller et al. 2002; Niemi et al. 2003; Zammit et al. 2004). The schizophrenia prodrome is most often defined retrospectively as a pre-psychotic state that represents a deviation from the usual behaviour of an individual (Yung & McGorry 1996). Patients in the prodromal phase have a gradual onset of symptoms (misperceptions, over-valued beliefs, ideas of reference) prior to the onset of psychotic symptoms. There is often a decline in cognitive, social, and vocational functioning during the prodromal phase (Ang & Tan 2004; Fuller et al. 2002; Zammit et al. 2004).

The psychotic symptoms that characterize the first episode of schizophrenia can have an acute or insidious onset (Harrison et al. 2001). The onset of psychotic symptoms occurs between 15 and 30 years of age for 75% of the patients with schizophrenia (an der Heiden & Hafner 2000). Women have a slightly older age of onset relative to men (Hafner et al. 1998; Jablensky & Cole 1997). Positive symptoms such as systematized delusions and hallucinations are most common during the earlier stage of the illness (Lieberman 1999). There is often a time-limited deterioration with the decline in level of functioning most apparent during the first three years of the illness (McGlashan & Fenton 1993). As the symptoms of schizophrenia emerge during the first episode, cognitive impairment leads to further deficits in social and vocational impairments (Green et al. 2000).

After this initial phase of deterioration, patients with schizophrenia have a chronic, plateau phase. The disease course during the chronic phase of schizophrenia is highly heterogeneous from complete recovery to chronic, disabling symptoms. Approximately one-third of the patients with schizophrenia have relatively good outcome characterized by mild symptoms and mild functional impairment. The remaining two-thirds of the patients have moderate to severe symptoms and severe functional impairment (Bottlender et al. 2002; Harrison et al. 2001; Kua et al. 2003; Mason et al. 1995; Svedberg et al. 2001 Wiersma et al 1998). About 10% of the patients with schizophrenia in the chronic phase have persistent, unremitting psychotic symptoms throughout the course of the illness (Thara et al 1994; Wiersma et al. 1998).

Duration of untreated psychosis, relapse, and disease progression

The original conceptualization that untreated psychosis is 'toxic' to the brain was based on clinical studies showing worsening outcomes with antipsychotic treatment delays or discontinuations (Wyatt 1991). These clinical studies generated the hypothesis that psychosis reduces neuronal connectivity (Norman & Malla 2001; Wyatt 1991). This topic has generated considerable debate. One of the original proponents of this hypothesis later acknowledged that this idea was 'speculative' (Wyatt 1997). Despite this ongoing debate, duration of untreated psychosis and psychotic relapses do appear to be associated with increased disability and treatment resistance (Bottlender et al. 2002).

Initiation of antipsychotic therapy for patients in the first episode of psychosis is often delayed. The delay in treatment is poorly understood but may be related to lack of recognition of the mental illness by the patient and significant others. Duration of untreated psychosis is defined as the time from the earliest manifestation of psychotic symptoms to initiation of treatment (Norman & Malla 2001). The average time from psychosis to initiation of treatment in most communities is greater than one year (Larsen et al. 2001). Duration of untreated psychosis has been extensively studied in the schizophrenia literature with retrospective and longitudinal designs (Norman & Malla 2001). Longitudinal studies assess patients for duration of untreated psychosis at their first presentation and then follow them up for possible outcomes. These studies have a more accurate estimation of the duration of untreated psychosis and allow for better control of possible confounds. A systematic review of 26 longitudinal studies found an association with long duration of untreated psychosis and worse outcomes with symptoms and quality of life in patients with schizophrenia (Marshall et al. 2005). Furthermore, the patients with the longer duration of untreated psychosis were less likely to achieve remission. Early treatment is crucial as studies of treatment–response in early psychosis suggest that the duration of psychosis prior to treatment is a predictor of response to medication (Szymanski et al. 1996; Wiersma et al. 1998). A few studies have documented that first-episode patients have a rate of response to typical antipsychotic drugs at least as good (70%) and perhaps better than in chronic patients (Sheitman et al. 1997).This analysis supports the importance of early intervention for first-episode patients.

Many patients will have a psychotic relapse after their first episode. In a five-year longitudinal study of 104 first-episode patients, the cumulative first relapse rate was 82%, and a second relapse rate was 78% (Robinson et al. 1999). Relapse often leads to a psychiatric readmission and decline in functioning. Recurrent episodes are also associated with symptom chronicity and increased disability (Wiersma et al. 1998). Relapses are also associated with development of treatment resistance in schizophrenia. Treatment-resistant, poor-outcome patients can have progressive functional deterioration and evidence of structural brain changes throughout the disease course (Mitelman & Buchsbaum 2007). Relapse prevention with maintenance antipsychotic treatment is essential to the successful long-term treatment of schizophrenia.

Antipsychotics and relapse prevention

Environmental factors such as community demands, available resources, and treatment significantly alter the disease course of schizophrenia (Lieberman et al. 2001). The effectiveness of antipsychotics drugs in reducing the risk of relapse is incontrovertible and consists of drug discontinuation studies and studies that compare continuous maintenance treatment with intermittent treatment. Multiple studies show that discontinuation of antipsychotic treatment is associated with increased risk of psychotic relapse (e.g. Almerie et al. 2007; Gilbert et al. 1995; Leucht et al. 2003). Gilbert et al. (1995) reviewed 66 discontinuation studies published between 1958 and 1993. The follow-up period ranged from two months to two years (mean 6.3 months). The mean rate of relapse in the patients on maintenance therapy was 16% in comparison with 53% in those withdrawn from medication. Relapse was most likely to occur within the first three months of antipsychotic discontinuation. Almerie et al. (2007) conducted a meta-analysis of clinical trials that compared withdrawal of chlorpromazine with continued treatment for patients with schizophrenia. Chlorpromazine withdrawal significantly increased the risk of relapse across all three periods assessed i.e. in the short term, medium term and long term. Leucht et al. (2003) conducted a systematic review and meta-analysis of randomized, controlled trials that assessed the efficacy of second-generation antipsychotic (SGA) drugs in relapse prevention in schizophrenia. An analysis of six placebo comparison studies, involving a total of 983 patients, showed a significantly lower relapse rate for SGAs versus placebo. It is interesting to note that a further analysis of studies that compared SGAs to first-generation antipsychotics (FGAs) showed that the relapse rate was significantly, although modestly, lower with SGAs (Leucht et al. 2003). It was unclear whether this reflected improved adherence or superior efficacy.

Discontinuation of antipsychotic treatment is associated with not only an increased risk of relapse but also poorer social adjustment, increased disability, and treatment resistance (e.g. Gilbert et al. 1995; Hogarty et al. 1976). The early discontinuation studies showed a relationship between a period of antipsychotic discontinuation and poor social adjustment after patients had resumed antipsychotic treatment (Curson et al. 1985; Johnson et al. 1983).

Studies of continuous treatment versus intermittent or targeted dosing also support the role of antipsychotics in the maintenance phase of schizophrenia (Davis et al. 1994; Kane 1996). Intermittent dosing strategies can be subdivided into fixed intermittent dosing, early warning sign interventions, and crisis interventions. Early warning sign interventions initiate antipsychotic treatment as the patient starts to show signs of a relapse (Herz et al. 1991). Crisis interventions initiate antipsychotic treatment after the patient has developed psychotic symptoms (Gaebel et al. 2002). These studies have repeatedly shown that intermittent therapies are less effective than maintenance treatment in preventing relapse (Gaebel 1994; Gaebel et al. 2002; Kane 1996; Schooler et al. 1997). The results of five such studies are shown in Figure 1.1. Intermittent therapies have also been associated with an increased risk of tardive dyskinesia (McCreadie et al. 1980). In a study of several lifetime medication variables, including cumulative amount of antipsychotics and of anticholinergics, only the number of antipsychotic interruptions was significantly related to tardive dyskinesia (van Harten et al. 1998).

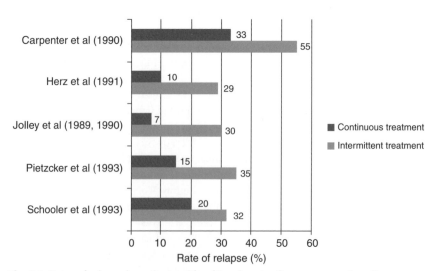

Fig. 1.1 Rates of relapse in patients with schizophrenia after one year of continuous or intermittent maintenance therapy in five studies. Most patients had had more than one prior psychotic episode. Reproduced from Kane (1996) Copyright © [1996] Massachusetts Medical Society. All rights reserved.

A recent study in the Netherlands (the MESIFOS study) assessed targeted treatment versus maintenance antipsychotic treatment in remitted first-episode psychosis (Wunderink et al. 2007). After six months of remission patients were randomized to gradually stop medication, with a view to restarting it should they show signs of relapse (targeted treatment), or to received maintenance treatment. During the 18-month follow-up period, twice as many relapses occurred in the discontinuation group compared to the maintenance group (43% vs. 21%, $p = .011$). The findings confirm earlier intermittent treatment studies in patients with established schizophrenia, namely that antipsychotic medication reduces the risk of relapse but is more effective when administered continuously in comparison to medication administered intermittently.

Antipsychotic treatment guidelines

Various treatment guidelines for schizophrenia are available including those of the American Psychiatric Association (Lehman et al. 2004), the National Institute of Clinical Excellence (2009a), the Canadian Psychiatric Association (2005), and the Royal Australian and New Zealand College of Psychiatrists (2005). These guidelines are more similar than different, and, in the interest of brevity, this section is limited to a review of the American Psychiatric Association guidelines regarding antipsychotic treatment for patients at different stages of the illness (Lehman et al. 2004).

The American Psychiatric Association treatment guidelines for the first-episode of psychosis emphasise diagnostic clarification (Lehman et al. 2004). A thorough and systematic effort at differential diagnosis is mandatory, not only for the identification of potentially reversible neurological and medical causes of psychosis but also because idiopathic forms of psychosis have important prognostic implications. First-episode patients are more sensitive to the therapeutic effects and side-effects of antipsychotic medications. It is therefore particularly important to consider the different side-effect profiles of antipsychotics when selecting a drug for the treatment of first-episode psychosis (Haddad & Sharma 2007).

More than 75% of the first-episode patients will achieve cross-sectional symptom remission within the first year of initiation of treatment (Lieberman et al. 1996). There is debate about how long antipsychotic medication should be continued in first-episode patients. However, first-episode patients who have at least one year of symptom remission while taking antipsychotic medications may be candidates for medication discontinuation. Clinicians working with remitted first-episode patients should engage them in a discussion of the risks and benefits associated with risks and benefits of long-term (indefinite) maintenance therapy (Tauscher-Wisniewski & Ziursky 2002) versus a gradual tapering and discontinuation of antipsychotic treatment and risk of relapse. If the patient elects medication discontinuation, the antipsychotic dosage should be gradually reduced at the rate of 10% per month. The treatment plan should also include additional precautions such as regular follow-ups with a physician even after medication discontinuation. Family members should be educated regarding the importance of identifying early warning signs of relapse (such as changes in sleep, anxiety, depression, ideas of reference) to maximize the likelihood of preventing a full psychotic relapse (Bustillo et al. 1995).

Psychotic relapses in multi-episode patients occur from medication non-adherence, substance use, psychosocial stressors, and the natural course of schizophrenia (Lehman et al. 2004). The patient's history of symptom response and side-effects guides the selection of antipsychotic medication during a relapse (Leucht et al. 1999; National Institute for Clinical Excellence 2009a). The time to onset of antipsychotic action has been debated but meta-analytic studies have shown that response to antipsychotic medication typically occurs shortly after initiation of therapy (Agid et al. 2003). If the patient is not improving, the clinician may consider increasing the dose gradually to the maximum licensed dose, assuming this is tolerated, and continuing this for a finite period such as two to four weeks. If dose adjustment does not improve clinical response, a different antipsychotic should be considered.

Treatment resistance has been defined in various ways. One of the most rigorous definitions is persistent illness and continuing psychotic symptoms despite adequate trials of three antipsychotics and a prospective failure of a high-dose haloperidol trial (Kane et al. 1988). Numerous controlled trials have demonstrated clozapine's superiority over other antipsychotics in treatment-resistant populations (Conley et al. 1998; Kane et al. 1988; Kumra et al. 1996; Pickar et al. 1992). The American Psychiatric Association guidelines recommend a consideration of clozapine for 'patients who have shown a poor response to other antipsychotic medications' (Lehman et al. 2004).

For patients with multiple episodes or two episodes of psychosis within five years, lifetime maintenance treatment with antipsychotics is recommended (Lehman et al. 2004). Some data suggest that second-generation antipsychotics may be associated with greater efficacy in relapse prevention (Csernansky & Schuchart 2002; Leucht et al. 2003). The goals of maintenance therapy include preventing a psychotic relapse and maximizing the quality of life and level of functioning (Lehman et al. 2004). Relapse in the context of a previous clear response to antipsychotic treatment should not necessarily be assumed to represent treatment resistance. A psychotic relapse may be attributable to the natural disease course of schizophrenia, co-morbidities such as substance abuse, and problems with adherence.

Defining adherence

Adherence is defined as the extent to which a person's behaviour matches the recommendations from a health care provider (Haynes et al. 1979). More specifically adherence with medication describes the extent to which the patient's medication intake matches that agreed with the prescriber. Adherence can be applied to health care recommendations other than medication intake. For example, one can consider adherence with dietary advice or adherence with an exercise regime. Adherence and compliance are synonymous but adherence is generally preferred. Adherence is often confused with concordance but the two terms describe different phenomena. Adherence describes a person's behaviour, whereas concordance usually refers to a consultation process in which the patient and health care professional agree on therapeutic decisions that incorporate their respective views (Haynes et al. 1979).

Despite widespread acceptance of the term, operational definitions and measurement of adherence have considerable variability from study to study (Velligan et al. 2006). Further clouding of this concept are the many shades of adherence. Adherence lies on a continuum from medication refusal to non-adherent to partially adherent to fully adherent (Velligan et al. 2006). Patients who immediately decline to take medications are 'medication refusers' to distinguish them from 'medication acceptors' (Velligan et al. 2006). Those who initially accept medications and continue to take them as prescribed are fully adherent. Most investigators define fully adherent patients as those who take their medications as prescribed at least 80% of the time.

Most patients with schizophrenia are partially adherent with their medications. This has been defined as adherence with treatment at least 50% to 80% of the time (Velligan et al. 2009). Partial adherence is difficult to assess and may be related to important outcome measures such as symptoms, relapse, and suicide. Patients may deviate from dosage or timing for unintentional or intentional reasons. Unintentional reasons include forgetting to take a dose, misunderstanding on medication directions, and environmental barriers such as lack of transportation (Velligan et al. 2006). The missed doses may be covert and kept away from staff. Unintentional dosage deviations and irregular adherence may further erode insight and therapeutic alliance resulting in the intentional discontinuation of antipsychotic treatment.

Measuring adherence

Percentage of medication taken, medication possession ratios, and medication event monitoring are used to measure adherence. In a comprehensive review of 161 studies on adherence, indirect methods such as self-report, provider report, significant other report, or chart review were used the majority of the time (77%) to measure adherence (Velligan et al. 2006). These subjective reports are prone to error. In one study, 55% of the participants reported that they were 'perfectly adherent' but blood level data showed that only 23% were adherent (Velligan et al. 2003). Another study compared clinician ratings of adherence with an electronic monitoring device (Byerly et al. 2005). The electronic monitoring device (objective) determined that 48% of the patients were non-adherent, whereas the Clinician Rating Scale (subjective) failed to detect a single, non-adherent patient. Subsequent studies have confirmed that both patients and clinicians overestimated adherence relative to electronic monitoring (Byerly et al. 2007; Velligan et al. 2007). The report from informants or significant others is largely dependent on their time and involvement spent with the patient (Velligan et al. 2006). Chart reviews are largely dependent on the patient's self-report. The inability of patients and clinicians to accurately gauge adherence is likely to have consequences for patient outcomes and argues for different methods of measuring adherence.

Direct or objective measures such as pill count, blood/urine analysis, electronic monitoring, and refill records are also available to measure adherence. Pharmacy-based measures include the medication possession ratio (Sajatovic et al. 2007). The medication possession ratio measures adherence by dividing the number of days' supply of medication by the number of days the patient needed to take the medication continuously. Retrospective reviews of pharmacy refill data have shown a direct correlation between estimated adherence and risk of psychiatric hospitalization (Karve et al. 2009; Weiden et al. 2004). Despite these correlations, the medication possession ratio or refill records may be confounded by the patient's use of samples or old medications that are still available to the patient (Velligan et al. 2006). Medication event monitoring records the time and date whenever the pill bottle is opened. Medication event monitoring is the most accurate measure of adherence and the 'gold standard' for adherence monitoring with other populations of chronic illness. However, studies with medication event monitoring in schizophrenia have high rates of missing data (Velligan et al. 2006). Medication event monitoring studies may be confounded by the cognitive impairment and unstable living situations common with schizophrenia.

The medication event monitoring studies may bias results towards higher level of adherence as the opening of the pill bottle does not necessarily mean that medication happened (Velligan et al. 2006). This is illustrated by a study that measured adherence to metered dose inhalers with a Nebulizer Chronologs (the metered dose inhaler equivalent of the medication event monitoring) in patients with chronic obstructive pulmonary disease (Simmons et al. 2000). Thirty per cent of the patients activated their inhalers more than 100 times in a three-hour interval shortly before a clinic follow-up visit. Self-reported inhaler usage, demographic variables, smoking status, pulmonary function tests, and respiratory symptoms were similar for 'dumpers' and 'non-dumpers'. The authors concluded that 'deception' among the non-adherent is common in clinical trials and often not revealed by the usual methods of monitoring adherence. Covert non-adherence most likely occurs in the psychiatric clinic as well.

The subjective ratings are still widely used in adherence studies despite the 'gold standard' of electronic monitoring. Researchers have improved the accuracy of self-reported medication adherence with the development and evolution of adherence scales such as The Dug Attitude Inventory, the Medication Adherence Rating Scale, and the Brief Evaluation of Medication Influences Scale (Dolder et al. 2004; Fialko et al. 2008; Hogan et al. 1983; Thompson et al. 2000). The Brief Adherence Rating Scale was the most recently developed scale to measure adherence (Box 1.1). This scale was validated with electronic monitoring, the preferred direct measure of medication adherence (Byerly et al. 2008; Osterberg & Blaschke 2005). The Brief Adherence Rating Scale provides a sensitive, reliable, and valid measure of antipsychotic adherence in patients with schizophrenia as compared to electronic monitoring. Furthermore, this scale is simple, quick, and easy to administer making it applicable for clinical settings. Expert consensus guidelines for measurement in adherence studies recommend the use of a subjective ratings and an objective direct measure such as electronic monitoring (Velligan et al. 2006, 2009).

Predictors of adherence

Predictors of adherence may be contextualized in the 'health belief model' (Bebbington 1995). The health belief model is based on four constructs or core beliefs—perceived susceptibility, severity, barriers, and benefits (Rosenstock 1966). This model emphasizes the collaboration between physician and patient in treatment decisions. The patient will weigh the benefits of antipsychotic treatment such as symptom reduction

Box 1.1 The Brief Adherence Rating Scale. This is a clinician-administered scale. The clinician should read aloud questions 1, 2, and 3 to the patient and translate the patient's responses to these questions in the right-hand column next to each question. The clinician then records an overall rating of adherence on the visual analogue scale (Byerly et al. 2008).

Patient Identification: _____   Date: _____

BRIEF ADHERENCE RATING SCALE

The following information is obtained by the clinician:

1. How many pills of _____ (name of antipsychotic) did the doctor tell you to take each day?	
2. Over the month since your last visit with me, on how many days did you NOT TAKE your _____ (name of antipsychotic)?	Few, if any (<7)
	7-13
	14-20
	Most (>20)
3. Over the month since your last visit with me, how many days did you TAKE LESS THAN the prescribed number of pills of your _____ (name of antipsychotic)?	Always/Almost Always (76-100% of the time) = 1
Note: 1 = poor adherence 4 = good adherence	Usually (51-75% of the time) = 2
	Sometimes (26-50% of the time) = 3
	Never/Almost never (0-25% of the time) = 4

Please place a single vertical line on the dotted line below that you believe best describes, out of the prescribed antipsychotic medication (_____) doses, the proportion of doses taken by the patient in the past month.

None					Half				All
0%	10%	20%	30%	40%	50%	60%	70%	80%	90%	100%

Response struck on above line (%) = _____

Rater's Initials: _____

Byerly M, Nakonezny P. (2008) The Brief Adherence Rating Scale (BARS) validated against Electronic Monitoring in assessing the Antipsychotic Medication Adherence of Outpatients with Schizophrenia and Schizoaffective Disorder, Schiz Res, 100 (1-3),60-9.

with the associated costs of antipsychotic treatment such as side-effects. Benefits of antipsychotic treatment are largely dependent on the patient's knowledge about their illness and belief the treatment may have on the severity of their symptoms. The health belief model emphasizes the patient's as opposed to the physician's understanding of illness and treatment (Perkins 2002).

Perceived benefits of treatment are largely dependent on the patient's illness awareness and insight. Insight has been one of the most common predictors of adherence problems (Lacro et al. 2002; Perkins 2002). Insight is not necessarily found in all patients who are adherent with antipsychotics (Garavan et al. 1998). Perceived benefits of treatment also include the therapeutic relationship. The quality of the therapeutic relationship is related to medication adherence (Fenton et al. 1997; Frank & Gunderson 1990). In a cross-sectional and longitudinal adherence study with 162 patients, working alliance was most consistently related to medication adherence (Weiss et al. 2002). Patient satisfaction in the physician–patient relationship may lead to a greater willingness to follow the physician's advice independent of the level of insight of the patient.

Costs of treatment include the patient's perception of medication side-effects. Extrapyramidal side-effects include akinesia, akathisia, dystonia, and dyskinesia. Extrapyramidal side-effects are frequently cited as a reason for medication discontinuation (McCann et al. 2008). Akinesia and akathisia are closely related to patient distress and a negative subjective response to antipsychotic medication (Buchanan 1992; Gervin et al. 1999). The negative subjective response or 'neuroleptic dysphoria' is closely related to non-adherence (Gervin et al. 1999). Other side-effects of antipsychotics include sedation, weight gain, sexual dysfunction, and various symptoms that reflect raised prolactin including galactorrhea and menstrual irregularities (Haddad & Sharma 2007). When patients perceive adverse effects as problematic or unacceptable they may lead to poor adherence (Fleischhacker et al. 1994). On the contrary patients will often continue to take medication despite unpleasant side-effects if they perceive the benefits of medication as outweighing the disadvantages caused by side-effects. A good example of this is clozapine, which is often associated with high adherence and continuation rates despite a range of adverse effects including weight gain, sedation, and hypersalivation (Gaszner & Makkos 2004). It is likely that this is partly owing to patients who were treatment resistant appreciating that they have gained symptomatic improvement since starting clozapine.

Other patient-related factors may contribute to poor adherence. Severity of psychopathology and a failure to respond to treatment are associated with adherence problems (Fenton et al. 1997; Perkins et al. 2008). Paranoia can be detrimental to the development of a successful working alliance. Co-morbid substance abuse is strongly associated with adherence problems (Olfson et al. 2000). Cognitive impairment, especially executive dysfunction, might also be associated with adherence problems (Perkins 2002). These factors are often present in the same patients and may synergistically complicate adherence.

The introduction of second-generation oral antipsychotics in the early 1990s led to speculation that the reduced risk of extrapyramidal side-effects would lead to less improved adherence in schizophrenia (Young et al. 1999). The results were unfortunately equivocal and did not live up to the initial expectations for second-generation antipsychotics (Diaz et al. 2004; Dolder et al. 2002; Gianfrancesco et al. 2006; Menzin et al. 2003). Aside from clozapine, second-generation oral antipsychotics do not have improved rates of adherence compared to first-generation oral antipsychotics. Interventions to improve adherence need to be considered irrespective of which antipsychotic is prescribed (Dolder et al. 2002).

Extent of poor adherence in schizophrenia

Poor adherence is common in schizophrenia. In a longitudinal study of 162 patients, the risk of becoming non-adherent was constant throughout the 22 months of this study (Weiss et al. 2002). The average time of treatment adherence was only 13.3 months. Another longitudinal study followed patients for a period of four years and calculated medication possession ratios to measure adherence (Valenstein et al. 2006). In each year 36%-37% of patient were poorly adherent whereas 61% of the patients had problems with adherence at some time in the four-year period. An often quoted review estimated a medication adherence rate in schizophrenia in 58% (Cramer & Rosenheck 1998). This is similar to another review that gave a median adherence rate of about 50% (Oehl et al. 2000). As mentioned previously, adherence is dynamic with up to 67% of patients being non-adherent for a month or more for some period during a 12-month period (Williams et al. 1999). Overall, about 80% of patients with schizophrenia will be non-adherent at some stage of their illness (Corrigan et al. 1990).

Problems with adherence are not unique to schizophrenia. Virtually all chronic illnesses, such as asthma and rheumatoid arthritis, have significant percentages of patients with partial or poor adherence to treatment (Kyngas 1999; Viller et al. 1999). The National Institute for Clinical Excellence (2009b) has established a set of guidelines for initiating a patient-centred approach that encourages 'informed adherence'. Patients with schizophrenia may have more pronounced problems with adherence compared to patients with other chronic diseases. This may be related to the illness itself. Schizophrenia often involves thought disorder and cognitive impairment, and there is a high prevalence of co-morbid substance abuse, which affects the symptom severity and directly adherence. Finally, the 'missed dose' in schizophrenia is often silent and will not lead to a psychotic relapse until months later.

Clinical consequences of non-adherence

Studies have repeatedly shown that non-adherence with antipsychotic medication has a range of negative consequences in schizophrenia (e.g. Law et al. 2008; Novick et al. 2010; Olfson et al. 2000). The association between adherence and clinical outcomes was recently investigated in a secondary analysis of data for nearly 7000 patients from the European Schizophrenia Health Outcomes (SOHO) study, a three-year, prospective, observational study of patients with schizophrenia (Novick et al. 2010). Non-adherence with antipsychotic medication, as rated by the assessing clinician, was significantly associated with an increased risk of future relapse, hospitalization, and suicide attempts. In another study, Olfson et al. (2000) found that non-adherence was associated with symptom exacerbation, emergency room visits, readmission, and homelessness within three months of medication discontinuation. Even a short period without medication has been associated with an increased risk of admission. An observational cohort study of patients with schizophrenia used pharmacy claims to define days without available medication. Individuals in the first 10 days following a missed prescription refill had a significantly increased risk for psychiatric hospitalization compared with those with available medication (Law et al. 2008).

The consequences of poor adherence can last beyond the psychotic relapse. Patients who have psychotic relapses also have a longer time to remission of symptoms (Lieberman et al. 1996). After the first relapse, patients take an average of 47 days to remission. After the third relapse, patients take an average of 130 days to get to remission. Non-adherence is also associated with increased costs related to both psychiatric and medical in-patient hospital days (Gilmer et al. 2004).

Missed dosages, or patients unilaterally reducing the dose of their antipsychotic, may have a greater impact with the current practice of treating patients with the lowest effective antipsychotic dosage during maintenance phases of treatment. In the past there was a tendency to use higher antipsychotic doses and some even advocated that patients in the acute phase were routinely dosed to the 'extrapyramidal symptom threshold' (the dose at which extrapyramidal symptoms begin to appear with minimal rigidity; McEvoy et al. 1991).

Economic consequences of non-adherence

Relapse is a major contributor to the costs of schizophrenia. In the past relapse usually led to in-patient care. The introduction of assertive outreach teams and crisis home treatment teams in many countries means that today many people with schizophrenia who relapse are managed in the community. Irrespective of this, relapse still leads to increased input from mental health services and as such is expensive. A UK study calculated costs and outcomes by relapse status over a six-month period in a random sample of patients with schizophrenia (Almond et al. 2004). The costs for those who relapsed were more than four times higher than for the non-relapse group.

Several studies have estimated the economic impact of non-adherence in schizophrenia (Knapp et al. 2004; Sun et al. 2007). Knapp et al. (2004) assessed the impact of various factors, including medication non-adherence, on the treatment costs for patients with schizophrenia in the United Kingdom. Non-adherent patients were estimated to be more than one-and-a-half times more likely than adherent patients to use in-patient services. Non-adherence predicted an excess annual cost per patient of approximately £2500 for in-patient services and more than £5000 for total services. Sun et al. (2007) conducted a systematic review of the economic impact of non-adherence in the treatment of schizophrenia. Inclusion criteria were that the studies were in English language, were published between 1995 and 2007, assessed patients with schizophrenia treated in the United States, and assessed the impact of antipsychotic non-adherence in terms of direct health care costs or in-patient days. Seven studies were identified. Despite different measures of adherence, all the studies found that antipsychotic non-adherence was associated with an increased risk of relapse, increased hospitalization rate, or higher hospitalization costs. When hospital costs were extrapolated to the national level it was estimated that the annual rehospitalization cost owing to antipsychotic non-adherence in the United States in 2005 was between $1392 million and $1826 million.

It follows that improving medication adherence in schizophrenia has the potential to reduce relapse rates and direct treatment costs. In the longer term it is possible that improved adherence may also reduce indirect costs. The published literature contains no high quality economic evaluations of antipsychotic long-acting injections (LAIs) and so the cost-effectiveness of LAIs compared to oral antipsychotic treatment remains unknown (Knapp et al. 2002). However several methodologically simpler studies at least suggest that LAIs have the potential to reduce cost. Modelling studies indicate that treatment with an FGA-LAI (Glazer & Ereshefsky 1996; Hale & Wood 1996) and RLAI (Haycox 2005) is cost-effective compared to oral antipsychotic treatment, at least in certain situations, owing to the potential to reduce relapse and in-patient bed usage. Mirror-image and observational studies for both FGA-LAIs (Haddad et al. 2009) and RLAI (Olivares 2009a, b; Olivares et al. 2008; Taylor et al. 2008) have reported reduced in-patient days, or a longer time to readmission, during LAI treatment compared to previous oral treatment suggesting an economic advantage for the LAI. The main weakness of these studies is that financial costs are either not estimated or if they are then only selected costs are assessed. In addition mirror-image studies have various methodological weaknesses, reviewed by Haddad et al. (2009), which include regression to the mean and the effect of confounders that significantly weaken this evidence.

Interventions to improve medication adherence

Interventions to improve adherence to antipsychotic medication include psychosocial interventions, programmatic treatments, and pharmacological strategies. These interventions should not be seen as competing and in practice will often be combined. For example irrespective of whether a patient or a clinician decides to use an LAI or an oral antipsychotic, adherence is likely to be better if the medication is accompanied by psychoeducation and is supervised by an appropriate clinical team/service.

Psychosocial interventions include psychoeducation, compliance therapy, and cognitive adaptation therapy. Psychoeducation incorporates strategies to teach patients and families about schizophrenia, medication benefits and side-effects, and relapse prevention. Psychoeducation and family intervention programmes reduce psychotic relapse and improve medication adherence (Mari & Streiner 1994; Pekkala & Merinder 2002; Pitschel-Walz et al. 2001). Compliance therapy is a cognitive behavioural therapy intervention that incorporates motivational interviewing and psychoeducation to improve treatment adherence. This intervention has also improved adherence to treatment (Kemp et al. 1996, 1998). Cognitive adaptation training targets the cognitive deficits in schizophrenia with environmental supports to improve medication adherence. In a nine-month study, patients continued to have improved adherence months after completing the training (Velligan et al. 2008). Psychosocial strategies may have problems regarding the persistence of their effects if regular 'top-ups' are not supplied, and not all authors agree that the benefits on improved adherence are clear (Nose et al. 2003; Zygmunt et al. 2002).

An example of programmatic interventions that have improved adherence is the assertive community treatment. Assertive community treatment is a team-based, intensive case management intended to reduce hospitalizations and improve the level of functioning in patients with schizophrenia. This form of intensive case management has also improved medication adherence (Bush et al. 1990; Marshall et al. 2000).

Pharmacological interventions to improve adherence include close monitoring for medication side-effects, simplification of medication regimens, considering agents with longer plasma half-lives, and switching to antipsychotic LAIs also known as 'depots'. The LAIs were developed to mitigate the widespread problem of non-adherence and partial adherence. Available antipsychotic LAIs include first-generation antipsychotics and second-generation antipsychotics. Several new, second-generation long-acting antipsychotics are in the later stages of development and are likely to be licensed in the coming years. Expert consensus guidelines for the treatment of schizophrenia including those of the American Psychiatric Association (Lehman et al. 2004), the National Institute of Clinical Excellence (2009a), the Canadian Psychiatric Association (2005), and the Royal Australian and New Zealand College of Psychiatrists (2005) recommend offering a long-acting injectable antipsychotic to patients in whom avoiding non-adherence is a priority. The decision to use an LAI should be made on an individual patient basis. Where possible, the patient should be fully involved in the decision-making process, even when community-treatment orders or other medico-legal constraints pertain.

Summary and conclusions

Schizophrenia follows a highly variable course but for most patients it is a chronic relapsing condition. The benefit of antipsychotic medication in preventing relapse is shown by both discontinuation studies and intermittent versus continuous maintenance studies. Despite this, poor adherence to antipsychotic medication is common in schizophrenia, as it is, with 'maintenance medication' in many chronic medical disorders such as hypertension and chronic obstructive airways disease. Adherence exists on a spectrum with most patients showing intermittent adherence. Non-adherence can be unintentional or intentional. Antipsychotic non-adherence leads to an increased risk of relapse, hospitalization, and self-harm. Relapse also worsens the longer-term prognosis of patients with schizophrenia; both relapse and duration of untreated psychosis are associated with increased disability and treatment resistance. Poor adherence is best understood in the context of a health belief model. Disease-related symptoms such as cognitive impairment and poor reality testing may limit a patient's ability to perceive the benefits of antipsychotic therapy; however side-effects may also promote non-adherence. The clinician can use a range of interventions to improve adherence including psychosocial interventions, programmatic treatments, and pharmacological strategies including an LAI. Often a combination of these approaches will be appropriate. The approach that is adopted will depend on the individual patient and should be made jointly by the patient and clinician.

References

Agid O, Kapur S, Arenovich T, Zipursky RB. (2003). Delayed-onset hypothesis of antipsychotic action: a hypothesis tested and rejected. *Arch Gen Psychiatry*, **60**(12), 1228–35.

Almerie MQ, Alkhateeb H, Essali A, Matar HE, Rezk E. (2007). Cessation of medication for people with schizophrenia already stable on chlorpromazine. *Cochrane Database Syst Rev*, **24**(1), CD006329.

Almond S, Knapp M, Francois C, Toumi M, Brugha T. (2004). Relapse in schizophrenia: costs, clinical outcomes and quality of life. *Br J Psychiatry*, **184**, 346–51.

an der Heiden W, Hafner H. (2000). The epidemiology of onset and course of schizophrenia. *Eur Arch Psychiatry Clin Neurosci*, **250**(6), 292–303.

Ang YG, Tan HY. (2004). Academic deterioration prior to first episode schizophrenia in young Singaporean males. *Psychiatry Res*, **121**(3), 303–7.

Bebbington PE. (1995). The content and context of compliance. *Int Clin Psychopharmacol*, **9** (Suppl 5), 41–50.

Bottlender R, Sato T, Jager M, Groll C, Strauss A, Moller HJ. (2002). The impact of duration of untreated psychosis and premorbid functioning on outcome of first inpatient treatment in schizophrenic and schizoaffective patients. *Eur Arch Psychiatry Clin Neurosci*, **252**(5), 226–31.

Buchanan A. (1992). A two-year prospective study of treatment compliance in patients with schizophrenia. *Psychol Med*, **22**(3), 787–97.

Bush CT, Langford MW, Rosen P, Gott W. (1990). Operation outreach: intensive case management for severely psychiatrically disabled adults. *Hosp Community Psychiatry*, **41**(6), 647–9; discussion 649–51.

Bustillo J, Buchanan RW, Carpenter WT, Jr. (1995). Prodromal symptoms vs. early warning signs and clinical action in schizophrenia. *Schizophr Bull*, **21**(4), 553–9.

Byerly M, Fisher R, Whatley K, Holland R, Varghese F, Carmody T, et al. (2005). A comparison of electronic monitoring vs. clinician rating of antipsychotic adherence in outpatients with schizophrenia. *Psychiatry Res*, **133**(2–3), 129–33.

Byerly MJ, Nakonezny PA, Rush AJ. (2008). The Brief Adherence Rating Scale (BARS) validated against electronic monitoring in assessing the antipsychotic medication adherence of outpatients with schizophrenia and schizoaffective disorder. *Schizophr Res*, **100**(1–3), 60–9.

Byerly MJ, Thompson A, Carmody T, Bugno R, Erwin T, Kashner M, et al. (2007). Validity of electronically monitored medication adherence and conventional adherence measures in schizophrenia. *Psychiatr Serv*, **58**(6), 844–7.

Canadian Psychiatric Association. (2005). Clinical and Practical Guidelines: treatment of schizophrenia. *Can J Psychiatry*, **50**(Suppl 1), 7S–56S.

Conley RR, Tamminga CA, Bartko JJ, Richardson C, Peszke M, Lingle J, et al. (1998). Olanzapine compared with chlorpromazine in treatment-resistant schizophrenia. *Am J Psychiatry*, **155**(7), 914–20.

Corrigan PW, Liberman RP, Engel JD. (1990). From noncompliance to collaboration in the treatment of schizophrenia. *Hosp Community Psychiatry*, **41**(11), 1203–11.

Cramer JA, Rosenheck R. (1998). Compliance with medication regimens for mental and physical disorders. *Psychiatr Serv*, **49**(2), 196–201.

Csernansky JG, Schuchart EK. (2002). Relapse and rehospitalisation rates in patients with schizophrenia: effects of second generation antipsychotics. *CNS Drugs*, **16**(7), 473–84.

Curson DA, Barnes TR, Bamber RW, Platt SD, Hirsch SR, Duffy JC. (1985). Long-term depot maintenance of chronic schizophrenic out-patients: the seven year follow-up of the Medical Research Council fluphenazine/placebo trial. III. Relapse postponement or relapse prevention? The implications for long-term outcome. *Br J Psychiatry*, **146**, 474–80.

Davis JM, Matalon L, Watanabe MD, Blake L, Metalon L. (1994). Depot antipsychotic drugs. Place in therapy. *Drugs*, **47**(5), 741–73.

Diaz E, Neuse E, Sullivan MC, Pearsall HR, Woods, SW. (2004). Adherence to conventional and atypical antipsychotics after hospital discharge. *J Clin Psychiatry*, **65**(3), 354–60.

Dolder CR, Lacro JP, Dunn, LB, Jeste DV. (2002). Antipsychotic medication adherence: is there a difference between typical and atypical agents? *Am J Psychiatry*, **159**(1), 103–8.

Dolder CR, Lacro JP, Warren KA, Golshan S, Perkins DO, Jeste, DV. (2004). Brief evaluation of medication influences and beliefs: development and testing of a brief scale for medication adherence. *J Clin Psychopharmacol*, **24**(4), 404–9.

Fenton WS, Blyler CR, Heinssen RK. (1997). Determinants of medication compliance in schizophrenia: empirical and clinical findings. *Schizophr Bull*, **23**(4), 637–51.

Fialko L, Garety PA, Kuipers E, Dunn G, Bebbington PE, Fowler D, et al. (2008). A large-scale validation study of the Medication Adherence Rating Scale (MARS). *Schizophr Res*, **100**(1–3), 53–9.

Fleischhacker WW, Meise U, Gunther V, Kurz, M. (1994). Compliance with antipsychotic drug treatment: influence of side effects. *Acta Psychiatr Scand*, **89**(Suppl 382), 11–15.

Frank AF, Gunderson JG. (1990). The role of the therapeutic alliance in the treatment of schizophrenia. Relationship to course and outcome. *Arch Gen Psychiatry*, **47**(3), 228–36.

Fuller R, Nopoulos P, Arndt S, O'Leary D, Ho BC, Andreasen NC. (2002). Longitudinal assessment of premorbid cognitive functioning in patients with schizophrenia through examination of standardized scholastic test performance. *Am J Psychiatry*, **159**(7), 1183–9.

Gaebel W. (1994). Intermittent medication—an alternative? *Acta Psychiatr Scand*, **89**(Suppl 382), 33–8.

Gaebel W, Janner M, Frommann N, Pietzcker A, Kopcke W, Linden M, et al. (2002). First vs multiple episode schizophrenia: two-year outcome of intermittent and maintenance medication strategies. *Schizophr Res*, **53**(1–2), 145–59.

Garavan J, Browne S, Gervin M, Lane A, Larkin C, O'Callaghan, E. (1998). Compliance with neuroleptic medication in outpatients with schizophrenia; relationship to subjective response to neuroleptics; attitudes to medication and insight. *Compr Psychiatry*, **39**(4), 215–19.

Gaszner P, Makkos Z. (2004). Clozapine maintenance therapy in schizophrenia. *Prog Neuropsychopharmacol Biol Psychiatry*, **28**(3), 465–69.

Gervin M, Browne S, Garavan J, Roe M, Larkin C, O'Callaghan, E. (1999). Dysphoric subjective response to neuroleptics in schizophrenia: relationship to extrapyramidal side effects and symptomatology. *Eur Psychiatry*, **14**(7), 405–9.

Gianfrancesco FD, Rajagopalan K, Sajatovic M, Wang, RH. (2006). Treatment adherence among patients with schizophrenia treated with atypical and typical antipsychotics. *Psychiatry Res*, **144**(2–3), 177–89.

Gilbert PL, Harris MJ, McAdams LA, Jeste, DV. (1995). Neuroleptic withdrawal in schizophrenic patients. A review of the literature. *Arch Gen Psychiatry*, **52**(3), 173–88.

Gilmer TP, Dolder CR, Lacro JP, Folsom DP, Lindamer L, Garcia P, et al. (2004). Adherence to treatment with antipsychotic medication and health care costs among Medicaid beneficiaries with schizophrenia. *Am J Psychiatry*, **161**(4), 692–9.

Glazer WM, Ereshefsky L. (1996). A pharmacoeconomic model of outpatient antipsychotic therapy in 'revolving door' schizophrenic patients. *J Clin Psychiatry*,**57**(8), 337–45.

Green MF, Kern RS, Braff DL, Mintz J. (2000). Neurocognitive deficits and functional outcome in schizophrenia: are we measuring the 'right stuff'? *Schizophr Bull*, **26**(1), 119–36.

Haddad PM, Sharma SG. (2007). Adverse effects of atypical antipsychotics: differential risk and clinical implications. *CNS Drugs*, **21**(11), 911–36.

Haddad PM, Taylor M, Niaz OM. (2009). First-generation antipsychotic long-acting injections v. oral antipsychotics in schizophrenia: systematic review of randomised controlled trials and observational studies. *Br J Psychiatry*, **195**, S20–8.

Hafner H, an der Heiden W, Behrens S, Gattaz WF, Hambrecht M, Loffler W, et al. (1998). Causes and consequences of the gender difference in age at onset of schizophrenia. *Schizophr Bull*, **24**(1), 99–113.

Hale AS, Wood C. (1996). Comparison of direct treatment costs for schizophrenia using oral or depot neuroleptics. *Br J Med Econ*, **10**, 37–45.

Harrison G Hopper K, Craig T, Laska E, Siegel C, Wanderling J, et al. (2001). Recovery from psychotic illness: a 15- and 25-year international follow-up study. *Br J Psychiatry*, **178**, 506–17.

Haycox A. (2005). Pharmacoeconomics of long-acting risperidone: results and validity of cost-effectiveness models. *Pharmacoeconomics*, **23**(Suppl 1), 3–16.

Haynes RB, Sackett DL, Taylor DW (eds.) (1979). *Compliance in Health Care*. Baltimore, MD: Johns Hopkins University Press.

Herz MI, Glazer WM, Mostert, MA, Sheard MA, Szymanski HV, Hafez H, et al. (1991). Intermittent vs maintenance medication in schizophrenia. Two-year results. *Arch Gen Psychiatry*, **48**(4), 333–9.

Hogan TP, Awad AG, Eastwood R. (1983). A self-report scale predictive of drug compliance in schizophrenics: reliability and discriminative validity. *Psychol Med*, **13**(1), 177–83.

Hogarty GE, Ulrich RF, Mussare F, Aristigueta N. (1976). Drug discontinuation among long term, successfully maintained schizophrenic outpatients. *Dis Nerv Syst*, **37**(9), 494–500.

Jablensky A, Cole SW. (1997). Is the earlier age at onset of schizophrenia in males a confounded finding? Results from a cross-cultural investigation. *Br J Psychiatry*, **170**, 234–40.

Johnson DA, Pasterski G, Ludlow JM, Street K, Taylor RD. (1983). The discontinuance of maintenance neuroleptic therapy in chronic schizophrenic patients: drug and social consequences. *Acta Psychiatr Scand*, **67**(5), 339–52.

Jolley AG, Hirsch SR, Morrison E, McRink A, Wilson L. (1990). Trial of brief intermittent neuroleptic prophylaxis for selected schizophrenic outpatients: clinical and social outcome at two years. *BMJ*, **301**(6756), 837–42.

Kane JM. (1996). Schizophrenia. *N Engl J Med*, **334**(1), 34–41.

Kane J, Honigfeld G, Singer J, Meltzer H. (1988). Clozapine for the treatment-resistant schizophrenic. A double-blind comparison with chlorpromazine. *Arch Gen Psychiatry*, **45**(9), 789–96.

Karve S, Cleves MA, Helm M, Hudson TJ, West DS, Martin BC. (2009). Good and poor adherence: optimal cut-point for adherence measures using administrative claims data. *Curr Med Res Opin*, **25**(9), 2303–10.

Kemp R, Hayward P, Applewhaite G, Everitt B, David A. (1996). Compliance therapy in psychotic patients: randomised controlled trial. *BMJ*, **312**(7027), 345–9.

Kemp R, Kirov G, Everitt B, Hayward P, David A. (1998). Randomised controlled trial of compliance therapy. 18-month follow-up. *Br J Psychiatry*, **172**, 413–19.

Knapp M, Ilson S, David A. (2002). Depot antipsychotic preparations in schizophrenia: the state of the economic evidence. *Int Clin Psychopharmacol*, **17**(3), 135–40.

Knapp M, King D, Pugner K, Lapuerta P. (2004). Non-adherence to antipsychotic medication regimens: associations with resource use and costs. *Br J Psychiatry*, **184**, 509–16.

Kua J, Wong KE, Kua EH, Tsoi WF. (2003). A 20-year follow-up study on schizophrenia in Singapore. *Acta Psychiatr Scand*, **108**(2), 118–25.

Kumra S, Frazier JA, Jacobsen LK, McKenna K, Gordon CT, Lenane MC, et al. (1996). Childhood-onset schizophrenia. A double-blind clozapine-haloperidol comparison. *Arch Gen Psychiatry*, **53**(12), 1090–7.

Kyngas HA. (1999). Compliance of adolescents with asthma. *Nurs Health Sci*, **1**(3), 195–202.

Lacro JP, Dunn LB, Dolder CR, Leckband SG, Jeste, DV. (2002). Prevalence of and risk factors for medication nonadherence in patients with schizophrenia: a comprehensive review of recent literature. *J Clin Psychiatry*, **63**(10), 892–909.

Larsen TK, Friis S, Haahr U, Joa I, Johannessen JO, Melle I, et al. (2001). Early detection and intervention in first-episode schizophrenia: a critical review. *Acta Psychiatr Scand*, **103**(5), 323–34.

Law MR, Soumerai SB, Ross-Degnan D, Adams AS. (2008). A longitudinal study of medication nonadherence and hospitalization risk in schizophrenia. *J Clin Psychiatry*, **69**(1), 47–53.

Lehman AF, Lieberman JA, Dixon LB, McGlashan TH, Miller AL, Perkins DO, et al. (2004). Practice guideline for the treatment of patients with schizophrenia, second edition. *Am J Psychiatry*, **161**(Suppl 2), 1–56.

Leucht S, Barnes TR, Kissling W, Engel, RR, Correll C, Kane JM. (2003). Relapse prevention in schizophrenia with new-generation antipsychotics: a systematic review and exploratory meta-analysis of randomized, controlled trials. *Am J Psychiatry*, **160**(7), 1209–22.

Leucht S, Pitschel-Walz G, Abraham D, Kissling W. (1999). Efficacy and extrapyramidal side-effects of the new antipsychotics olanzapine, quetiapine, risperidone, and sertindole compared to conventional antipsychotics and placebo. A meta-analysis of randomized controlled trials. *Schizophr Res*, **35**(1), 51–68.

Lieberman JA. (1999). Is schizophrenia a neurodegenerative disorder? A clinical and neurobiological perspective. *Biol Psychiatry*, **46**(6), 729–39.

Lieberman JA, Alvir JM, Koreen A, Geisler S, Chakos M, Sheitman B, et al. (1996). Psychobiologic correlates of treatment response in schizophrenia. *Neuropsychopharmacology*, **14** (Suppl 3), 13S–21S.

Lieberman JA, Koreen AR, Chakos M, Sheitman B, Woerner M, Alvir JM, et al. (1996). Factors influencing treatment response and outcome of first-episode schizophrenia: implications for understanding the pathophysiology of schizophrenia. *J Clin Psychiatry*, **57** (Suppl 9), 5–9.

Lieberman JA, Perkins D, Belger A, Chakos M, Jarskog F, Boteva K, et al. (2001). The early stages of schizophrenia: speculations on pathogenesis, pathophysiology, and therapeutic approaches. *Biol Psychiatry*, **50**(11), 884–97.

Mari JJ, Streiner DL. (1994). An overview of family interventions and relapse on schizophrenia: meta-analysis of research findings. *Psychol Med*, **24**(3), 565–78.

Marshall M, Lewis S, Lockwood A, Drake R, Jones P, Croudace T. (2005). Association between duration of untreated psychosis and outcome in cohorts of first-episode patients: a systematic review. *Arch Gen Psychiatry*, **62**(9), 975–83.

Marshall M, Lockwood A, Bradley C, Adams C, Joy C, Fenton M. (2000). Unpublished rating scales: a major source of bias in randomised controlled trials of treatments for schizophrenia. *Br J Psychiatry*, **176**, 249–52.

Mason P, Harrison G, Glazebrook C, Medley I, Dalkin T, Croudace T. (1995). Characteristics of outcome in schizophrenia at 13 years. *Br J Psychiatry*, **167**, 596–603.

McCann TV, Boardman G, Clark E, Lu S. (2008). Risk profiles for non-adherence to antipsychotic medications. *J Psychiatr Ment Health Nurs*, **15**(8), 622–9.

McCreadie RG, Dingwall JM, Wiles DH, Heykants JJ. (1980). Intermittent pimozide versus fluphenazine decanoate as maintenance therapy in chronic schizophrenia. *Br J Psychiatry*, **137**, 510–17.

McEvoy JP, Hogarty GE, Steingard S. (1991). Optimal dose of neuroleptic in acute schizophrenia. A controlled study of the neuroleptic threshold and higher haloperidol dose. *Arch Gen Psychiatry*, **48**(8), 739–45.

McGlashan TH, Fenton WS. (1993). Subtype progression and pathophysiologic deterioration in early schizophrenia. *Schizophr Bull*, **19**(1), 71–84.

Menzin J, Boulanger L, Friedman M, Mackell J, Lloyd JR. (2003). Treatment adherence associated with conventional and atypical antipsychotics in a large state Medicaid program. *Psychiatr Serv*, **54**(5), 719–23.

Mitelman SA, Buchsbaum MS. (2007). Very poor outcome schizophrenia: clinical and neuroimaging aspects. *Int Rev Psychiatry*, **19**(4), 345–57.

National Institute for Clinical Excellence. (2009a). *Clinical Guideline 82. Core interventions in the treatment and management of schizophrenia in primary and secondary care*, Issue Date March 2009, from http://www.nice.org.uk/nicemedia/pdf/CG82QuickRefGuide.pdf (accessed 7 May, 2010).

National Institute for Clinical Excellence. (2009b): Medicines Adherence [Electronic (2009). Version], *NICE Clinical Guideline 76* from www.nice.org.uk (accessed 7 May, 2010).

Niemi LT, Suvisaari JM, Tuulio-Henriksson A, Lonnqvist JK. (2003). Childhood developmental abnormalities in schizophrenia: evidence from high-risk studies. *Schizophr Res*, **60**(2–3), 239–58.

Norman RM, Malla AK. (2001). Duration of untreated psychosis: a critical examination of the concept and its importance. *Psychol Med*, **31**(3), 381–400.

Nose M, Barbui C, Gray R, Tansella M. (2003). Clinical interventions for treatment non-adherence in psychosis: meta-analysis. *Br J Psychiatry*, **183**, 197–206.

Novick D, Haro JP, Suarez D, Perez V, Dittmann R, Haddad PM. (2010). Predictors and consequences of adherence with antipsychotic medication in the outpatient treatment of schizophrenia. *Psychiatry Res*, **176**(2–3), 109–13.

Oehl M, Hummer M, Fleischhacker WW. (2000). Compliance with antipsychotic treatment. *Acta Psychiatr Scand*, **102**(Suppl 407), 83–6.

Olfson M, Mechanic D, Hansell S, Boyer CA, Walkup J, Weiden PJ. (2000). Predicting medication noncompliance after hospital discharge among patients with schizophrenia. *Psychiatr Serv*, **51**(2), 216–22.

Olivares JM, Peuskens J, Pecenak J, Resseler S, Jacobs A, Akhras KS; e-STAR Study Group. (2009a). Clinical and resource-use outcomes of risperidone long-acting injection in recent and long-term diagnosed schizophrenia patients: results from a multinational electronic registry. *Curr Med Res Opin*, **25**(9), 2197–206.

Olivares JM, Rodriguez-Martinez A, Burón JA, Alonso-Escolano D, Rodriguez-Morales A; e-STAR Study Group (2008). Cost-effectiveness analysis of switching antipsychotic medication to long-acting injectable risperidone in patients with schizophrenia: a 12- and 24-month follow-up from the e-STAR database in Spain. *Appl Health Econ Health Policy*, **6**(1), 41–53.

Olivares JM, Rodriguez-Morales A, Diels J, Povey M, Jacobs A, Zhao Z, et al. (2009b). Long-term outcomes in patients with schizophrenia treated with risperidone long-acting injection or oral antipsychotics in Spain: results from the electronic Schizophrenia Treatment Adherence Registry (e-STAR). *Eur Psychiatry*, **24**(5), 287–96.

Osterberg L, Blaschke T. (2005). Adherence to medication. *N Engl J Med*, **353**(5), 487–97.

Pekkala E, Merinder, L. (2002). Psychoeducation for schizophrenia. *Cochrane Database Syst Rev* (**2**), CD002831.

Perkins, DO. (2002). Predictors of noncompliance in patients with schizophrenia. *J Clin Psychiatry*, **63**(12), 1121–8.

Perkins DO, Gu H, Weiden PJ, McEvoy JP, Hamer RM, Lieberman JA. (2008). Predictors of treatment discontinuation and medication nonadherence in patients recovering from a first episode of schizophrenia, schizophreniform disorder, or schizoaffective disorder: a randomized, double-blind, flexible-dose, multicenter study. *J Clin Psychiatry*, **69**(1), 106–13.

Pickar D, Owen RR, Litman RE, Konicki E, Gutierrez R, Rapaport MH. (1992). Clinical and biologic response to clozapine in patients with schizophrenia. Crossover comparison with fluphenazine. *Arch Gen Psychiatry*, **49**(5), 345–53.

Pitschel-Walz G, Leucht S, Bauml J, Kissling W, Engel RR. (2001). The effect of family interventions on relapse and rehospitalization in schizophrenia—a meta-analysis. *Schizophr Bull*, **27**(1), 73–92.

Robinson D, Woerner MG, Alvir JM, Bilder R, Goldman R, Geisler S, et al. (1999). Predictors of relapse following response from a first episode of schizophrenia or schizoaffective disorder. *Arch Gen Psychiatry*, **56**(3), 241–7.

Rosenstock IM. (1966). Why people use health services. *Milbank Mem Fund Q*, **44**(3), S94–S127.

Royal Australian and New Zealand College of Psychiatrists clinical practice guidelines for the treatment of schizophrenia and related disorders. (2005). *Aust N Z J Psychiatry*, **39**, 1–30.

Sajatovic M, Valenstein M, Blow F, Ganoczy D, Ignacio R. (2007). Treatment adherence with lithium and anticonvulsant medications among patients with bipolar disorder. *Psychiatr Serv*, **58**(6), 855–63.

Schooler NR, Keith SJ, Severe JB, Matthews SM, Bellack AS, Glick ID, et al. (1997). Relapse and rehospitalization during maintenance treatment of schizophrenia. The effects of dose reduction and family treatment. *Arch Gen Psychiatry*, **54**(5), 453–63.

Sheitman BB, Lee H, Strous R, Lieberman JA. (1997). The evaluation and treatment of first-episode psychosis. *Schizophr Bull*, **23**(4), 653–61.

Simmons MS, Nides MA, Rand CS, Wise RA, Tashkin DP. (2000). Unpredictability of deception in compliance with physician-prescribed bronchodilator inhaler use in a clinical trial. *Chest*, **118**(2), 290–5.

Sun SX, Liu GG, Christensen DB, Fu AZ. (2007). Review and analysis of hospitalization costs associated with antipsychotic nonadherence in the treatment of schizophrenia in the United States. *Curr Med Res Opin*, **23**(10), 2305–12.

Svedberg B, Mesterton A, Cullberg J. (2001). First-episode non-affective psychosis in a total urban population: a 5-year follow-up. *Soc Psychiatry Psychiatr Epidemiol*, **36**(7), 332–7.

Szymanski SR, Cannon TD, Gallacher F, Erwin RJ, Gur RE. (1996). Course of treatment response in first-episode and chronic schizophrenia. *Am J Psychiatry*, **153**(4), 519–25.

Tauscher-Wisniewski S, Ziursky R. (2002). The role of maintenance pharmacotherapy in achieving recovery from a first episode of schizophrenia. *Int Rev Psychiatry*, **14**, 284–92.

Taylor M, Currie A, Lloyd K, Price M, Peperell K. (2008). Impact of risperidone long acting injection on resource utilization in psychiatric secondary care. *J Psychopharmacol*, **22**(2), 128–31.

Thara R, Henrietta M, Joseph A, Rajkumar S, Eaton WW. (1994). Ten-year course of schizophrenia—the Madras longitudinal study. *Acta Psychiatr Scand*, **90**(5), 329–36.

Thompson K, Kulkarni J, SergejewAA. (2000). Reliability and validity of a new Medication Adherence Rating Scale (MARS) for the psychoses. *Schizophr Res*, **42**(3), 241–7.

Valenstein M, Ganoczy D, McCarthy JF, Myra Kim, H, Lee, TA, Blow FC. (2006). Antipsychotic adherence over time among patients receiving treatment for schizophrenia: a retrospective review. *J Clin Psychiatry*, **67**(10), 1542–50.

van Harten PN, Hoek HW, Matroos GE, Koeter M, Kahn RS. (1998). Intermittent neuroleptic treatment and risk for tardive dyskinesia: Curacao Extrapyramidal Syndromes Study III. *Am J Psychiatry*, **155**(4), 565–7.

Velligan DI, Diamond PM, Mintz J, Maples N, Li X, Zeber J, et al. (2008). The use of individually tailored environmental supports to improve medication adherence and outcomes in schizophrenia. *Schizophr Bull*, **34**(3), 483–93.

Velligan DI, Lam F, Ereshefsky L, Miller AL (2003). Psychopharmacology: Perspectives on medication adherence and atypical antipsychotic medications. *Psychiatr Serv*, **54**(5), 665–7.

Velligan DI, Lam YW, Glahn DC, Barrett JA, Maples NJ, Ereshefsky L, et al. (2006). Defining and assessing adherence to oral antipsychotics: a review of the literature. *Schizophr Bull*, **32**(4), 724–42.

Velligan DI, Wang M, Diamond P, Glahn DC, Castillo D, Bendle S, et al. (2007). Relationships among subjective and objective measures of adherence to oral antipsychotic medications. *Psychiatr Serv*, **58**(9), 1187–92.

Velligan DI, Weiden PJ, Sajatovic M, Scott J, Carpenter D, Ross R, et al. (2009). The expert consensus guideline series: adherence problems in patients with serious and persistent mental illness. *J Clin Psychiatry*, **70** (Suppl 4), 1–46; quiz 47–48.

Viller F, Guillemin F, Briancon S, Moum T, Suurmeijer T, van den Heuvel W. (1999). Compliance to drug treatment of patients with rheumatoid arthritis: a 3 year longitudinal study. *J Rheumatol*, **26**(10), 2114–22.

Weiden PJ, Kozma C, Grogg A, Locklear J. (2004). Partial compliance and risk of rehospitalization among California Medicaid patients with schizophrenia. *Psychiatr Serv*, **55**(8), 886–91.

Weinberger DR. (1987). Implications of normal brain development for the pathogenesis of schizophrenia. *Arch Gen Psychiatry*, **44**(7), 660–9.

Weiss KA, Smith TE, Hull JW, Piper AC, Huppert JD. (2002). Predictors of risk of nonadherence in outpatients with schizophrenia and other psychotic disorders. *Schizophr Bull*, **28**(2), 341–9.

Wiersma D, Nienhuis FJ, Slooff CJ, Giel R. (1998). Natural course of schizophrenic disorders: a 15-year followup of a Dutch incidence cohort. *Schizophr Bull*, **24**(1), 75–85.

Williams CL, Johnstone BM, Kesterson JG, Javor KA, Schmetzer AD. (1999). Evaluation of antipsychotic and concomitant medication use patterns in patients with schizophrenia. *Med Care*, **37**(4 Suppl Lilly), AS81–6.

Wunderink L, Nienhuis FJ, Sytema S, Slooff CJ, Knegtering R, Wiersma D. (2007). Guided discontinuation versus maintenance treatment in remitted first-episode psychosis: relapse rates and functional outcome. *J Clin Psychiatry*, **68**(5), 654–61.

Wyatt RJ (1991). Neuroleptics and the natural course of schizophrenia. *Schizophr Bull*, **17**(2), 325–51.

Wyatt RJ (1997). Research in schizophrenia and the discontinuation of antipsychotic medications. *Schizophr Bull*, **23**(1), 3–9.

Young JL, Spitz RT, Hillbrand M, Daneri G. (1999). Medication adherence failure in schizophrenia: a forensic review of rates, reasons, treatments, and prospects. *J Am Acad Psychiatry Law*, **27**(3), 426–44.

Yung AR, McGorry PD. (1996). The prodromal phase of first-episode psychosis: past and current conceptualizations. *Schizophr Bull*, **22**(2), 353–70.

Zammit S, Allebeck P, David AS, Dalman C, Hemmingsson T, Lundberg I, et al. (2004). A longitudinal study of premorbid IQ Score and risk of developing schizophrenia, bipolar disorder, severe depression, and other nonaffective psychoses. *Arch Gen Psychiatry*, **61**(4), 354–60.

Zygmunt A, Olfson M, Boyer CA, Mechanic D. (2002). Interventions to improve medication adherence in schizophrenia. *Am J Psychiatry*, **159**(10), 1653–64.

Chapter 2

Pharmacology of antipsychotic long-acting injections

Tim Lambert and David Taylor

Correspondence: tim.lambert@sydney.edu.au

Introduction

In this chapter we discuss the applied pharmacology of antipsychotic long-acting injections (LAIs). We begin with an overview of the basic pharmacology of first-generation antipsychotic (FGA) and second-generation antipsychotic (SGA) LAIs, review the clinical applications of working with LAI kinetics, examine dosing equivalence between the LAIs and the common frequencies of administration, review initiation and loading strategies to achieve rapid plasma level changes, consider some of the pharmacodynamics of the various LAI formulations, and finally conclude with a brief overview of the pharmacology of switching to and from LAI antipsychotics. The objective of this chapter is to present sufficient material for the general clinician to understand the main differences between agents and to set the scene for an evidence-based approach to prescribing (see Chapter 10).

The LAIs have evolved both in terms of the class of antipsychotic delivered and the technology used to promote the 'depot' effect. Arguably there have been three phases of development of LAIs with respect to the latter (Table 2.1). These are the use of oil-based depots, the use of microsphere preparations, and the use of crystal-based technologies. These phases can be differentiated principally on the initiation and release kinetics, arguably one of the determining factors in a clinician's choice of an LAI antipsychotic in modern therapy. Clinicians may make choices based on other factors including the class of embedded antipsychotic (FGA, SGA), the patient's previous experience of antipsychotics in terms of response and tolerability, and cost. For further discussion on factors associated with LAI use, see Chapter 10.

Overview of FGA-LAIs

Chemically, the FGA-LAIs are esters of the parent FGA combined with a long chain fatty acid. Of the latter, the principal one is decanoic acid, a 10-carbon straight-chain fatty acid, although the enanthate (C8), undecylenate (C11), and palmitate (C16) esters of some agents are available in several countries.

Once esterified, the FGA becomes fat-soluble and can be dissolved in an oily base, such as sesame, coconut, or Viscoleo (a synthetic vegetable oil). The resulting solution

Table 2.1 Classification of LAIs by phase of development based on delivery mechanism

Class	Delivery	Agent
FGA	Oil	Fluphenazine decanoate
		Haloperidol decanoate
		Flupentixol/zuclopenthixol decanoates
		Pipotiazine palmitate
		Perphenazine decanoate
SGA	Microspheres	Risperidone LAI
	Crystal	Olanzapine pamoate
		Paliperidone palmitate

Flupentixol and flupenthixol are used in a region-specific manner

is delivered by deep intramuscular injection. The ester slowly leaves the oil from the reservoir formed in the muscle tissue. The active hydrophilic antipsychotic component of the ester orients itself to the interstitial fluid compartment and the hydrophobic fatty acid 'tails' orient themselves to the oily globule. This ensures that the release of the ester from the depot store is slow, leading to the long apparent half-lives of LAI antipsychotics. A discussion on the kinetics of the various LAI agents follows.

Once the esterified antipsychotic has left the globule, it is rapidly hydrolysed by plasma esterases allowing the antipsychotic component to diffuse to its target tissue (the brain) (Barnes & Curson 1994; Dencker & Axelsson 1996; Ereshefsky et al. 1984).

The clinical pharmacokinetics are somewhat complex (see below) but in summary antipsychotics delivered in depot form take some weeks to months to reach steady state with regular injections and have a correspondingly slow elimination period (Barnes & Curson 1994; Ereshefsky et al. 1984; Jann et al. 1985).

The long period to elimination may be critical in the clinical aspects of relapse prevention. Their pharmacokinetics and route of administration confers a number of other benefits, which are further discussed in Chapter 11.

A range of FGA-LAIs has been manufactured and nine common FGA-based agents are reviewed in Adams et al.'s synthesis of the systematic Cochrane reviews (Adams et al. 2001. See also table 1 in Dencker & Axelsson 1996). Their availability varies in different countries. In Australia, four FGA-LAI antipsychotics are available: fluphenazine decanoate, haloperidol decanoate, flupenthixol decanoate, and zuclopenthixol decanoate. In New Zealand and in the United Kingdom, in addition to these LAIs, pipotiazine palmitate is also available (Humberstone et al. 2004). In general, the range is broader than in the United States where only two FGA-LAI agents are available for prescription (fluphenazine and haloperidol decanoates).

Overview of SGA-LAIs

Risperidone LAI

Risperidone long-acting injection (RLAI) can be described as the first of the non-oil based LAIs. Rather than being an ester of the parent antipsychotic with a long chain fatty acid, risperidone is encapsulated in, and then delivered from a biodegradable microsphere preparation.

The RLAI formulation contains risperidone encapsulated into polymeric microspheres that require cold storage to retain the intended release characteristics. These microspheres are made up of biodegradable copolymers that are slowly hydrolysed *in vivo* to release risperidone (Ramstack et al. 2003). After intramuscular injection, a small but clinically insufficient amount of risperidone is released from the surface of the microspheres; however, further release is delayed for 2 to 3 weeks, during which time erosion of the microspheres takes place. The peak release is at about 28 days with minimally adequate levels being present from about the middle third week post-injection. In 2-weekly dosing, peak plasma levels continue to be seen at around 4 weeks after the injection.

The plasma half-life is of the order of 4 to 6 days when examining single-shot kinetics (Gefvert et al. 2005). The apparent half-life approximations are more complicated when examining RLAI owing to the initial absence of release for some weeks and then the progressive release as the microspheres break down. In practical terms, steady-state plasma levels are obtained after 8 weeks, at which time peak-to-trough levels vary threefold (Gefvert et al. 2005). When RLAI is ceased there is maintenance of adequate plasma level for 4 to 5 weeks before there is a rapid reduction. By 8 weeks following the last injection, there is no residue of RLAI left in the system (see Wilson 2004 for visual representations of RLAI kinetics).

Olanzapine LAI

Olanzapine LAI (OLAI) is the first of the crystal-based LAIs. It is a salt of pamoic acid and olanzapine (olanzapine pamoate) suspended in water (Taylor, 2009). Following injection, peak plasma levels occur some 2 to 4 days later and exhibit an apparent plasma half-life of about 26 days (range 2–4 weeks; Kurtz et al. 2008). Following injection of the suspension of the micron-sized crystals into muscle tissue, the pamoate salt slowly dissolves releasing free olanzapine and pamoic acid. The slow rate of dissolution of the crystalline salt gives OLAI its long-acting properties (Citrome 2009).

Plasma levels obtained are directly proportional to whatever dose is given and expected equivalences to oral preparations have been described (see Table 2.2). With regular injections, the time to steady state is approximately 2 to 3 months (Figure 2.1). Depending on the target equivalent dose required, the OLAI can be injected 2- or 4-weekly. In 2-weekly dosing, trough levels are approximately 50% of peak level; in monthly dosing, trough levels are 75% lower than peak (Kurtz et al. 2008). Although the OLAI crystals are somewhat insoluble in the muscle tissue, if they come in contact with blood, there is a more rapid dissolution and release of free olanzapine. It is thought that damage of vessels during injection with the extravasation of blood into or near the depot site may account for the post-injection syndrome seen with this agent (discussed further in Chapter 6).

Recommendations for prior olanzapine use state that a patient receiving OLAI should be stabilized prior to the first injection with oral olanzapine (Eli Lilly 2009). The definition of 'stabilized' is still open to some interpretation. At the time of writing,

Table 2.2 Equivalence for specific SGAs in oral and LAI form

SGA-LAI Drug	Target oral-equivalent dose[a]	LAI dose and frequency	References
Risperidone[b]	<3 mg oral	25 mg 2-weekly	Bai et al (2007)
	3 mg to 5mg oral	37.5 mg 2-weekly	
	> 5mg oral	50 mg 2-weekly	
Paliperidone[b]	6 mg	117 mg 4-weekly	Citrome, (2010);
	9 mg	156 mg 4-weekly	Janssen, (2009); Samtani et al., (2009a, b)
Olanzapine	10 mg	150 mg 2-weekly	Citrome (2009);
		300 mg 4-weekly	Eli Lilly (2009)
	15 mg	210 mg 2-weekly	
		405 mg 4-weekly	
	20 mg	300 mg 2-weekly	
		no 4-weekly equivalent	

[a] Equivalent doses at or approaching LAI steady state.
[b] Different views exist regarding dose equivalence of oral risperidone and RLAI (see the section below on pharmacodynamics as well as Chapter 5 for discussion).
[c] The actual doses marketed reflect the paliperidone palmitate entity and so are 39 mg, 78 mg, 117 mg, 156 mg, and 234 mg; these doses are equivalent to 25 mg, 50 mg, 75 mg, 100 mg, and 150 mg of paliperidone respectively.

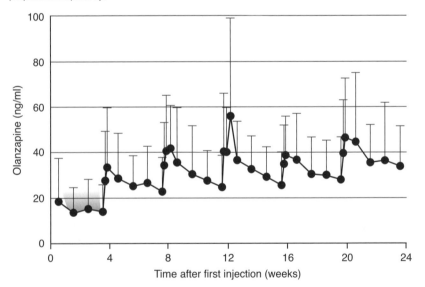

Fig. 2.1 Mean ±SD olanzapine plasma concentrations for 405 mg 4-weekly in LOBE patients.
Taken from Fig LOBE 11.7, ASSESSMENT REPORT FOR ZYPADHERA European Medicines Agency, Ref: EMEA/608654/2008.

OLAI has been approved for use in Australia, New Zealand, parts of Europe, and the United States with other regions likely to follow in the near future.

Paliperidone palmitate

Paliperidone palmitate is the second of the crystal-based LAIs to become available. The crystal salt (based on 'NanoCrystal' technology) is supplied in an aqueous suspension in pre-filled syringes. As shown in Table 2.2, dose equivalence has been established between the long-acting form and the oral form of paliperidone (note that the marketed doses are for the paliperidone palmitate, and in this chapter we discuss the equivalent doses of paliperidone itself; see footnote to Table 2.2). As can be seen, it is suggested that 9 mg of paliperidone oral (a typical dose in some public psychiatry settings, see Citrome 2009) is approximately equivalent to 100 mg eq. 4-weekly of the long-acting form (Janssen 2009).

Figure 2.2 shows the kinetic profile of paliperidone palmitate based on an initiation strategy of 150/100 mg eq. per day 1 and day 8 (discussed below). The peak plasma concentration occurs some 13 days following injection, although as with

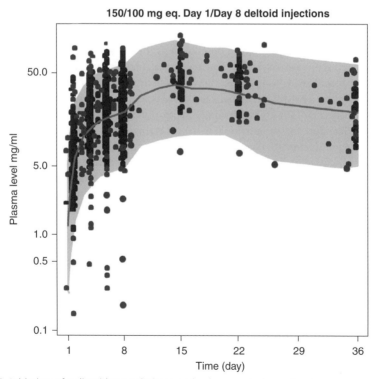

Fig. 2.2 Initiation of paliperidone palmitate and subsequent plasma levels. Source: Samtani et al. (2009a).

OLAI, there is an immediate release of clinically active levels of paliperidone with the first injection. As paliperidone palmitate is largely insoluble in the muscle tissue, there is slow release of the parent paliperidone antipsychotic, with a long apparent half-life of between 25 and 49 days for dose of between 25 and 150 mg eq. of paliperidone (Citrome 2009).

Kinetics: clinical applications

Pharmacokinetics

Optimal use of LAIs requires that clinicians are aware of their pharmacokinetic profiles. This knowledge is helpful in particular when assessing an individual's need for oral supplementation at the commencement of treatment, how long it might take to reach steady state, how long it will take for blood levels to decline once an LAI is stopped, how long one would need to wait for the effect of dose increases or decreases to become clinically apparent, and so on.

For all LAIs, apparent plasma half-life is determined by rate of drug release rather than drug metabolism. That is, the rate of release from the depot determines the persistence of the drug in the system: all drugs available as LAIs have plasma half-lives of 1 to 2 days at most when not given as depot formulations. For most LAIs, the apparent half-life after repeated use is between 14 and 27 days. Therefore, time to steady state is also prolonged in those receiving LAIs. Steady state is usually achieved after four to five half-lives. At this point, rate of drug removal equals rate of release, and plasma profile does not change between dose intervals. Before steady state is achieved, mean plasma levels increase over time. The lowest peak plasma level is what is obtained after the first dose. The highest peak plasma level will usually be that obtained after the fifth or sixth dose. The difference between these peak plasma levels can be severalfold (Ereshefsky et al. 1984). This obviously makes difficult the determination of the most appropriate dose for an individual patient. Loading doses (giving larger doses at the beginning of treatment) allow steady state levels to be achieved earlier than in normal dosing (discussed further below). It is notable that newer SGA-LAIs incorporate loading dose schedules into their official dosing recommendations (Eli Lilly 2009; Janssen 2009).

The long half-life of LAIs also means that after cessation of treatment plasma levels remain therapeutic (Nyberg et al. 1997; Wistedt 1981) and perhaps toxic (Harasko-van der Meer et al. 1993) for many weeks or, more usually, months. Further information on some comparative aspects of LAI formulations can be found in Taylor (2009).

Dosing equivalence

FGA-LAIs

The concept of equivalent doses for antipsychotics is a fraught one. However, based on the various combinations of mean doses in large populations, knowledge of relationships between plasma dose and effect, and similarly for dose/plasma level and positron emission tomography (PET) occupancy and effect, basic equivalent doses have been proposed. Table 2.3 lists current equivalent doses for FGA-LAIs that have some practical utility in daily clinical practice. As discussed in the section on plasma

Table 2.3 Equivalent doses for different FGA-LAIs

FGA-LAI Drug	LAI dose and frequency[a,b,c]	Comment
Flupentixol	40 mg 2-weekly	The thioxanthine LAI equivalences mainly stem from a Lundbeck monograph (Johnson & Dencker, 1997), although are consistent with most clinicians' views
Zuclopenthixol	200 mg 2-weekly	
Haloperidol	90-110 mg 4-weekly	Bazire (1999) summarizes the various views and an oral equivalence of 15× is considered. Given that 300 mg/day CPZe is about 6 mg of haloperidol, 100 mg 4-weekly would approximate this
Fluphenazine	25 mg 2-weekly	The starting point comes with Galletly and Tsourtos (1997) with a 25 mg 2-weekly equivalence of 293 mg/day CPZe
Pipotiazine	80 mg 4-weekly	A wide range of equivalences have been proposed (50 to 100 mg 4-weekly). Based on clinicians' comments, 80 mg 4-weekly is a good starting point
Perphenazine	70 -100 2-weekly[d]	For the decanoate, the actual injection frequency and thus dose can be optimised through therapeutic drug monitoring (where available) (Larsen & Hansen 1989). Plasma levels may be less stable across time with this depot (Tuninger & Levander 1996)

[a] Equivalent doses at or approaching LAI steady state.
[b] Equivalent to 300 mg/day CPZe.
[c] FGA-LAI conversion references: Johnson and Dencker (1997), Bazire (1999), Galletly and Tsourtos (1997), Simpson and Egan (1993), Larsen and Hansen (1989).
[d] Estimated from published data.
CPZe = Chlorpromazine equivalents.

dose variations, there is usually a wide variation in an individual's C_{max}/C_{min}; therefore the general precepts of using the smallest possible dose in the maintenance phase needs to be tempered with knowledge of an individual's peak to trough ratio so that there are not long periods of suboptimal treatment during long interval injection cycles. However, this does rely on therapeutic drug monitoring being more readily available than is currently in clinical practice. The conversions in Table 2.3 were used to determine the CPZ daily doses listed for the 'real world' in Table 2.4. As shown in Table 2.4, the highest daily doses are consonant with the agents' time since introduction—fluphenazine has the highest dose and was the first agent introduced in 1966, initially as fluphenazine enanthate and 18 months later as fluphenazine decanoate. It is followed by haloperidol with the second highest dose.

SGA-LAIs

The dosing equivalence of SGAs in oral and LAI formulations is shown in Table 2.2. Notwithstanding the remarks in the pharmacodynamics section, oral-LAI equivalence with the SGA-LAIs has benefited from the more robust use of PET studies. However, like those for FGA-LAIs, many of the PET studies have small numbers of subjects.

Table 2.4 LAI doses in stabilized community treated patients with schizophrenia

LAI	N	Percent	Typical dose/ injection	Modal injection frequency	CPZe mg/day, all[d]	CPZe mg/day monotherapy[e]
Flupentixol[a]	547	37.9	46.1±32.5	2-weekly	310±241	290±221
Haloperidol[a]	214	14.8	95.3 ±70.9	4-weekly	386±331	332±275
Fluphenazine[a]	245	17.0	43.0±25.4	2-weekly	456±323	460±327
Zuclopenthixol[a]	436	30.2	196.5±108.7	2-weekly	300±189	290±183
Total	1442	100				
Pipotiazine[b]	61	–	49.2±29.3	2-weekly	303±225	264±198
Perphenazine[c]	19	–	–	2-weekly	331±137	–

[a] Australian data for schizophrenia patients (Lambert 2005).
[b] for NZ doses, all psychoses (Humberstone et al. 2004). Doses don't differ appreciably for those for schizophrenia alone. Doses for other LAI antipsychotics are similar to Australian data in this table.
[c] Swedish data (Tuninger et al., 1994). Injection dose is imputed from daily dose ×14.
[d] Based on equivalences in Tables 2.2 and 2.3. These are for all cases of LAI prescription, whether in mono- or polyantipsychotic therapy.
[e] These converted doses are for patients with schizophrenia on monotherapy with FGA-LAIs.

The equivalence ranges for RLAI appear to be robust when one considers average doses. In Australia e.g. in stabilized community settings, the mean dose of oral risperidone for adult patients with schizophrenia is approximately 4 mg/day (Lambert 2005). Since its introduction in 2004, RLAI doses have gradually crept up in this same population with an estimated mean of between 45 and 50 mg 2-weekly being common at the time of writing. The relatively recent introduction into clinical practice of the crystal-based LAIs (paliperidone and olanzapine), suggests that their 'practical' equivalence, determined from what works with real patients at the coal-face, will evolve in the next few years.

Average doses in clinical practice

Typical doses employed for LAIs may differ regionally and alter with time as clinicians become aware of the clinically effective dose. In Table 2.4 pooled data from 1998 to 2002 for community-treated persons with schizophrenia from various countries are presented (Lambert 2005). The doses, converted to chlorpromazine equivalents (CPZe; based on the equivalences of the LAI to oral forms, shown in Table 2.3) indicate that in terms of CPZe the mean lies about 300 mg/day for zuclopenthixol, flupentixol, and pipotiazine, with higher doses found for fluphenazine decanoate (456 mg/day CPZe) and haloperidol decanoate (386 mg/day CPZe).

However, these average doses need to be considered in the context of whether the patient receives mono- or poly-antipsychotic therapy. The last column in Table 2.4 indicates that when FGA-LAIs are used in antipsychotic monotherapy, the actual doses of LAI antipsychotic are lower than the LAI doses used in a polyantipsychotic context. In the latter, higher LAI doses, plus additional oral antipsychotics result in a high total equivalent daily dose. Indeed some patients on the combination of oral plus

LAI may receive an above 'maximum licensed combined dose' (i.e. percentage of maximum licensed dose of first drug plus percentage of maximum licensed dose of second drug >100%). If such doses are prescribed there should be a good clinical reason, and the prescribing and monitoring should be in keeping with guidance of high dose prescribing (Royal College of Psychiatrists 2006). The different doses on LAIs when used as monotherapy and polytherapy need to be kept in mind when considering anecdotal views that those treated with LAIs receive higher doses—they may well, but it appears to be in situations suggesting treatment of difficult cases to help patients who differentially require poly-antipsychotic treatment. For example, this dataset indicates that the mean total daily dose for patients treated with mono-therapy with LAIs is considerably lower than the total daily dose when LAI+oral therapy is employed (325 ± 249 vs. 711 ± 391 mg/day CPZe, $p = .0001$). The differences may be an artefact of the conversion equivalences, or they could reflect that these agents have been in use for the longest period and may reflect slow development of supersensitivity requiring higher doses over time (e.g. as found with oral haloperidol). This is supported by the significantly older ages of those on fluphenazine and haloperi-dol decanoates when compared to flupentixol ($p < .001$), although this suggests that such patients have had long periods of stable prescribing on the older agents. The apparent equivalent dose has good face validity as doses around 400 mg/day CPZe are common for maintenance with oral antipsychotics, perhaps reflecting the likely peri-ods of partial adherence. The AUC_∞ may be equivalent for lower doses of (continu-ously given) LAI therapy when compared to somewhat higher doses of oral.

Injection interval

For the dataset in Table 2.4, the modal frequency of injection is 2-weekly, except for haloperidol decanoate (4-weekly). There is some difference between agents in clinical settings. Considering frequencies of less than 2-weekly, 2-weekly, 3-weekly, 4-weekly, and more than 4-weekly for each of the common FGA-LAIs, we find fluphenazine decanoate is administered at these intervals in 1.5%, 57.3%, 21.9%, 15.8%, 3.4%; for haloperidol decanoate the rates are 0.8%, 17.8%, 13.5%, 67.8%, and 0.0%; for flupen-tixol decanoate 1.2%, 61.5%, 23.5%, 13.5%, and 0.4%; for zuclopenthixol 3.6%, 79.3%, 8.9%, 7.5%, and 0.6%; and for pipotiazine palmitate 0.8%, 47.5%, 20.3%, 30.5%, and 0.8%, respectively (Lambert unpublished data).

Risperidone LAI is licensed for administration every 2 weeks partly owing to the somewhat invariable kinetic profile of the microsphere-based delivery mechanism. Some clinicians, used to prescribing FGA-LAIs at monthly intervals have been interested in the possibility of extending the injection interval. To date there is some preliminary evidence that 4-weekly injections may be effective in relapse prevention in a stable patient population, with 12-month relapse rates approximately in the range seen with FGA-LAIs (Gharabawi et al. 2007). However, it is not known whether in more unstable or unwell patients the period of low risperidone active moiety concentrations inherent in the 4-week cycle would predispose to relapse. Based on what we know of occupancy at various doses (Remington et al. 2006), periods of the cycle would have adequate D2-receptor occupancy, whereas periods of up to a week are likely to have periods of inadequate occupancy. These periods may confer an increased risk of replase but until formal studies are carried out in a double blind fashion, it will be prudent to carefully monitor any patients on longer than the recommended and licensed 2-week injection cycle. Based on the current evidence, the authors do not recommend that RLAI is used with an injection cycle other than 2 weeks.

Olanzapine pamoate injections are recommended for either 2- or 4-weekly cycles. The decision as to the appropriate frequency will depend on a number of factors including the target equivalent olanzapine dose and the need for more or less frequent visits if tied to the injection. Notwithstanding the initiation strategy (discussed below), if the maintenance target dose is the equivalent of 20 mg of olanzapine oral, then 2-weekly injections of 300 mg are required to reach the equivalent plasma level range. With maintenance olanzapine oral doses in many countries being somewhere between 15 and 20 mg/day, and given that there may be some degree of partial adherence for many patients, the 4-weekly injection of 405 mg—achieving an equivalence of 15 mg/day of olanzapine—may well be sufficient.

Paliperidone palmitate LAI is designed for 4-weekly administration during the maintenance phase. As discussed below, an initiation or loading strategy is proposed to take advantage of the immediate release kinetics and achieve plasma levels approximating those found at steady state within a brief interval.

Plasma level variations

There has been an indication that over time there are both within and between patient variations in the plasma concentration per given dose (C/D). Zuclopenthixol e.g. has a broad range of ratios of the plasma concentration at day 7 (C_{max}) compared with day 14 (C_{min}), with a mean of 2 but a range of up to 4 (Poulsen et al. 1994). Other zuclopenthixol studies have shown a C_{max}/C_{min} ratio of about 1.6 for a 2-week cycle and 2.8 for a 3-week cycle. These values lead to disparate assessments of apparent half-life (in these cases, ranging from 8 to 19 days). However, wide fluctuations may be related to the development of extrapyramidal symptoms (EPS) in one extreme and insufficient antipsychotic coverage at the other, with breakthrough symptoms possible towards the end of a cycle; in addition, responders are more likely to have smaller C_{max}/C_{min} ratios compared with non-responders. Similar conclusions were drawn from perphenazine LAI studies, where optimal treatment was more likely to occur when C_{max}/C_{min} ratios were of the order of 1.5 (Dencker & Axelsson 1996). The C_{max}/C_{min} has been estimated to be 2.5 for haloperidol decanoate and 3.1 for flupentixol decanoate (Dencker & Axelsson 1996).

Studies of RLAI show that peak-to-trough fluctuations in plasma levels of the active moiety (risperidone and 9-hydroxyrisperidone) and C max are reduced when compared to oral risperidone (Eerdekens et al. 2004 ; Mannaert et al. 2005). Chapter 5 provides further details of these and related studies. As noted above, lengthening the injection cycle beyond 2 weeks is likely to result in suboptimal plasma levels at the end of the cycle for some patients.

For paliperidone the C_{max}/C_{min} for those prescribed 150 mg 4-weekly is 1.8 and 2.2 for the gluteal and deltoid muscles, respectively (Janssen 2009). This broadly corresponds to the range seen with FGA-LAIs. There may be an argument for having low ratios in maintenance; therefore this suggests that clinicians may wish to consider moving from deltoid to gluteal injections in some circumstances. At this point, these suggestions apply only to the gluteal versus deltoid injections of paliperidone palmitate.

There is limited information on plasma level variation with olanzapine pamoate. In a study in which patients were switched from oral olanzapine 5 mg/day to 20 mg/day to 300 mg/month olanzapine pamoate, plasma levels rose from approximately 10 ng/ml one week after the first injection to 14 ng/ml after 4 weeks (plasma level at time zero was 37.4 ng/ml) (Mamo et al. 2008). At the time of the third injection, plasma level was 26.5 ng/ml, 26.5 ng/ml two weeks later, and 28.6 ng/ml before the fourth injection. There were no data on peak plasma levels (achieved after about three days), but these results suggest very limited variability in olanzapine plasma levels.

Loading or initiation strategies

A loading or initiation strategy aims to allow a drug to reach steady levels in the target tissue(s) more quickly than would be achieved if the normal maintenance dose was initiated and continued. With a LAI this effect can be achieved by using a higher initial dose, or initially increasing the frequency of injections of a standard dose, or combining both approaches i.e. using a higher initial dose and a shorter injection interval. Loading or initiation strategies can be used with FGA-LAIs and are recommended when starting treatment with olanzapine pamoate and paliperidone palmitate (see respective Summary of Product Characteristics). With regard to terminology, 'loading' strategy is often used in the literature on FGA-LAIs while 'initiation' strategy is used in the Summary of Product Characteristics for paliperidone palmitate. The two terms, loading strategy and initiation strategy, are synonymous and which is used is a matter of personal preference.

Loading strategies with oil-based LAIs often involve increasing the frequency of injections of a standard dose e.g. giving haloperidol decanoate injections weekly for 6 weeks rather than monthly. In such situations the plasma levels may quadruple over this short time frame (Ereshefsky et al. 1984), whereas if given at a standard monthly frequency and anticipating reaching steady state in 3 to 5 months, plasma changes will be relatively marginal. Loading strategies are possible with each of the FGA-LAIs, although one might anticipate that without vigilance, there may be issues of developing extrapyramidal side-effects in some cases. In particular, the known pharmacokinetic properties of fluphenazine decanoate (see below) might predict the likelihood of EPS being more common, owing to the high peak levels released within the first 8 to 24 hours post-injection. Ereshefsky et al. (1984) showed that a loading dose of 50 mg weekly of fluphenazine decanoate led to steady state in about 10 weeks (Figure 2.3). Clinically, loading strategies with FGA-LAIs can be very useful where there is concern over the ability to slowly wait for steady state to be achieved using the standard delivery frequencies and/or the need to use early adjunctive oral antipsychotics while antipsychotic levels slowly rise. However, the use of techniques to ensure the minimal effective dose, such as determining the neuroleptic threshold, have not been rigorously tested in those receiving FGA-LAIs and of course the long periods between injections make fine-tuning, based on this principle, a slow matter.

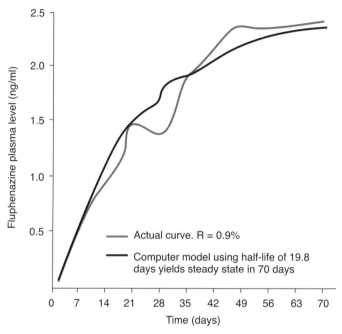

Fig. 2.3 Loading dose strategy for Fluphenazine decanoate: predicted and actual plasma levels.
Source: Figure 4, Ereshefsky et al. (1984).

With respect to the microsphere-based risperidone LAI, loading strategies to achieve higher initial plasma levels of the antipsychotic are not possible. As discussed in the kinetics section of this chapter there is scant release before about 24 days or so after injection and increasing the frequency of injections will lead to higher plasma levels down the track but cannot alter the fact that there is a gap of about 3 weeks before release from each injection, even if given weekly (see Figure 2.4 in the kinetics section; also Wilson 2004). The Summary of Product Characteristics for RLAI recommends oral antipsychotic supplementation for 3 weeks after the first injection of RLAI (Janssen 2009). Based on the pharmacokinetic data it is clear that this 3 week period is a minimum and in practice oral supplementation may be required for up to 6 weeks after starting RLAI i.e. until the RLAI has established plasma levels of the active moiety that approach steady state.

The most recently introduced LAIs, olanzapine pamoate, and paliperidone palmitate at the time of writing, are crystal-based and release effective and sustained levels of antipsychotic immediately after injection. This profile is in contrast to FGA-LAI agents, such as fluphenazine decanoate, which has a brief release spike within the first 24 hours but otherwise a standard FGA-LAI profile of a mild peak at about 7 days (Ereshesfky 1984). However, they require some months to attain a steady state, and in both cases initiation strategies have been developed to increase immediate blood levels, such that oral supplementation is not required.

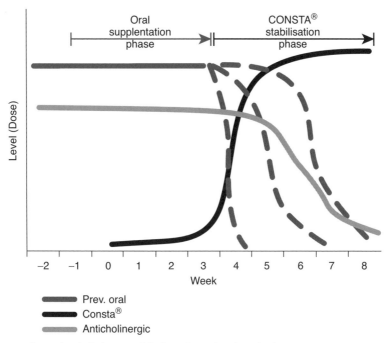

Fig. 2.4 Planned switch from anticholinergic oral antipsychotic to RLAI.
Image source: Switcha software package overview. http://www.open4media.com/
WebApps/Switcha/Switcha_intro.html; accessed 20 December 2009.

For paliperidone palmitate to achieve higher plasma levels at initiation, deltoid injections are favoured over gluteal injections, achieving a 28% higher plasma level, although at steady state there seems little difference in plasma levels between groups injected at the two sites (Hough et al. 2009). The initiation strategy also calls for an initial injection followed by one more injection a week later before proceeding to monthly injections (Citrome 2010; see also Figure 2.2). The proposed initiation doses are 150 mg eq[1] at the commencement, with 100 mg eq. after one week and thereafter a maintenance dose based on therapeutic needs but likely to be centred around 75 mg eq. 4-weekly. For patients with more chronic conditions, doses might be expected to be closer to 100 mg eq. 4-weekly based on current oral paliperidone use in those populations and perhaps less for patients of less chronicity (Citrome 2010). Based on the initial experiences of previously introduced SGA oral and LAI agents (Citrome et al. 2009), following paliperidone palmitate's more widespread introduction in years to come, the initiation and maintenance doses are likely to change somewhat.

---

[1] The equivalence between the paliperidone dose and the palmitate dose can be found in the footnote of Table 2.2. For example, 100 mg eq. of paliperidone equates to the commercially available dose of 156 mg of the palmitate.

Olanzapine pamoate is also an LAI with a crystal-based delivery system. If standard doses are given at regular intervals it takes about 2 to 3 months to come to a steady state. As with paliperidone palmitate, to achieve plasma levels approximating those that steady state, a loading strategy has been proposed. For example, doses of 300 mg 2-weekly for the first four injections will rapidly establish plasma levels equivalent 20 mg of oral olanzapine. In an acute study of the effectiveness of olanzapine in relapsing patients, no oral supplementation was provided, and no initiation strategy was purposefully implemented (Lauriello et al. 2008). Onset of action was as early as 3 days in this study, a finding that would be consistent with modern views of the time to onset of action of oral antipsychotics (Agid et al. 2003). Following the loading or initiations strategy, the clinician has the choice of prescribing OLAI 2- or 4-weekly depending on the target equivalent dose required (see Table 2.2). For example, 405 mg 4-weekly would be equivalent to 15 mg/day of oral olanzapine. In order to achieve higher target equivalent doses e.g. the equivalence of 20 mg/day of oral olanzapine, the prescription would need to be 300 mg 2-weekly. Other variations in the target dose can be achieved by varying either the frequency of injections or the dose given at each injection (Table 2.2).

Changing treatment paradigms: LAIs as acute and maintenance agents

In the previous paragraphs it was shown that owing to the novel formulation of the crystal-based LAIs, the rapidity of their onset is markedly different from either oil- based or microsphere-based LAIs, which will have a natural propensity to take some time to come to steady state. The crystal-based LAIs, used with recommended initiation strategies, open up the possibility for these agents to be used in both the acute setting and in longer-term maintenance. It is a common problem to find that those responsible for inpatient care are not those also responsible for community-based care. Decisions about *when* to start an FGA-LAI or an SGA-LAI are critical. Given the short lengths of stay afforded to those in acute relapse nowadays (Alwan et al. 2008), planning the use of an LAI is problematical. Does one wait until the patient is stabilized and then give the first dose prior to discharge? Alternatively, does one make the argument for critical non-adherence, treat the acute episode with standard procedures, but suggest in a discharge plan that the community staff commence the LAI *in situ*? Both may lead to ineffective use of LAIs if there is no tight integration between inpatient and community (Meadows & Singh 2001). Owing to the nature of the kinetic profile of the phase III LAIs, they may be able to bridge both acute and maintenance settings. Using the suggested initiation doses, paliperidone palmitate will be set by day 8 of treatment. Although the olanzapine initiation strategy takes a little longer to stabilize patients on the higher oral-equivalent doses, for those on lower-target trajectories ample and likely sufficient plasma levels can still be achieved in a short-duration acute admission (Lauriello et al. 2008). In both cases, at discharge the pharmacological maintenance of the patient is pretty well set and there is— one hopes—less opportunity for the future LAI therapy to founder. As both agents have been available only briefly in clinical practice, this potential windfall from the pharmacokinetic profile needs to be examined closely in the coming years.

Pharmacodynamics

Both FGAs and SGAs administered by any route are presumed to exert their antipsy-chotic action by blocking central dopamine receptors of the D2 receptor subtype. All LAIs are potent *in vitro* antagonists of D2 receptors. *In vivo*, potency in humans is usually determined by measuring striatal D2 occupancy using methods such as PET and single photon emission computerized tomography (SPECT). Therapeutic response seems to be associated with striatal D2 occupancies of 65% or more, whereas hyperprolactinaemia and extrapyramidal side-effects occur at occupancies of 72% and 78%, respectively (Kapur et al. 2000); however, these observations are based on a single study including a limited number of individuals.

Antipsychotic action may be derived from activity in the mesolimbic striatum, and striatal occupancies correlate closely with response to antipsychotic treatment, at least with respect to positive symptoms and adverse motor effects (Agid et al. 2007). Few studies have examined striatal D2 occupancy afforded by the use of LAIs. The earliest PET study found occupancies of 50% to 80% for patients receiving 50 to 200 mg a month of haloperidol decanoate, 100 mg a month of pipotiazine palmitate, and 200 mg a month of fluphenazine decanoate (Baron et al. 1989).

Occupancy levels appeared to increase in the 20 days following injection. A later study of four patients receiving 30 to 50 mg haloperidol decanoate a month showed that peak D2 occupancies were in the range 66% to 82% a week after injection (Nyberg et al. 1997).

In an extension of this study (*n* = 8, including two patients who participated in the previous study), D2 occupancies peaked from 60% to 82% a week after injection (doses 30–50 mg every 4 weeks; Nyberg et al. 1995). Four weeks later occupancies were in the range 20% to 74%. The patients remained healthy despite these low occupancies. Note however, that a fixed-dose randomized study showed 50 mg every 4 weeks to be significantly less effective than higher doses (Kane et al. 2002).

A relatively recent study of patients responding to perphenazine decanoate found that at plasma levels of 1.8 to 9 nmol/l striatal D2 occupancy ranged from 66% to 82% (Talvik et al. 2004). Doses used were in the range 38 to 108 mg per 2 weeks.

One study has examined D2 occupancy produced by olanzapine pamoate (Mamo et al. 2008). Participants were switched from oral olanzapine to the LAI (300 mg every 4 weeks) and followed up for 6 months. Dopamine D2 receptor occupancy averaged 69% for oral olanzapine (5–20 mg per day) but then fell to approximately 55% in the first month before rising to a little more than 60% (all trough samples). There was no change in patients' clinical condition over the study period. These occupancies will be consistent with an equivalence of about 10 mg/day of oral olanzapine (Eli Lilly 2009; Pilowsky et al. 1996).

Two studies have determined D2 occupancy associated with the use of risperidone LAI. In the first study, 28 patients received 2-weekly injections of 25 mg, 50 mg, or 75 mg risperidone, and D2 occupancy was estimated 2 weeks after the fifth injection (i.e. at steady-state trough plasma levels): the D2 occupancies were 25% to 48% for 25 mg, 59% to 83% for 50 mg and 62% to 72% for 75 mg (Gefvert et al. 2005; see Table 2.2).

In the second study, D2 occupancies were determined for nine participants up to 3 days after injection and less than 5 days before the next injection (Remington et al. 2006).

All participants had at least five injections before PET determinations were carried out. Occupancies were 53% to 75% for two patients receiving 25 mg, 59% to 85% for five patients receiving 50 mg, and 71% to 85% for two patients receiving 75 mg. Table 2.2 indicates a consensus approach to equivalence (see also Chapter 5). Based on comparisons of plasma levels for risperidone in its oral and IM formulations (Eerdekens 2004; Gefvert et al 2005) and matching this to PET occupancy data (Gefvert et al. 2005; Remington et al. 2006; Kapur et al.1995) it is common in countries such as Australia to accept the equivalence of oral to IM risperidone of 2/25, 3/37.5, 4/50. Our consensus view of using the figures suggested by Bai et al. (2007), which were based on a modest study in Taiwanese patients, allows for flexibility in calculating equivalence. Of course monitoring of target symptoms will drive final doses in any one individual.

The pharmacokinetics and dynamics of paliperidone palmitate has received comprehensive review by Citrome (2010). Following an injection, Tmax for paliperidone release is about 13 days with the release starting immediately after injection and continuing up to 126 days. Based on pharmacokinetic data presented in poster form a suggested minimum effective level of paliperidone is 7.5 ng/ml, equating approximately to 60% D2R occupancy on PET (Samtani et al. 2009a). This minimum plasma level threshold is achieved in 84% of patients within 8 to 36 days using the 150/100 mg eq. initiation regime (above). It is worth noting that it has been argued that plasma levels of SDA antipsychotics may be more effective (at least with respect to positive symptoms) if D2R occupancy is in the 65% to 78% range (Arakawa et al. 2008; Pani et al. 2007), which will be approximately within the 7.5 to 50 ng/ml range for paliperidone. For further information on paliperidone palmitate kinetics see Samtani et al. (2009a, b).

Data on D2 occupancies associated with the use of FGA-LAIs are somewhat perplexing. They appear to show apparently sub-therapeutic D2 occupancies associated with some doses, at least at some time points, without attendant relapse. This may mean that persistently high striatal D2 receptor occupancy is not required for full therapeutic effect or that other D2 activities outside the striatum or other receptor activities are relevant. On the other hand, the low occupancies seen with low doses of haloperidol and risperidone do fit with clinical data suggesting that these doses are suboptimal (Bai et al. 2007; Eklund & Forsman 1991; Kane et al. 2002; Taylor et al. 2006;). The experience of many clinicians is that the mean time to relapse after ceasing LAIs is in terms of many months (as opposed to weeks), consistent with their long apparent half-lives (Wistedt 1981).

Genetic or drug-induced variability in drug metabolizing enzyme activity has received relatively little study with respect to LAIs. Although the apparent half-life is determined by drug release rather than drug metabolism, when free drug is made available, it is still subject to the same influences that the oral form experiences. For example, there are some instances where an increase in metabolic activity may result in the need for higher depot doses—smoking (by inducing CYP1A2) significantly reduces fluphenazine levels (Jann et al. 1985); coprescribing of fluoxetine increases risperidone levels, presumably in both oral and long-acting forms (Spina et al. 2002).

Clearly more research is required in this area as polypharmacy is of growing concern in modern practice (Mojtabai & Olfson 2010).

However, it is always wise to consider a patient's ethnicity (and thereby the potential for pharmacokinetic and pharmacodynamic differences) when prescribing any psychotropic. For example, LAI doses may be lower in persons from Asia primarily owing to reduced body mass rather than because of any primary effect of carrying slow metabolizing genes such as those that code for the *10 allele of *CYP2D6* (Lambert & Norman 2008). In such cases one makes the assumption that plasma levels are correlated with target receptor occupancy.

Switching to and from LAIs

In this section we consider the pharmacological issues that relate to switching from oral antipsychotics to LAIs, the converse, and switching between different LAIs. When switching antipsychotics, clinicians need to be aware of the pitfalls that can arise when a switch is inexpertly planned, or unexpected vagaries arise in the switch process (Lambert et al. 2007). The kinetics of LAIs, in the main, makes switching more stable and with due consideration, should avoid some of the classic switch-withdrawal phenomena such as supersensivity rebound psychosis or withdrawal-emergent dyskinesias (Lambert et al. 2007). When switching from one LAI to another, the most parsimonious approach is simply to substitute the new LAI for the previous one at a planned injection appointment. It would be anticipated that this would create the equivalent of a cross-taper oral switch—the previous LAI plasma levels falling over a number of months, with a corresponding slow rise to steady state of the new agent. The anticipation is of no large dips or troughs in blood levels as this occurs. However, as the washout phase of some FGA-LAIs may be much longer than the initial period from initiation to steady state, there may be a period of effective dual therapy, which may confer either benefits or side-effects, depending on the individual's particular clinical state. If the LAI that is stopped was prescribed at the maximum licensed dose, then the prescriber should consider starting the new LAI at a relatively low dose or the patient may receive a combined antipsychotic dose during the cross-over phase that places them in an above licensed dose range. This should be avoided owing to the higher risk of adverse effects and the potential for significant QTc prolongation (Haddad & Anderson 2002).

Switching from an LAI to an oral antipsychotic is usually a straightforward process. The LAI is ceased and its natural plasma level decay provides ample antipsychotic cover, whereas the new oral builds to steady state. An issue that arises here is that of potential dual therapy again. Whereas it may take weeks to months for the LAI to wash out, most oral antipsychotics achieve steady state within 5 to 10 days. If the oral is instigated immediately after the last depot injection, there will be active effects from both medications for a variable period. Despite their being scant evidence to support any form of polyantipsychotic therapy in routine clinical use, in switching from LAIs some clinicians report that the new oral drug loses its initial effectiveness some months after its instigation. This suggests that the patient's initial response may have been because of combination therapy, and the subsequent relapse reflects them being progressively exposed to single rather than dual antipsychotic therapy. The corollary is that having two agents at work may lead to an increased side-effect burden. On occasion this leads the clinician to discontinue the new oral agent because of 'unexpected side effects'. Clearly, it is important to anticipate an interaction in some cases and monitor the effectiveness of treatment during the switch period, which may be over a period of months when LAIs are involved. In principle, combined antipsychotic therapy has little evidence to support it and any dual therapy during a switch should be minimized where possible.

A switch to LAIs from an oral antipsychotic requires consideration of the relevant kinetics once again. Planning a switch to an FGA-LAI should incorporate the following: what are the equivalent doses? What is the expected time to steady state of the LAI? What is the period before it will achieve a minimally effective plasma level? Is a loading strategy planned to bring plasma levels up more rapidly? What are the anticipated potential interactions that might occur between the previous drug and the LAI? These questions might help determine how the previous antipsychotic is discontinued (abrupt, gradual taper, step, or hybrid taper); the period between starting the LAI and starting to discontinue the oral; and planning to observe for potential switch consequences.

Of course in any of the above scenarios, the general precepts of switching antipsychotics need to be observed; For example, being careful to avoid cholinergic rebound, sedative-withdrawal rebound, or any of the less common switching/withdrawal motor syndromes (Lambert et al. 2007).

Figure 2.4 shows a planned switch to RLAI for a patient treated with an anticholinergic oral antipsychotic. In this scenario an anticholinergic agent such as benztropine is added when the previous anticholinergic antipsychotic is withdrawn relatively quickly. This is to prevent cholinergic rebound. As RLAI does not release appreciable amounts of free risperidone until about the fourth week after the 2-weekly injection, oral supplementation with the previous agent is suggested for at least 3 weeks before tapering. It is when this tapering is fast that an anticholinergic might be added and is probably not required where the prior anticholinergic antipsychotic is very slowly withdrawn. These precautions occur as risperidone and others such as paliperidone, fluphenazine, and haloperidol have negligible intrinsic anticholinergic properties themselves. Prior to switching it can be helpful to select patients who might be appropriate for LAI therapy. Ostensibly this would imply patients with issues of relapse or poor outcomes relating to non-adherence. Second, a switch might be from an FGA to an SGA-LAI because of the inherently better properties of the latter. Such switches have been shown to be effective, at least from the perspective of symptom improvements (Lasser et al. 2004). A number of patient 'ideal types' other than those mentioned have been identified for switching to SGA-LAIs (Lambert 2006). Of the various types of suggested patients, the benefits of an overt injection on kinetics and metabolism form an integral component of the switch logic. Although these ideal types were derived from early clinical service experience with SGA-LAIs, their utility in a broader range of settings requires further empirical testing.

Finally, switching choices are often formed by ease of use of the target medication and ensuring that pharmacological benefits are not offset by practical delivery factors.

Table 2.5 Practical issues concerning LAI administration

Drug	Injection site	Storage	Reconstitution and administration
FGAs	Gluteal	Oil in vial	z-tracking injection technique to avoid post-injection leakage; concentrates—where available—may reduce injection volume; nodule formation with repeated injections; essential to rotate injection sites; possibility of subcutaneous injections[a]; evidence base for differing injection techniques slim[b]
Risperidone	Gluteal or deltoid	Powder; Special kits	Requires cold chain storage (unique among LAIs); special kits and training; fractional use of drawn-up material to achieve low or intermediate doses not recommended; evidence on deltoid use slim (new preparation); z-tracking not required
Paliperidone	Deltoid or gluteal	Pre-filled syringe kit	Choice of needle size based on weight (longer needle for >90 Kg); deltoid achieves more rapid uptake; z-tracking not required
Olanzapine	Gluteal	Powder; special kits	Special kits and training required; reconstitution for smaller doses requires some special calculations by nursing staff; getting powder into suspension can be time consuming; large volumes at top dose; z-tracking not required; 3-hour observation in a health care facility required due to possibility of post-injection syndrome.

[a] Elsom and Kelly (2009).
[b] Cocoman and Murray (2008). For further information of injection site pain, see Chapter 3.

Some of the issues that should be considered are shown in Table 2.5. As this table shows, although medication choice may be made on clinical effectiveness and tolerability grounds, there is still an important requirement to consider the practical issues of storage, reconstitution, and administration and to ensure that nursing and other relevant staff have adequate support and training to deliver the LAI effectively.

Conclusions

In this chapter we have reviewed some of the key aspects of the psychopharmacology of FGA and SGA-LAIs. The LAIs have had three principal development phases based on the vehicle used for the 'depot' store and each having particular pharmacokinetics associated with the formulation. The oil-based LAIs (all FGAs) have, compared to their oral counterparts, a long period before they achieve clinical effective levels, many months to steady state, and correspondingly, many months to 'wash out'. Wide pharmacokinetic variation both within and between patients' suggests that optimizing clinical use of FGA-LAIs remains both an art and a science. RLAI has unique kinetics that stem from its microsphere-based technology. Its kinetics are more predictable, albeit with some limitations in the sense of having a 3-week interregnum of no release following injection. The crystal-based LAIs offer sustained delivery of clinically effective doses from the first day of injection and have well-defined pharmacokinetic profiles. Given their very recent introduction, their clinical utility will be an evolving story in the coming months and years.

With average target doses in mind we examined dose equivalence between the orals and their LAI counterparts, and between LAIs in a comparative fashion. Having a clear idea of how doses can translate into optimal antipsychotic efficacy with good tolerability is aided by considering equivalencies. There is little doubt that inaccurate equivalencies may account for relative 'overdoses' or 'inadequate response', so often seen throughout the antipsychotic field. We note that when adherence is assured through LAI use, average daily doses in maintenance appear to be of the order of 300 mg/day CPZe for the more recently introduced agents and somewhat higher for agents that were first brought into clinical practice (fluphenazine, haloperidol).

In reviewing injections intervals there appears a wide choice available to clinicians between 1 and 6 weeks. For the FGA-LAIs—although many may be given 4-weekly—the mode for fluphenazine, flupentixol, zuclopenthixol, and pipotiazine is 2-weekly and for haloperidol 4-weekly. There may be a need for clinicians in certain treatment settings to consider longer treatment intervals, which may reduce the burden on patients and staff in some cases. RLAI is licensed only for 2-weekly injections by its manufacturer, although some preliminary evidence suggests longer injection intervals may be possible in some patients individuals. Paliperidone palmitate is given solely as a 4-weekly injection after its initiation (day 1 and day 8 loading). Olanzapine pamoate has 2- or 4-weekly injections intervals possible, with the target oral olanzapine equivalent dose driving the choice.

In order to rapidly achieve clinically meaningful plasma levels of the active antipsychotic component of LAIs, a number of initiation or loading strategies were presented. Such protocols overcome the slow time to steady state of some of the agents and reduce the need for complicated reducing regimes of oral supplementation when LAIs are first prescribed.

The pharmacodynamics were reviewed, indicating that there is a considerable dearth of studies examining LAIs, both for FGAs and surprisingly for SGA-LAIs. As PET studies are complex, many studies to date are limited by small patient numbers from selected populations, making generalizability difficult. However, this is an important area of scientific understanding of the LAIs, and it is hoped that more studies will be carried out in the coming years.

The chapter concludes with an overview of the pharmacology of switching LAIs. In general switching from and between LAIs is simple to carry out and carries few risks. When switching to and from oral antipsychotics, it is important to plan the switch carefully and to take into account the relative pharmacology of agents on both sides of the switch equation. Of course one should always be clear about why one would wish to cease an LAI if it effective in forestalling relapse and keep in mind the adage 'if it ain't broke, don't fix it'.

References

Adams CE, Fenton MK, Quraishi S, David AS. (2001). Systematic meta-review of depot antipsychotic drugs for people with schizophrenia. *Br J Psychiatry*, **179**, 290–9.

Agid O, Kapur S, Arenovich T, Zipursky RB. (2003). Delayed-onset hypothesis of antipsychotic action: a hypothesis tested and rejected. *Arch Gen Psychiatry*, **60**(12), 1228–35.

Agid O, Mamo D, Ginovart N, Vitcu I, Wilson AA, Zipursky RB, et al. (2007). Striatal vs extrastriatal dopamine D2 receptors in antipsychotic response—a double-blind PET study in schizophrenia. *Neuropsychopharmacology*, **32**(6), 1209–15.

Alwan NA, P , Johnstone , G Zolese, . (2008). 'Length of hospitalisation for people with severe mental illness.'. *Cochrane Database Syst Rev*, (1), CD000384.

Arakawa R, Ito H, Takano A, Takahashi H, Morimoto T, Sassa T, et al. (2008). Dose-finding study of paliperidone ER based on striatal and extrastriatal dopamine D2 receptor occupancy in patients with schizophrenia. *Psychopharmacology (Berl)*, **197**(2), 229–35.

Bai YM, Ting Chen T, Chen JY, Chang WH, Wu B, Hung CH, et al. (2007). Equivalent switching dose from oral risperidone to risperidone long-acting injection: a 48-week randomized, prospective, single-blind pharmacokinetic study. *J Clin Psychiatry*, **68**(8), 1218–25.

Barnes TRE, Curson DA. (1994). Long-term depot antipsychotics: a risk-benefit assessment. *Drug Safety*, **10**, 464–79.

Baron JC, Martinot JL, Cambon H, Boulenger JP, Poirier MF, Caillard V, et al. (1989). Striatal dopamine receptor occupancy during and following withdrawal from neuroleptic treatment: correlative evaluation by positron emission tomography and plasma prolactin levels. *Psychopharmacology (Berl)*, **99**(4), 463–72.

Bazire S. (1999). *Psychotropic Drug Directory 1999: The Professionals Pocket Handbook and Aide Memoire*, (Dinton: Quay Books Division Mark Allen Publishing).

Citrome L. (2009). Olanzapine pamoate: a stick in time? A review of the efficacy and safety profile of a new depot formulation of a second-generation antipsychotic. *Int J Clin Pract*, **63**(1), 140–50.

Citrome L. (2010). Paliperidone palmitate—review of the efficacy, safety and cost of a new second-generation depot antipsychotic medication. *Int J Clin Pract*, **64**(2), 216–39.

Citrome L, Reist C, Palmer L, Montejano L, Lenhart G, Cuffel B, et al. (2009). Dose trends for second-generation antipsychotic treatment of schizophrenia and bipolar disorder. *Schizophr Res*, **108**(1–3), 238–44.

Cocoman A, Murray J. (2008). Intramuscular injections: a review of best practice for mental health nurses. *J Psychiatr Ment Health Nurs*, **15**(5), 424–34.

Dencker SJ, Axelsson R. (1996). Optimising the use of depot antipsychotics. *CNS Drugs*, **6**(5), 367–81.

Eerdekens M, Van Hove I, Remmerie B, Mannaert E. (2004). Pharmacokinetics and tolerability of long-acting risperidone in schizophrenia. *Schizophr Res*, **70**(1), 91–100.

Eklund K, Forsman. (1991). Minimal effective dose and relapse—double-blind trial: haloperidol decanoate vs. placebo. *Clin Neuropharmacol*, **14**(Suppl 2), S7–S12.

Eli Lilly Australia Pty Ltd. (2009). *Product Information: Zyprexa relprevv*. 9 October 2009.

Elsom S, Kelly T. (2009). Need for clinical practice guidelines for im injections *Aust N Z J Psychiatry*, **43**(9), 877–8.

Ereshefsky L., Saklad SR, Jann MW, Davis CM, Richards A, Seidel DR. (1984). Future of depot neuroleptic therapy: pharmacokinetic and pharmacodynamic approaches. *J Clin Psychiatry*, **45** (5 Pt 2), 50–9.

Galletly CA, Tsourtos G. (1997). Antipsychotic drug doses and adjunctive drugs in the outpatient treatment of schizophrenia. *Ann Clin Psychiatry*, 9(2), 77–80.

Gefvert O, Eriksson B, Persson P, Helldin L, Björner A, Mannaert E, et al. (2005). Pharmacokinetics and D2 receptor occupancy of long-acting injectable risperidone (Risperdal Consta) in patients with schizophrenia. *Int J Neuropsychopharmacol*, **8**(1), 27–36.

Gharabawi GM, Gearhart NC, Lasser RA, Mahmoud RA, Zhu Y, Mannaert E, et al. (2007). Maintenance therapy with once-monthly administration of long-acting injectable risperidone in patients with schizophrenia or schizoaffective disorder: a pilot study of an extended dosing interval. *Ann Gen Psychiatry*, **6**, 3.

Haddad PM, Anderson IM. (2002). Antipsychotic-related QTc prolongation, torsade de pointes and sudden death. *Drugs*, **62**(11), 1649–71.

Harasko-van der Meer, C, T, Brucke S , Wenger, P Fischer, L Deecke, I Podreka (1993). 'Two cases of long term dopamine D2 receptor blockade after depot neuroleptics.'. *J Neural Transm Gen Sect*, **94**(3), 217–21.

Hough D, Lindenmayer JP, Gopal S, Melkote R, Lim P, Herben V, et al. (2009). Safety and tolerability of deltoid and gluteal injections of paliperidone palmitate in schizophrenia. *Prog Neuropsychopharmacol Biol Psychiatry*, **33**(6), 1022–31.

Humberstone V, Wheeler A, Lambert T. (2004). An audit of outpatient antipsychotic usage in the three health sectors of Auckland, New Zealand. *Aust N Z J Psychiatry*, **38**(4), 240–5.

Jann MW, Ereshefsky L, Saklad SR. (1985). Clinical pharmacokinetics of the depot antipsychotics. *Clin Pharmacokinet*, **10**(4), 315–33.

Janssen, Division of Ortho-McNeil-Janssen Pharmaceuticals. (2009). *Product Information. Paliperidone palmitate* http://www.invegasustenna.com/invegasustenna/shared/pi/invegasustenna.pdf (accessed 18 December 2009).

Johnson D, Dencker S. (1997). *Maintenance Treatment of Chronic Schizophrenia*. Copenhagen: Lundbeck.

Kane JM, Davis JM, Schooler N, Marder S, Casey D, Brauzer B, et al. (2002). A multidose study of haloperidol decanoate in the maintenance treatment of schizophrenia *Am J Psychiatry*, **159**(4), 554–60.

Kapur S, Remington G, Zipursky RB, Wilson AA, Houle S. (1995). The D2 dopamine receptor occupancy of risperidone and its relationship to extrapyramidal symptoms: a PET study. *Life Sci*, **57**(10), PL103–7.

Kapur S, Zipursky R, Jones C, Remington G, Houle S. (2000). Relationship between dopamine D(2) occupancy, clinical response, and side effects: a double-blind PET study of first-episode schizophrenia. *Am J Psychiatry*, **157**(4), 514–20.

Kurtz D, Bergstrom R, McDonnell DP, Mitchell M, et al. (2008). Pharmacokinetics (PK) of multiple doses of olanzapine long acting injection (OLAI), an intramuscular (IM) depot formulation of olanzapine (OLZ), in stabilized patients with schizophrenia. *Biol Psychiatry*, **63** S 288.

Lambert T (2006). Selecting patients for long-acting novel antipsychotic therapy. *Australas Psychiatry*, **14**(1), 38–42.

Lambert T, de Castella A, Kulkarni J, Ong AN, Singh B. (2007). One year estimate of depot antipsychotic adherence and readmission in Australian community mental health settings [abstract]. *Schizophr Bull*, **33**, 485.

Lambert T, Norman T. (2008). Ethnic differences in psychotropic drug response and pharmacokinetics. In: CH Ng, K-M Lin, BS Singh (eds.), *Ethno-psychopharmacology: Advances in Current Practice*. Cambridge, New York: Cambridge University Press, pp. 38–61.

Lambert TJR. (2005). *The Use of Depot Antipsychotics in Community Psychiatry* (Doctoral dissertation, University of Melbourne, 2005).

Larsen NE, and LB Hansen . (1989). 'Prediction of the optimal perphenazine decanoate dose based on blood samples drawn within the first three weeks.'. *Ther Drug Monit*, **11**(6), 642–46.

Lasser RA, Bossie CA, Gharabawi GM, Turner M. (2004). Patients with schizophrenia previously stabilized on conventional depot antipsychotics experience significant clinical improvements following treatment with long-acting risperidone. *Eur Psychiatry*, **19**(4), 219–25.

Lauriello J, Lambert T, Andersen S, Lin D, Taylor CC, McDonnell D. (2008). An 8-week, double-blind, randomized, placebo-controlled study of olanzapine long-acting injection in acutely ill patients with schizophrenia. *J Clin Psychiatry*, **69**(5), 790–9.

Mamo David, Kapur S, Keshavan M, Laruelle M, Taylor CC, Kothare PA, et al. (2008). D2 receptor occupancy of olanzapine pamoate depot using positron emission tomography: an open-label study in patients with schizophrenia. *Neuropsychopharmacology*, **33**(2), 298–304.

Mannaert E, Vermeulen A, Remmerie B, Bouhours P, Levron JC, . (2005). Pharmacokinetic profile of long-acting injectable risperidone at steady-state: comparison with oral administration. *Encephale* , **31**(5 Pt 1), 609 –15.

Meadows G, and B, Singh(eds) (2001). *Mental health in Australia: collaborative community practice*. Melbourne: Oxford University Press.

Mojtabai R, Olfson, M. (2010). National trends in psychotropic medication polypharmacy in office-based psychiatry. *Arch Gen Psychiatry*, **67**(1), 26–36.

Nyberg S, Farde L, Halldin C. (1997). Delayed normalization of central D2 dopamine receptor availability after discontinuation of haloperidol decanoate. Preliminary findings. *Arch Gen Psychiatry*, **54**(10), 953–8.

Nyberg S, Farde L, Halldin C, Dahl ML, Bertilsson L. (1995). D2 dopamine receptor occupancy during low-dose treatment with haloperidol decanoate. *Am J Psychiatry*, **152**(2), 173–8.

Pani L, Pira L, Marchese G. (2007). Antipsychotic efficacy: relationship to optimal D2-receptor occupancy. *Eur Psychiatry*, **22**(5), 267–75.

Pilowsky LS, Busatto GF, Taylor M, Costa DC, Sharma T, Sigmundsson T, et al. (1996). Dopamine D2 receptor occupancy in vivo by the novel atypical antipsychotic olanzapine—a 123I IBZM single photon emission tomography (SPET) study. *Psychopharmacology* 124, 148–53.

Poulsen JH, Olesen OV, Larsen NE. (1994). Fluctuation of serum zuclopenthixol concentrations in patients treated with zuclopenthixol decanoate in viscoleo. *Ther Drug Monit*, **16**(2), 155–9.

Ramstack M, Grandolfi G, Mannaert E, D'Hoore P, Lasser R. (2003). Long-acting risperidone: Prolonged-release injectable delivery of risperidone using medisorbò microsphere technology. *Schizophr Res*, **60**(1), 314.

Remington G, Mamo D, Labelle A, Reiss J, Shammi C, Mannaert E, et al. (2006). A PET study evaluating dopamine D2 receptor occupancy for long-acting injectable risperidone. *Am J Psychiatry*, **163**(3), 396–401.

Royal College of Psychiatrists. (2006). *Consensus statement on high-dose antipsychotic medication. Council Report CR138.* http://www.rcpsych.ac.uk/files/pdfversion/CR138.pdf (accessed 25 January 2010).

Samtani MN, Kern-Sliwa J, Haskins JT. (2009a). Initiation Dosing of Deltoid Intramuscular Paliperidone Palmitate in Schizophrenia: Pharmacokinetic Rationale Based on Modeling and Simulation *Annual Meeting of The College of Psychiatric and Neurologic Pharmacists*, Jacksonville, FL, 19–22 April 2009.

Samtani MN, Vermeulen A, Stuyckens K. (2009b). Population pharmacokinetics of intramuscular paliperidone palmitate in patients with schizophrenia: a novel once-monthly, long-acting formulation of an atypical antipsychotic. *Clin Pharmacokinet*, **48**(9), 585–600.

Simpson S, Egan T. (1993). Prescribers update: antipsychotics. *New Ethicals*, **30**(2), 29.

Spina E, Avenoso A, Scordo MG, Ancione M, Madia A, Gatti G, et al. (2002). Inhibition of risperidone metabolism by fluoxetine in patients with schizophrenia: a clinically relevant pharmacokinetic drug interaction. *J Clin Psychopharmacol*, **22**(4), 419–23.

Talvik M, Nordström AL, Larsen NE, Jucaite A, Cervenka S, Halldin C, et al. (2004). A cross-validation study on the relationship between central D 2 receptor occupancy and serum perphenazine concentration *Psychopharmacology*, **175**(2), 148–53.

Taylor DM. (2009). Psychopharmacology and adverse effects of antipsychotic long-acting injections: a review. *Br J Psychiatry*, **195**, S13–S19.

Taylor DM, Young C, Patel MX. (2006). Prospective 6-month follow-up of patients prescribed risperidone long-acting injection: factors predicting favourable outcome. *Int J Neuropsychopharmacol*, **9**(6), 685–94.

Tuninger E, Axelsson R, Levander S. (1994). A 3-year study of maintenance therapy with depot neuroleptics. Clinical characteristics and medication at study entry. *Nord J Psychiatry*, **48**, 409–9.

Tuninger E, Levander S. (1996). Large variations of plasma levels during maintenance treatment with depot neuroleptics. *Br J Psychiatry*, **169**, 618–21.

Wilson WH (2004). A visual guide to expected blood levels of long-acting injectable risperidone in clinical practice. *J Psychiatr Pract*, **10**(6), 393–401.

Wistedt B. (1981). A depot neuroleptic withdrawal study. A controlled study of the clinical effects of the withdrawal of depot fluphenazine decanoate and depot flupenthixol decanoate in chronic schizophrenic patients. *Acta Psychiatr Scand*, **64**, 65–84.

Chapter 3

Adverse effects and antipsychotic long-acting injections

Peter Haddad and W. Wolfgang Fleischhacker

Correspondence: peter.haddad@gmw.nhs.uk

Introduction

Antipsychotic drugs can cause a wide range of adverse effects (Table 3.1) irrespective of whether they are administered as oral medication or as a long-acting injection (LAI; Haddad & Sharma 2007). Clinicians need to be familiar with these effects to minimize their occurrence and recognize and manage them when they arise. The adverse effects listed in Table 3.1 are not considered in detail in this chapter as they are reviewed in other chapters of this book in relation to specific LAIs, namely Chapter 4 on first-generation antipsychotic LAIs (FGA-LAIs), Chapter 5 on risperidone long acting-injection (RLAI), and Chapter 6 on olanzapine long-acting injection (OLAI) and paliperidone long-acting injection (PLAI). This chapter concentrates on aspects of tolerability and safety that have special relevance to LAIs compared to oral medication.

We start by considering whether non–injection-related adverse effects are more frequent with LAIs than with oral medication. This is a common clinical question with a good pharmacological rationale; the pharmacokinetic profiles of oral medication and LAIs are very different. We then review injection-related adverse effects including pain, injection-site problems, and the olanzapine post-injection syndrome. Next we consider how the pharmacokinetics of LAIs can lead to the delayed appearance and resolution of adverse effects compared with those seen with oral medication following initiation and termination of treatment and dose adjustment. The clinical implications for the assessment and management of adverse effects and use of LAIs are reviewed. The chapter concludes with a short summary.

Incidence of adverse effects with oral antipsychotics and LAIs

Background

Kane et al. (1998) reported that some psychiatrists believe that LAIs are associated with a greater risk of certain side-effects than oral medication. Two surveys of psychiatrists in the United Kingdom, conducted in 2001 and 2006–2007, found that 38% and 39% of respondents, respectively believed that 'major side-effects' were more common with

Table 3.1 Examples of adverse effects caused by antipsychotics irrespective of route of administration

◆ **Antimuscarinic symptoms**	◆ **Hyperprolactinaemia**
Dry mouth	Decreased bone mineral density
Blurred vision	Galactorrhoea
Cognitive impairment	Gynaecomastia
Constipation	Menstrual abnormalities
Urinary retention	Sexual dysfunction[a]
◆ **Cardiovascular effects**	◆ **Metabolic effects**
Arrhythmias	Weight gain
Cardiomyopathy	Hyperglycaemia
Myocarditis	Dyslipidaemia
Oedema	◆ **Sexual dysfunction**[a]
Postural hypotension	Decreased libido
◆ **Extrapyramidal syndromes**	Decreased arousal including erectile dysfunction
Akathisia	Impaired orgasm
Dystonia	◆ **Miscellaneous adverse effects**
Parkinsonism	Cerebrovascular events
Tardive dyskinesia	Blood dyscrasias
	Neuroleptic malignant syndrome
	Photosensitivity
	Seizures
	Sedation

[a] Sexual dysfunction may be secondary to raised prolactin or may result from other pharmacological effects of medication

typical depots than typical oral antipsychotics (Patel et al. 2003, 2009). This view was also held by 54% of UK community psychiatric nurses surveyed in 2003 (Patel et al. 2005) and by 65% of psychiatric nurses surveyed in Hong Kong in 2006 (Patel et al. 2008). In this section we consider whether this view is supported by evidence.

Broad statements comparing the tolerability of oral antipsychotics versus LAIs are misleading, as are comparisons of first-generation antipsychotics (FGAs) versus second-generation antipsychotics (SGAs). This is because these questions are too broad to answer; it depends on what side-effect is considered and the specific antipsychotic drugs that are compared. Meta-analyses (e.g. Leucht et al. 2009) and narrative reviews (e.g. Haddad & Sharma 2007) show significant differences in the adverse-effect profiles of different oral antipsychotics. For example, mean weight gain is greater with olanzapine than with risperidone, whereas the prevalence of hyperprolactinaemia is higher with risperidone than olanzapine (Haddad & Sharma 2007). Consequently it is more meaningful to make comparisons between specific drugs and in relation to specific adverse effects (Haddad & Sharma 2007). Thus the key question is whether specific adverse effects differ when equivalent doses of the same antipsychotic are administered in oral and LAI preparations.

Several studies indicate that LAIs compared to oral medication show less fluctuation in plasma antipsychotic levels (Eerdekens et al. 2004; Mannaert et al. 2005; Tavacar et al. 2000). Based on the finding that LAIs result in lower peak plasma levels some commentators have suggested that they may show a better side-effect profile than the same drug in oral form. Few commentators discuss whether the evidence supports this or consider the opposite possibility i.e. that reduced plasma troughs with an LAI may aggravate side-effects. To determine whether pharmacokinetic differences between oral and LAI formulations of an antipsychotic affect tolerability, a study should compare bioequivalent doses of the two drugs in a double-blind randomized design and assess tolerability, and ideally efficacy, using validated rating scales. We are not aware of any study that fulfils these criteria. Furthermore such a study would be relevant only to the specific antipsychotic studied; the different pharmacokinetic and tolerability profiles of antipsychotics mean it would be invalid to generalize the results to all antipsychotic LAIs and their equivalent oral formulations.

LAIs are not always associated with narrow fluctuations in plasma antipsychotic levels. A large variation in plasma levels has been reported during long-term treatment with constant doses of FGA-LAIs (Tuninger & Levander 1996). This may reflect the pharmacokinetics of the LAI, poor injection technique, or pharmacokinetic interactions with smoking or co-prescribed medication. Poor technique may result in retrograde seepage along the injection track, leakage of the medication onto the skin surface, and an effective reduction in the administered dose (Hay 1995). Poor technique can result in injection into the subcutaneous tissue rather than muscle but whether this alters antipsychotic absorption from the injection site is unclear. By inducing cytochrome enzymes and increasing metabolism, cigarette smoking can reduce the plasma levels of several antipsychotics, including haloperidol (Nayak et al. 1987), fluphenazine (Jann et al. 1985; Tuninger & Levander 1996), and olanzapine (Carrillo et al. 2003) irrespective of whether these drugs are administered orally or intramuscularly. Jann et al. (1985) reported that cigarette smoking led to a 2.3-fold increase in the clearance of fluphenazine decanoate. Co-administered drugs can alter plasma antipsychotic levels by either inducing or inhibiting cytochrome enzymes involved in antipsychotic metabolism.

In the rest of this section we consider some key studies that have compared the pharmacokinetic and/or side-effect profiles of antipsychotics in oral and LAI forms.

First-generation antipsychotic LAIs

Pharmacokinetics studies measuring plasma antipsychotic level were not possible when the FGA-LAIs were introduced in the 1960s owing to the inability to measure sub-nanomolar plasma concentrations accurately (Jann et al. 1985). Subsequent studies comparing FGAs in oral and LAI formulations, including fluphenazine and haloperidol, found that at steady state there was less variability in the range of plasma concentration with the LAI compared with oral medication (Tavacar et al. 2000).

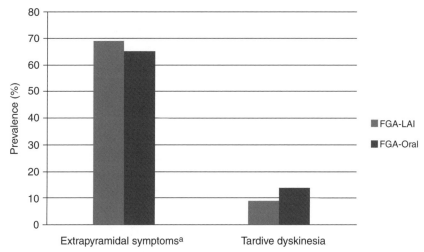

Fig. 3.1 Prevalence of extrapyramidal symptoms and tardive dyskinesia in patients treated with first generation antipsychotics in oral and LAI preparations (data from Adams et al. 2001).
[a] prevalence based on prescription of anticholinergic medication.

Some studies showed lower mean plasma concentrations for the LAI than for clinically equivalent dose of the oral drug.

Little data compare the tolerability of FGAs in oral and depot forms (Haddad et al. 2009). A meta-analysis by Adams et al. (2001) compared adverse effects in patients randomized to FGA-LAIs and FGA oral drugs. There was no significant difference between the two groups in the rate of prescribing of anticholinergic medication, a proxy marker for the presence of extrapyramidal symptoms (EPS; 69% FGA-LAI cohort; 65% FGA-oral cohort), or in the prevalence of tardive dyskinesia (TD) assessed by rating scales (9.0% FGA-LAI cohort; 14.1% FGA-oral cohort; Figure 3.1). It should be noted that this meta-analysis showed that LAIs were at least as effective as oral medication; relapse rates did not differ between the two groups but global improvement was more likely with an LAI. The main strength of this analysis is that it is based on randomized data yet one has to critically note that it included some short-term studies that are unlikely to demonstrate an efficacy advantage for LAIs over oral medication. In addition, not all the studies in the meta-analysis compared the same drug in oral and LAI forms, which complicates interpretation.

Some observational studies, including the Schizophrenia Outpatient Heath Outcomes (SOHO) study (Haro et al. 2007), have reported higher rates for adverse effects, including EPS, in patients treated with FGA-LAIs versus FGA-orals. However, the lack of randomization means that the differences may reflect selection bias rather than differences between drugs. Furthermore, it is possible that an excess of adverse effects with an LAI in an observational study may reflect better adherence compared to that seen with oral medication rather than an intrinsic difference between the two drugs.

In summary, the available data suggest an equivalent rate of EPS and TD for FGAs in oral and long-acting injectable formulations.

Risperidone LAI

Eerdekens et al. (2004) compared the pharmacokinetics and tolerability of RLAI versus oral risperidone in a 15-week open-label study of 86 patients with schizophrenia. Patients stabilized on 2, 4, or 6 mg of oral risperidone once daily for a minimum period of 4 weeks were switched to receive 25, 50, or 75 mg of RLAI 2-weekly, respectively, for 10 weeks. Pharmacokinetic analyses were based on the active moiety (i.e. risperidone plus its active metabolite 9-hydoxyrisperidone) and were calculated on day 7 of oral dosing and on values obtained during the 14 days after the fifth injection of RLAI. The mean steady-state C_{min} concentrations of the active moiety did not differ for oral risperidone and RLAI but the mean steady-state C_{max} concentrations were 25% to 32% lower for RLAI than for oral risperidone depending on the dose considered. Percentage fluctuations in plasma active moiety concentrations were 32% to 42% lower with RLAI than with oral risperidone (see Figure 3.2). The 90% confidence intervals for RLAI/oral risperidone ratios for (i) the mean steady-state plasma-AUC (area under curve) corrected for dosing interval, and (ii) the average plasma concentration were within the bioequivalence range of 80% to 125% for the active moiety. Severity of EPS, assessed by the Extrapyramidal Symptom Rating Scale (ESRS), were low at the end of the oral phase but fell further following the switch to RLAI. Symptoms of schizophrenia, assessed by the mean total Positive and Negative Syndrome Scale (PANSS) score, improved during treatment with all three doses of RLAI. To summarize, this study shows that bioequivalent doses of oral risperidone and RLAI have a different

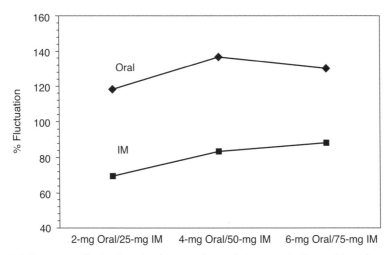

Fig. 3.2 Percentage fluctuations in plasma active-moiety concentrations with oral risperidone and RLAI [% fluctuation = 100 × (C_{max}–C_{min})/$C_{average}$] (reprinted from Schizophrenia Research, Maiëlle Eerdekens, Ilse Van Hove, Bart Remmerie, and Erik Mannaert, Pharmacokinetics and tolerability of long-acting risperidone in schizophrenia. Copyright 2004 with permission from Elsevier).

pharmacokinetic profile with RLAI showing less fluctuations in plasma levels and a lower C_{max}. The next question is whether this has a tolerability advantage for RLAI.

The fall in EPS following the switch from oral risperidone to RLAI (Eerdekens et al. 2004) may reflect smoother plasma levels but methodological issues, including the open assessment and switch design of the study, mean that other factors may explain the improvement. Two controlled studies have compared the side-effect profile of RLAI and oral risperidone (Bai et al. 2006; Chue et al. 2005), and both suggested a possible tolerability advantage for RLAI compared to oral risperidone.

Chue et al. (2005) conducted a 12-week, double-blind study of RLAI and oral risperidone in 640 patients with schizophrenia. All patients were initially treated with open-label oral risperidone (1–6 mg) for 8 weeks. At the end of this period, symptomatically stable patients were randomly switched to RLAI (active injections, placebo oral) or made to continue oral risperidone (placebo injections, active oral) for 12 weeks. Both groups showed a significant improvement from baseline to endpoint in PANSS total scores. There was a significantly greater fall from baseline to end point in prolactin levels in the RLAI-group compared with the oral-group, although in both groups the mean prolactin at endpoint was above the upper limit of the normal range. There were no significant differences from baseline to endpoint between the two groups in weight increase, various measures of extrapyramidal symptoms, QTc, vital signs, or laboratory values other than prolactin.

Bai et al. (2006) compared RLAI to oral risperidone in a 12-week randomized, single-blind study. Fifty patients, treated with oral risperidone for more than 3 months, were randomized to switch to RLAI or to continue oral risperidone. The dose of RLAI (25, 37.5, or 50 mg 2-weekly) was determined by the previous dose of oral risperidone. The RLAI and oral risperidone groups did not differ in terms of baseline to endpoint change on the PANSS total, negative, and general psychopathology scores but the RLAI group did show a significant increase in the PANSS positive score. In comparison to the oral group the RLAI group showed a significant reduction in adverse effects measured by the Udvalg for Kliniske Undersogelser (UKU) Scale and improved social life domains on the Short-Form Health Survey (SF-36) at the end of the study. The only specific adverse effect on the UKU that was significantly lower in the RLAI group was 'lassitude, increased fatiguability'. From baseline to both week 6 and week 12 serum prolactin decreased in the RLAI group but increased slightly in the oral risperidone group; at both times points the change in prolactin between the two groups was statistically significant. As there is no simple relationship between prolactin levels and symptoms, it is unclear whether the fall in prolactin following a switch to RLAI in the Chue et al. (2005) and Bai et al. (2006) studies was of clinical benefit.

Olanzapine LAI

Kane et al. (2010) compared the efficacy and tolerability of olanzapine LAI (OLAI) to oral olanzapine in the maintenance treatment of schizophrenia. Patients who had maintained stability on an oral olanzapine (10, 15, or 20 mg/day) for 4 to 8 weeks were randomized to 24 weeks of double-blind treatment with 'low' (150 mg every 2 weeks; $N = 140$), 'medium' (405 mg every 4 weeks; $N = 318$), or 'high' (300 mg every 2 weeks;

$N = 141$) doses of OLAI; a very low reference dose of OLAI (45 mg every 4 weeks; $N = 144$); or to continue their stabilized dose of oral olanzapine ($N = 322$). The very low dose of OLAI can be regarded as an active placebo. In terms of time to exacerbation, the three standard OLAI doses (i.e. low, medium, and high) were superior to the very low reference dose. Two patients treated with OLAI experienced post-injection syndrome reflecting possible accidental intravascular injection (discussed later in the chapter). With the exception of injection-related adverse events, the safety and side-effect profile of OLAI and oral olanzapine was comparable suggesting that pharmacokinetic differences between the two preparations are irrelevant to the side-effect profile. There were no significant differences in the rate of the six most common treatment-emergent adverse events between the oral olanzapine arm and three standard OLAI doses (see Figure 3.3). The only significant difference in the data shown in Figure 3.3 is that the incidence of weight increase was greater in the high-dose OLAI group than in the medium-dose OLAI group.

Adverse effects secondary to poor adherence

Antipsychotic withdrawal or discontinuation symptoms typically commence within days of stopping an oral antipsychotic and resolve rapidly if the drug is restarted (Dilsaver & Alessi 1988). Such symptoms are varied and can include motor phenomenon, including a temporary exacerbation of TD, nausea, insomnia, and anxiety. Withdrawal phenomena are particularly well recognized with clozapine and include a severe rebound psychosis (Shiovitz et al. 1996). In patients who adhere poorly to oral

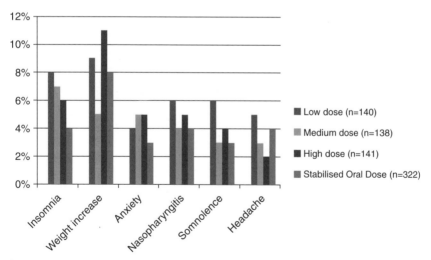

Fig. 3.3 Most common treatment-emergent adverse effects in patients randomized to different doses of OLAI or oral olanzapine (data from Kane et al. 2010).
Note: Rates do not differ significantly between the oral olanzapine cohort and three OLAI dose cohorts.
Low dose = 150 mg every 2-weeks; Medium dose = 405 mg every 4 weeks;
High dose = 300 mg every 2-weeks; Stabilized oral dose = 10, 15, or 20 mg/day.

medication withdrawal symptoms may be a repeated phenomenon. In this population an LAI may improve adherence, prevent withdrawal effects, and thus improve tolerability.

There is some evidence that intermittent antipsychotic treatment may increase the overall risk of TD. Van Harten et al. (1998) examined the association between three lifetime medication variables (cumulative antipsychotic dose, number of interruptions in antipsychotic treatment of longer than 3 months each, cumulative anticholinergic dose) and the occurrence and severity of TD. The number of antipsychotic interruptions was the only one of the three lifetime medication variables significantly related to TD, which was as assessed using the Abnormal Involuntary Movement Scale. Patients with more than two antipsychotic interruptions had a threefold higher risk of TD than those with two or less interruptions. The number of interruptions of antipsychotic treatment was associated with the severity as well as the occurrence of TD. The main weakness of the study is the retrospective design. Nevertheless the findings raise the possibility that by improving adherence an LAI may reduce the risk of TD compared to that seen with long-term erratic adherence with oral medication. However, no study has investigated this possibility.

Summary

Several studies show that LAIs are associated with smoother plasma levels than the same drug in oral form (e.g. Eerdekens et al. 2004; Tavacar et al. 2000). However, there is no convincing evidence that this translates into better tolerability. A meta-analysis of FGAs showed no difference between oral and LAIs in terms of EPS and TD (Adam et al. 2001). In a 24-week maintenance study the safety and side-effect profile of OLAI and oral olanzapine was comparable, injection-related events apart (Kane et al. 2010). Two randomized studies found that RLAI caused less prolactin elevation than oral risperidone but the clinical significance is unclear (Bai et al. 2006; Chue et al. 2005). Bai et al. (2006) found that adverse effects, measured by total UKU score, improved in RLAI-treated patients compared to oral risperidone-treated patient, but the single-blind nature of the study and poorer efficacy on one outcome measure for RLAI weaken the impact of this finding. Adverse effects, other than serum prolactin, did not differ between RLAI and oral risperidone in the second study (Chue et al. 2005). In patients who adhere poorly with oral medication an LAI may prevent the occurrence of antipsychotic withdrawal symptoms. Improved adherence with an LAI may decrease the long-term risk of TD compared to that seen in patients who adhere erratically with oral antipsychotics but this is yet to be investigated.

There is no evidence to support the belief, voiced in several surveys, that adverse effects are more common with LAIs than the corresponding oral medications (Patel et al. 2003, 2005, 2008, 2009). This view may reflect LAIs leading to better adherence and therefore more adverse effects occurring in 'real world' clinical practice than with oral medication. Furthermore, in clinical practice the proportion of patients with severe and difficult to manage illnesses who receive high doses of antipsychotics may be higher among LAI users than among those treated with oral medication alone. This selection bias may lead to a higher rate of adverse effects being seen in some patients treated with LAIs but the comparison with the oral group is not valid as the two groups are not comparable. The view that LAIs intrinsically cause more non–injection-related adverse effects than the same drug given orally is not supported by the evidence and appears a myth. Where comparisons exist, rates of non–injection-related adverse events are generally comparable between oral and LAI formulations. Some evidence suggests improved tolerability of RLAI compared to oral risperidone but the data are methodologically weak and of uncertain clinical significance.

Injection-related adverse effects

Injection-related adverse events comprise injection-site pain, a range of local injection-site complications (swelling, induration, redness, nodules, and occasionally abscesses), and post-injection syndrome. The first two problems can occur with any injectable antipsychotic, whereas post-injection syndrome is unique to OLAI. These problems are considered in turn.

Injection-site pain

Two observational studies (Hay 1995; Jones et al. 1998) of FGA-LAIs found pain to be the most common of a range of injection-site complications. Bloch et al. (2001) investigated the time course of pain in 34 consecutive outpatients who had been treated with an FGA-LAI at a stable dose and injection frequency for at least 2 months. A visual analogue scale (VAS) was used to assess the patient's pain with 0 representing no pain and 10 the maximum imaginable pain. To minimize the effect of injection technique all patients had their injections administered by a single nurse. Five VAS assessments were made at the following time-points: 5 minutes before the injection, 5 minutes after the injection, 2 days after the injection, 10 days after the injection, and immediately prior to the next injection.

Mean pain increased markedly 5 minutes after the injection but was still comparatively low, approximately 3 on the 0 to 10 VAS scale for the total sample (Figure 3.4). Pain had reduced 2 days later and returned to baseline by 10 days. The acute nature of the pain suggests that a local anaesthetic cream administered prior to injection may reduce it. Approximately 90% of patients reported no pain (VAS = 0) before the injection or 10 days after the injection. The time course of pain was similar for the different LAIs. Zuclopenthixol caused significantly greater pain than haloperidol and fluphenazine 5 minutes post-injection although the reliability of this finding is unclear given the small numbers of patients treated with each LAI. Pain 5 minutes post-injection was significantly correlated with patients' depressive (HAM-D) and anxiety symptoms (HAM-A) and overall symptomatology (BPRS). This may reflect affective symptoms influencing the perception of pain. Pain assessed 2 days after the LAI correlated significantly with the patient's report of the effect of injection-site pain and attitudes towards LAIs.

Injection-site pain with RLAI, given by gluteal injection, has been assessed in RCTs and observational studies using investigator and patient pain ratings (Chue et al. 2005; Fleischhacker et al. 2003; Kane et al. 2003). Patient ratings were made using a 100-mm VAS (0 = no pain; 100 = unbearably painful). Kane et al. (2003) reported patients' VAS pain ratings from a 12-week double-blind randomized trial. The pain ratings at

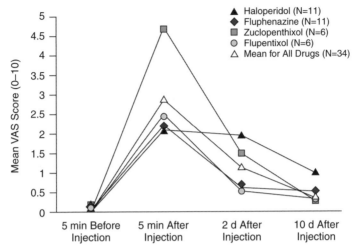

Fig. 3.4 Mean VAS scores according to time before and after injection (Bloch et al. 2001. Copyright 2001, Physicians Postgraduate Press. Reprinted by permission).

the first and sixth injection are shown in Figure 3.5. It can be seen that patients' mean pain ratings were low at the start of the trial, decreased during the study, and were similar for placebo and all doses of RLAI. A 12-week RCT by Chue et al. (2005) reported mean scores of 18 to 20 on a VAS (0–100) and noted that scores were similar after injections containing RLAI and placebo. In a 12-month open-label study, pain was low at the start of the study and decreased as the study progressed (Fleischhacker et al. 2003).

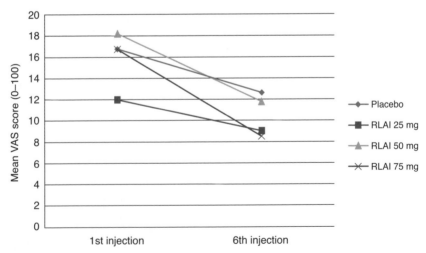

Fig. 3.5 Patient rating of injection-site pain in 12-week RCT (data from Kane et al. 2003).
VAS = Visual Analogue Scale from 0 to 100 (0 = no pain, 100 = unbearably painful).

The median VAS score was 10 at the first injection and 5 at the twenty-fifth injection. On investigator ratings, no injection-site pain was recorded in 68% of patients at the first injection and in 80% at the last injection. Recently RLAI has been licensed for deltoid injection and available data suggest that injection-site tolerability is good (Thyssen et al. 2010).

At the time of writing only limited data on injection-site pain with OLAI and PLAI were available. Data for OLAI indicate that injection-site pain is not a major problem (Kane et al. 2010; Lauriello et al. 2008). Data on injection-site pain with PLAI are available from a maintenance study that comprised a 9-week open-label transition phase followed by a 24-week double-blind placebo-controlled phase when PLAI was administered at the gluteal site (Hough et al. 2010). Investigator-rated injection-site pain was similar for the placebo and PLAI groups. Most patients reported an absence of injection-site pain in the transition phase and at the end of the double-blind period (81% PLAI vs. 82% placebo). PLAI is licensed for both gluteal and deltoid injections and a cross-over study has compared the safety and tolerability of administration at the two sites (Hough et al. 2009). The gluteal site was slightly better tolerated with lower rates of both observer- and patient-rated pain and observer-rated swelling and induration. The overall proportion of patients who withdrew from the study for all adverse effects, systemic and local, was similar for both treatment sequences (<9%).

In summary, data on injection-site pain are available for several antipsychotic LAIs. Taken overall it indicates that injection-site pain is short-lived, related to the immediate injection, and generally mild. Studies with RLAI show that pain reduces with successive injections. Pain does not appear to be a significant problem for most patients receiving LAIs. The most important aspect of reducing pain is a good injection technique. If pain is still a problem, it can be reduced with a local anaesthetic cream (Bloch et al. 2004).

Injection-site complications

Jones et al. (1998) conducted a cross-sectional study of 318 patients receiving an FGA-LAI from two centres in England. The mean age was 43 years and approximately two-thirds were treated with flupentixol decanoate. A range of potential complications were assessed including skin thickening, infection and erythema, nodules and lumps, bleeding, pain, and tenderness. Severity was rated by the nurse who administered the LAI using a 4-point Likert scale ranging from 0 (none) to 4 (severe). Reactions rated as 2 or above were regarded as clinically significant. The total prevalence of clinically significant reactions was 17%. Pain and bleeding were the two most common reactions (Figure 3.6). There were no cases of clinically significant erythema.

Jones et al. (1998) found that local reactions were associated with increased volume of injections and a greater frequency of injections in the preceding 12 months. There was no relationship with the concentration of the FGA-LAI after controlling for the volume received in the preceding 12 months. Reactions were unrelated to the dose of the depot (in chlorpromazine equivalents), body mass index, gender, or age. The authors suggested that the incidence of local reactions may be reduced by increasing the interval between injections and using low-volume, high-concentrated preparations to reduce the total volume administered.

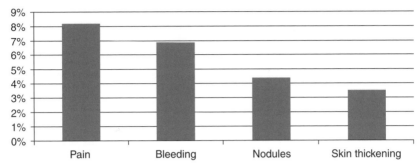

Fig. 3.6 Prevalence of clinically significant injection-site reactions (observer-rated) with FGA-LAIs (data from Jones et al. 1998).

Hay (1995) assessed 221 patients receiving FGA-LAIs for a variable period (2 to 38 weeks, mean 21.8 weeks). The mean age of the patients was 48 years. The study did not describe how reactions were rated and no details are given on the severity threshold required to achieve a rating. A total of 19% of patients experienced a local complication of any type, 13% experienced an acute local reaction (i.e. a discrete episode), and 8% a chronic local reaction (i.e. recurrent induration or nodules present during most of the observation period). The two most frequent acute problems were pain followed by bleeding or haematoma which is consistent with the findings of Jones et al. (1998). The third most frequent complication in Hay's study was clinically important leakage of drug from the injection site.

Hay (1995) found that injection-site complications were more common in patients treated with concentrated versus standard FGA-LAI preparations and in those who had received higher doses (chlorpromazine equivalents), weekly injections, and injection volumes greater than 1 ml and injections for more than 5 years. However, no analysis was conducted to see whether these were independent factors. Animal experiments suggest that both the volume and concentration of FGA- LAIs are related to the degree of muscle damage (Svendsen & Blom 1984).

Case reports have described various injection-site problems with FGA-LAIs. Hamann et al. (1990) reported four patients treated with haloperidol decanoate in whom the injection sites, including the deltoid muscle, became red, pruritic, oedematous, and tender within 1 to 3 days of the injection. In each case a palpable nodule developed and remained for up to 3 months but infection was not believed to be responsible for these problems. Abscesses have been reported as complications of flupentixol decanoate (Andrade 2002) and perphenazine enantate (Starmark et al. 1980) but are likely to reflect poor injection technique including injection into the subcutaneous tissue leading to local irritation.

In a 1-year study of RLAI reported by Fleischhacker et al. (2003) investigator ratings reported no redness in 95% and 100% of patients at the first and last injections, no swelling in 98% and 100%, and no induration in 100% and 93%, respectively. In a 12-week RCT of RLAI (Chue et al. 2005) redness at the injection site was mild and reported by 3.7% to 6.8% of patients in the RLAI group and was less frequent after the third injection. Induration was absent in almost all patients in both the RLAI and placebo groups. A review of two studies of RLAI by Lindernmayer et al. (2005) found no association between local reactions or pain and RLAI dose.

Published data on injection-site complications with OLAI and PLAI are limited as both drugs were first licensed in 2009. An 8-week placebo controlled trial of OLAI noted few injection-site reactions, and those that were reported were mild or moderate in severity (Lauriello et al. 2008). In a 24-week double-blind maintenance trial of OLAI, the incidence of local injection-site reactions, including pain, was low (3%; Kane et al. 2010). The data in both studies are based on patient reports and were not systematically collected and so may underestimate the frequency of problems.

A recent review of four short-term RCTs of PLAI reported that injection-site reactions occurred at a rate ranging from 4% to 10%, depending on the dose regimen, versus 2% for the pooled placebo arms (Citrome 2010). A cross-over trial that compared the tolerability of gluteal and deltoid injections of PLAI found that swelling and induration were slightly more common at the deltoid compared with the gluteal site, although redness scores were similar at both sites (Hough et al. 2009). As already discussed, pain was also more intense at the deltoid site in this study. Nevertheless, the overall proportion of patients who withdrew from the study was similar for both treatment sequences, and 77% of patients in the United States preferred the deltoid to the gluteal site. Interestingly patient preference for injection site showed a marked geographic variation as 30% of patients from non-US countries preferred the deltoid to the gluteal site.

A case report described a patient who experienced a reduction in injection-site nodules following a switch from an FGA-LAI to RLAI (Saxena et al. 2008). It is impossible to determine whether this reflected improved injection technique, spontaneous resolution of the nodules, or a genuine difference between the two LAIs in the risk of causing local complications. It is possible that incidence and severity of pain and injection-site problems may vary between LAIs owing to differences in the drug and other elements of the injecteded material; e.g. RLAI is composed of microsphere in an aqueous solution, whereas FGA-LAIs are esters dissolved in oil. In addition, the gauge or bore of needle supplied with the different SGA-LAIs varies (the smallest gauge is with PLAI) which may affect pain. Unfortunately, methodological differences impede cross-study comparisons (Hamer & Haddad 2007) and make it impossible to state whether injection-site complications and pain differ between specific LAIs. It is an area that warrants further research.

Injection-site complications and injection technique

Injection-site complications are more likely following injection into the subcutaneous tissues e.g. owing to use of too short a needle or seepage of the drug into the subcutaneous tissues from the original intramuscular injection site. This is probably because adipose tissue has a poorer blood supply than muscle with the result that injected material persists for longer and is therefore likely to lead to irritation and inflammation. The z-track technique is recommended for intramuscular injections as it minimizes leakage from the intramsuscular injection site into the subcutaneous tissue and onto the skin surface (UKPPG 2009). This is because when the needle is withdrawn, after the LAI has been administered, there is not a straight pathway from the injection site to the skin surface, rather there is a z-shaped injection pathway.

There is marked individual variation in the thickness of subcutaneous fat, particularly in the buttocks. Studies have repeatedly shown that in many patients, particularly those who are overweight, standard length needles will result in an inadvertent subcutaneous rather than intramuscular injection (e.g. Burbridge 2007; Chan et al. 2006; Nisbet et al. 2006). Chan et al. (2006) used computerized tomographic scans to determine the true injection site in patients given intramuscular injections at the dorsogluteal site ('upper outer quadrant'). Only one-third of patients received intramuscular injections, whereas the remainder received subcutaneous injections. Significantly more women than men received a subcutaneous injection reflecting the greater gluteal fat thickness in women. The thickness of subcutaneous fat is less at the ventrogluteal site than the dorsogluteal site (Nisbet et al. 2006). Consequently it has been recommended that nurses use the ventrogluteal site in preference to the dorsogluteal site when administering LAIs in overweight patients or use a longer needle (Dougherty & Lister 2004).

Further research is required to determine whether the deltoid injection site is associated with a reduced risk of subcutaneous injection. Currently RLAI and PLAI are the only antipsychotic LAIs licensed for deltoid injection in addition to gluteal injection. OLAI is only licensed for gluteal injection. All FGA-LAIs are licensed for gluteal injection, although zuclopenthixol and flupentixol are also licensed for injection into the lateral thigh (UKPPG 2009).

Strategies to minimize the risk of injection-site problems are summarized in Table 3.2. In addition to appropriate injection technique, these include rotating injection sites, avoiding excessive injection volume, and increasing the injection interval where feasible (Table 3.2).

Post-injection syndrome with OLAI

Post-injection syndrome is unique to OLAI. It is considered only briefly here as it is dealt with in detail in Chapter 6. It occurs in less than 0.1% of injections and presents with signs and symptoms of an olanzapine overdose including sedation and delirium

Table 3.2 Strategies to minimize the risk of injection-site complications

---

- ◆ Meticulous injection technique
  - • Appropriate infection control procedures
  - • Use needle of sufficient length to reach muscle
  - • Z-track technique: minimize tracking from muscle into subcutaneous tissue
- ◆ Avoid excessive injection volume
- ◆ Rotate injection sites
- ◆ Increase injection interval where feasible (no rationale for any patient to have 1-week injections)
- ◆ If pain is a problem then consider use of local anaesthetic cream

---

(ZypAdhera®: Summary of Product Characteristics, SPC). OLAI is an ionic salt of olanzapine and pamoic acid (olanzapine pamoate monohydrate) with microscopic crystals of the salt suspended in water. After intramuscular injection, the salt slowly dissolves and dissociates into olanzapine and pamoic acid that enter the circulation continuously over more than 4 weeks. Post-injection syndrome is believed to occur when the salt inadvertently comes into contact with a large amount of blood or serum, either owing to accidental injection into a blood vessel or capillary bed or if there is bleeding around the injection track. This leads to rapid dissociation and a large release of olanzapine into the circulation.

Citrome (2009) summarized safety data on the post-injection syndrome collected from completed and ongoing trials of OLAI. As of 31 May 2008 the overall incidence of the syndrome was 0.07% of injections and 29 cases had been reported. Symptoms included sedation, dizziness, confusion, slurred speech, altered gait, weakness, and unconsciousness. The median time from injection to symptom onset was 25 minutes; 80% of the cases started within 1 hour of injection and only 3% (i.e. 1 case) began after 3 hours. The syndrome can start with milder symptoms and progress with time with confusion and sedation appearing only later on in the clinical course. All patients made a full recovery between 1.5 and 72 hours. The syndrome has important practical implications that include the requirements that after each injection of OLAI a patient is observed in a health care facility by an appropriately qualified person for a minimum period of 3 hours for features consistent with olanzapine overdose and that patients should be accompanied home and should not drive or operate machinery on the day they receive OLAI (ZypAdhera®: SPC).

LAIs and time course of adverse effects

This section considers the time course of 'general' adverse effects of antipsychotics e.g. those listed in Table 3.1, and not injection-related adverse effects i.e. pain, injection-site complications, and post-injection syndrome with OLAI. The pharmacokinetics of LAIs can delay the appearance and resolution of adverse effects, compared to that seen with oral medication, following initiation and termination of treatment, and dose adjustment. This has important clinical implications.

It takes 2 to 3 months for steady-state plasma levels to be reached after starting an LAI, assuming the dose and injection interval remains constant. With some LAIs this period can be reduced with a loading or initiation strategy. In one study, patients who received fluphenazine decanoate 50 mg each week showed a fourfold increase in plasma levels during the first six weeks of treatment despite no change in dose during this time (Ereshefsky et al. 1984). Patients should be monitored for 2 to 3 months after starting an LAI or increasing the dose to determine whether adverse effects develop. This is in addition to the routine monitoring for adverse effects that should continue throughout the duration of antipsychotic treatment, whether this be an oral medication or an LAI.

Adverse effects may persist for several months after an LAI is reduced in dose or stopped. Owing to differences in apparent half-life (see Chapter 2) adverse effects may persist for longer after stopping/reducing the dose of an FGA-LAI than after altering the dose of RLAI. If a patient develops EPS during treatment with an LAI and benefits from the prescription of a drug to treat this, e.g. an anticholinergic drug to treat

Parkinsonism or a beta-blocker to treat akathisia, then the 'anti-EPS' drug may need to continued for some months after the LAI is stopped or reduced in dose (Lambert 2007). When an LAI is switched to another drug because of adverse effects, it may be several months before the true tolerability of the new drug can be assessed owing to carry-over effects from the previous LAI. For example, raised prolactin may persist for up to 6 months after stopping an FGA-LAI (Haddad & Wieck 2004).

The potential persistence of adverse effects is one reason why it is recommended to give an initial small 'test dose' of FGA-LAIs (Maudsley Prescribing Guidelines 2009). A test dose does not make sense with RLAI owing to the 3-week lag period before the drug is released. With all three SGA-LAIs (i.e. OLAI, RLAI, PLAI) we recommend that, where possible, tolerability be assessed by first prescribing the oral equivalent. This is also consistent with the SPC for OLAI and RLAI, which state that each is indicated for maintenance treatment of schizophrenia in patients previously stabilized on the oral equivalent (British National Formulary 2009; ZypAdhera®: Summary of Product Characteristics). Just because a test dose of an LAI, or a few days of the equivalent oral antipsychotic, is tolerated does not mean that adverse effects will not occur with repeated higher doses of an LAI.

Positron emission tomography (PET) studies that assess D2 occupancy are consistent with the persistence of adverse effects seen after stopping LAIs and sustained antipsychotic efficacy throughout the injection interval at steady state. Therapeutic response to antipsychotics is usually regarded as requiring a striatal D2 receptor occupancy above a 60% threshold with adverse events, including EPS, being more likely at higher occupancy levels (Grunder et al. 2003). D2 receptor occupancy returns to pre-treatment levels within 5 to 15 days after stopping oral antipsychotic medication (Baron et al. 1989). In contrast, D2 striatal occupation with FGA-LAIs remains stable over a 4-week injection interval (Baron et al. 1989). Mamo et al. (2008) reported that mean D2 receptor occupancy was more than 60% immediately prior to the sixth consecutive injection of OLAI 300 mg 4-weekly, which is consistent with antipsychotic efficacy. Similarly, Remington et al. (2006) reported that mean pre-injection D2 occupancy after stabilization with RLAI 50 mg 2-weekly was approximately 65%.

Nyberg et al. (1997) reported on four patients with schizophrenia who had repeated PET scans for 1 year after stopping low-dose treatment with haloperidol decanoate (30–50 mg every 4 weeks). D2 receptor occupancy was highest 1 week after depot injection but subsequently decreased slowly. Six months after discontinuation of treatment, three of the four patients showed D2 receptor occupancy in the approximate range of 25% to 33%. Harasko-van der Meer et al. (1993) reported two patients with schizophrenia who developed severe Parkinsonism and TD during treatment with fluphenazine decanoate. D2 receptor occupancy assessed by single photon emission tomography (SPECT) 6 weeks after stopping the LAI was 83% and 50%, respectively. This was despite no oral antipsychotic being administered to either patient in the 4 weeks before the scan.

Barnes and Wiles (1983) investigated whether the plasma level fluctuations that occur during the injection cycle with FGA-LAIs could influence the severity of TD and Parkinsonism. TD can be suppressed temporarily by increasing the dose of an antipsychotic drug, whereas lowering the dose can transiently worsen the condition.

Conversely, the severity of antipsychotic induced Parkinsonism is proportional to the drug dose. Six patients receiving fluphenazine decanoate and two patients receiving flupentixol decanoate were assessed using standard rating scales for TD and Parkinsonism at repeated points during the injection cycle. With both LAIs, changes were observed in the severity of TD, and to a lesser degree of Parkinsonism, that were consistent with the expected fluctuation of plasma antipsychotic levels. More specifically, TD ratings showed a drop within 24 hours of the injection of fluphenazine decanoate and a slow rise towards the end of the injection interval. This is consistent with the one-day post-injection peak in plasma levels with fluphenazine decanoate and the subsequent slow decline in plasma levels (Wiles & Gelder 1979). In contrast, both patients treated with flupentixol decanoate showed the lowest severity of TD 1 week after the injection followed by a subsequent increase in severity. This is consistent with the pharmacokinetics of the flupentixol decanoate, which shows a maximal plasma level about 1 week post-injection in contrast to the 1-day post-injection peak seen with fluphenazine decanoate. Fluctuations in the severity of Parkinsonism were less marked but as expected showed the converse pattern to TD with the maximal severity of Parkinsonism occurring soon after the injection at the time that antipsychotic plasma levels would be predicted to be maximal.

Chouinard et al. (1982) reported that TD was more severe towards the end of a 4-week injection interval with fluphenazine decanoate. In summary both studies (Barnes & Wiles 1998; Chouinard et al. 1982) suggest that the severity of TD during the injection cycle is a mirror image of plasma antipsychotic levels. One implication is that repeated assessments of TD e.g. aimed at assessing the progress of the disorder, should occur at a standard time relative to administration of an LAI.

Cautions and contraindications to LAIs

Antipsychotic naïve patients

Antipsychotic naïve patients are more sensitive to adverse effects of drugs yet their tolerability to specific antipsychotic agents is unknown. Both factors, plus the risk of persistence of adverse effects with an LAI, mean that LAIs should be avoided in patients who have *never* received treatment with an oral antipsychotic drug. The importance of these points is illustrated by a case report of a 14-year-old female who developed severe neuroleptic malignant syndrome (NMS) following a single dose of zuclopenthixol LAI 200 mg (Erermis 2007). LAIs can be appropriately used in a first episode of psychosis and may lead to excellent outcomes in this group (see Chapter 7). However their role, as in other patient groups, is primarily in maintenance and not acute treatment. When an antipsychotic LAI is prescribed for a person with first-episode schizophrenia it is particularly important that tolerability is assessed with the equivalent antipsychotic in oral form and that the LAI is then started at a low dose.

Neuroleptic malignant syndrome

A history of NMS is usually regarded as a contraindication to treatment with an LAI. NMS is a potentially fatal syndrome consisting of four key components: alteration of consciousness, autonomic disturbance, elevated temperature, and muscular rigidity (Haddad & Dursun 2008). It has been reported with all classes of antipsychotic drugs including low- and high-potency FGAs and all SGAs including clozapine as well as various non-antipsychotic drugs. The risk appears highest with haloperidol, a high-potency FGA. NMS has been reported with several LAIs including fluphenazine decanaote (Aruna & Murungi 2005; Wilson et al. 1998), pipotiazine palmitate (Montoya et al. 2003), and zuclopenthixol decanoate (Erermis 2007). NMS caused by an LAI is likely to be more serious than when it occurs with oral antipsychotic medication because after medication is stopped (a key part of the treatment of NMS) plasma and central nervous system (CNS) antipsychotic levels will remain high for weeks with an LAI reflecting continued slow release of the antipsychotic from the 'depot' site. In contrast, plasma and CNS levels will fall to zero within days of stopping an oral antipsychotic.

Epilepsy

Most antipsychotic drugs lower the seizure threshold and should therefore be used with caution in patients with a history of seizures. The risk is dose related and among oral antipsychotics, clozapine, zotepine, and chlorpromazine are regarded as having greater risk (Haddad & Dursun 2008). LAIs should be used with caution in patients with epilepsy, not because they are of higher epileptogenic risk than oral antipsychotics, but because their long apparent half-life means that the antipsychotic cannot be quickly withdrawn if seizures occur. We would generally recommend that an LAI is avoided in a patient with epilepsy unless the patient has received treatment for 2 to 4 weeks with the oral equivalent.

Prior allergic reaction

A prior allergic reaction to a drug is a contraindication to future use. With oral medication an allergic reaction may be to the drug itself or one of the other constituents in the tablet e.g. the filler. Similarly with an antipsychotic LAI a patient may develop a reaction to the antipsychotic itself or to another constituent in the LAI. A case report has described the rapid onset of generalized pruritic rash following administration of an initial injection of RLAI despite the patient tolerating oral risperidone (Reeves & Mack 2005). The rash settled over a few days. The authors suggested that the patient had an allergic reaction to the copolymer complex of the formulation and not to risperidone itself. A case report described a possible allergic reaction to coconut oil used in flupentixol decanoate with the patient developing intense local irritation at the injection site and a generalized pruritus within one hour of the injection with the systemic symptoms starting to resolve within 24 hours (Reeves & Howard 2002).

Summary

It is reassuring that the common belief among clinicians that LAIs cause more adverse effects than their oral counterparts appears unfounded. LAIs appear to carry the same risk of non-injection-related adverse effects as their oral equivalents. Initial speculation that smoother plasma levels may reduce the incidence of adverse effects is only supported by very preliminary evidence and further studies are needed to investigate this.

Pharmacokinetics dictate that the appearance of side-effects may be delayed for weeks after starting or increasing the dose of an LAI. Conversely, resolution of adverse effects may take months after an LAI is stopped or the dose decreased. A small test dose of an FGA-LAI is advisable to test tolerability, not only of the antipsychotic but also of the oily vehicle. With the SGA-LAIs, tolerability can be tested with the oral equivalent. LAIs should be avoided in those who are antipsychotic naïve or have a history of NMS and used with caution in those with epilepsy.

A key difference between oral antipsychotics and LAIs is that the latter are associated with injection-related adverse events. With the exception of post-injection syndrome with olanzapine these are not especially serious. Pain associated with LAIs is short-lived, is not severe in most patients, diminishes with successive injections, and its severity is comparable to that associated with placebo injections. In individual patients where pain is a problem it can be reduced by the use of a topical anaesthetic cream. Injection-site problems seen in observational studies of FGA-LAIs include redness, swelling, induration, nodules, and occasionally abscesses. The prevalence of these problems with SGA-LAIs, at least in clinical trials, is low. Whether this reflects a genuine difference in the risk of these problems, or the effect of confounders, is unclear owing to the absence of randomized head-to-head comparison studies. Injection-site problems can be minimized by meticulous injection technique. Post-injection syndrome is a serious adverse effect that is unique to OLAI and is believed to be due to inadvertent intravascular injection with olanzapine. It presents with signs and symptoms of an olanzapine overdose. To date, all patients have recovered. Its occurrence has led to special safeguards being required for the use of OLAI.

Extrapolating from data on oral antipsychotics it is reasonable to expect that different antipsychotic LAIs will show different side-effect profiles (Sharma & Haddad 2008). To date, the only randomized trial of an FGA-LAI and an SGA-LAI compared RLAI to zuclopenthixol decanoate (Rubio et al. 2006). It showed a reduced risk of EPS and superior efficacy with RLAI. However, the study was relatively small, single-blind and was conducted in patients with schizophrenia and co-morbid substance misuse. More head-to-head trials are required to compare different LAIs in terms of efficacy as well as their side-effect profiles. The recent increase in the range of LAIs is welcome as it allows greater choice for clinicians and patients. This is important as patients show marked individual variation in their tolerability and response to antipsychotics.

References

Adams CE, Fenton MKP, Quraishi S, David AS. (2001). Systematic meta-review of depot antipsychotic drugs for people with schizophrenia. *Br J Psych*, **179**, 290–9.

Andrade C. (2002). Flupenthixol decanoate and injection site abscesses in an obese patient. *Aust N Z J Psychiatry*, **36**(4), 561–2.

Aruna AS, Murungi JH. (2005). Fluphenazine-induced neuroleptic malignant syndrome in a schizophrenic patient. *Ann Pharmacother*, **39**(6), 1131–5.

Ayd FJ. (1967). Drug holidays: intermittent pharmacotherapy for psychiatric patients. *Medical Science*, 59–62.

Bai YM, Chen TT, Wu B, Hung CH, Lin WK, Hu TM, et al. (2006). A comparative efficacy and safety study of long-acting risperidone injection and risperidone oral tablets among hospitalized patients: 12-week randomized, single-blind study. *Pharmacopsychiatry*, **39**(4), 135–41.

Barnes TR, Wiles DH. (1983). Variation in oro-facial tardive dyskinesia during depot antipsychotic drug treatment. *Psychopharmacology (Berl)*, **81**(4), 359–62.

Baron JC, Martinot JL, Cambon H, Boulenger JP, Poirier MF, Caillard V, et al. (1989). Striatal dopamine receptor occupancy during and following withdrawal from neuroleptic treatment: correlative evaluation by positron emission tomography and plasma prolactin levels. *Psychopharmacology (Berl)*, **99**(4), 463–72.

Bloch Y, Levkovitz Y, Atshuler A, Dvoretzki V, Fenning S, Ratzoni G. (2004). Use of topical application of lidocaine-prilocaine cream to reduce injection-site pain of depot antipsychotics. *Psychiatr Serv*, **55**(8), 940–1.

Bloch Y, Mendlovic S, Strupinsky S, Altshuler A, Fennig S, Ratzoni G. (2001). Injections of depot antipsychotic medications in patients suffering from schizophrenia: do they hurt? *J Clin Psychiatry*, **62**(11), 855–9.

British National Formulary. (2009). No. 58. British Medical Association and Royal Pharmaceutical Society of Great Britain.

Burbridge BE. (2007). Computed tomographic measurement of gluteal subcutaneous fat thickness in reference to failure of gluteal intramuscular injections. *Can Assoc Radiol J*, **58**(2), 72–5.

Carrillo JA, Herráiz AG, Ramos SI, Gervasini G, Vizcaíno S, Benítez J. (2003). Role of the smoking-induced cytochrome P450 (CYP)1A2 and polymorphic CYP2D6 in steady-state concentration of olanzapine. *J Clin Psychopharmacol*, **23**(2), 119–27.

Chan VO, Colville J, Persaud T, Buckley O, Hamilton S, Torreggiani WC. (2006). Intramuscular injections into the buttocks: are they truly intramuscular? *Eur J Radiol*, **58**(3), 480–4.

Chouinard G, Annable L, Ross-Chouinard A. (1982). Fluphenazine enanthate and fluphenazine decanoate in the treatment of schizophrenic outpatients: extrapyramidal symptoms and therapeutic effect. *Am J Psychiatry*, **139**(3), 312–18.

Chue, P, Eerdekens M, Augustyns I, Lachaux B, Molcan P, Eriksson L, et al. (2005). Comparative efficacy and safety of long-acting risperidone and risperidone oral tablets. *Eur Neuropsychopharmacol*, **15**, 111–17.

Citrome L. (2009). Olanzapine pamoate: a stick in time? A review of the efficacy and safety profile of a new depot formulation of a second-generation antipsychotic. *Int J Clin Pract*, **63**(1), 140–50.

Citrome L. (2010). Paliperidone palmitate— review of the efficacy, safety and cost of a new second-generation depot antipsychotic medication. *Int J Clin Pract*, **64**(2), 216–39.

Dilsaver SC, Alessi NE. (1988). Antipsychotic withdrawal symptoms: phenomenology and pathophysiology. *Acta Psychiatr Scand*, **77**(3), 241–6.

Dougherty L, Lister S. (2004). *The Royal Marsden Hospital Manual of Clinical Nursing Procedures*, Sixth Edition (Royal Marsden NHS Trust). Blackwell Publishing.

Eerdekens M, Van Hove I, Remmerie B, Mannaert E. (2004). Pharmacokinetics and tolerability of long-acting risperidone in schizophrenia. *Schizophr Res*, **70**(1), 91–100.

Erermis S, Bildik T, Tamar M, Gockay A, Karasoy H, Ercan ES. (2007). Zuclopenthixol-induced neuroleptic malignant syndrome in an adolescent girl. *Clin Toxicol (Phila,)* **45**(3), 277–80.

Ereshefsky L, Saklad SR, Jann MW, Davis CM, Richards A, Seidel DR. (1984). Future of depot neuroleptic therapy: pharmacokinetic and pharmacodynamic approaches. *J Clin Psychiatry*, **45**(5 Pt 2), 50–9.

Fleischhacker WW, Eerdekens M, Karcher K, Remington G, Llorca PM, Chrzanowski W, et al. (2003). Treatment of schizophrenia with long-acting injectable risperidone: a 12-month open-label trial of the first long-acting second-generation antipsychotic. *J Clin Psychiatry,* **64**(10), 1250–7.

Gefvert O, Eriksson B, Persson P, Helldin L, Björner A, Mannaert E, et al. (2005). Pharmacokinetics and D2 receptor occupancy of long-acting injectable risperidone (Risperdal Consta) in patients with schizophrenia. *Int J Neuropsychopharmacol,* **8**(1), 27–36.

Grunder G, Carlsson A, Wong DF. (2003). Mechanism of new antipsychotic medications: occupancy is not just antagonism. *Arch Gen Psychiatry,* **60**(10), 974–7.

Haddad PM, Dursun SM. (2008). Neurological complications of psychiatric drugs: clinical features and management. *Hum Psychopharmacol,* **23** (Suppl 1), 15–26.

Haddad PM, Sharma SG. (2007). Adverse effects of atypical antipsychotic drugs: differential risk and clinical implications. *CNS Drugs.* **21**(11), 911–36.

Haddad PM, Taylor M, Niaz OM. (2009). First-generation antipsychotic long-acting injections v. oral antipsychotics in schizophrenia: systematic review of randomised controlled trials and observational studies. *Br Jl Psychiatry.* **195**, S20–8.

Haddad PM, Wieck A. (2004). Antipsychotic-induced hyperprolactinaemia: mechanisms, clinical features and management. *Drugs.* **64**(20), 2291–314.

Hamann GL, Egan TM, Wells BG, Grimmig JE. (1990). Injection site reactions after intramuscular administration of haloperidol decanoate 100 mg/mL. *J Clin Psychiatry,* **51**(12), 502–4.

Hamer S, Haddad PM. (2007). Adverse effects of antipsychotics as outcome measures. *Br J Psychiatry Suppl,* **50**, S64–S70.

Harasko-van der Meer C, Brücke T, Wenger S, Fischer P, Deecke L, Podreka I. (1993). Two cases of long term dopamine D2 receptor blockade after depot neuroleptics. *J Neural Transm Gen Sect,* **94**(3), 217–21.

Haro JM, Suarez D, Novick D, Brown J, Usall J, Naber D; SOHO Study Group. (2007). Three-year antipsychotic effectiveness in the outpatient care of schizophrenia: observational versus randomized studies results. *Eur Neuropsychopharmacol,* **17**(4), 235–44.

Hay J. (1995). Complications at site of injection of depot neuroleptics. *BMJ,* **311**(7002), 421.

Hough D, Gopal S, Vijapurkar U, Lim P, Morozova M, Eerdekens M. (2010). Paliperidone palmitate maintenance treatment in delaying the time-to-relapse in patients with schizophrenia: a randomized, double-blind, placebo-controlled study. *Schizophr Res,* **116**(2–3), 107–17.

Hough D, Lindenmayer JP, Gopal S, Melkote R, Lim P, Herben V, et al. (2009). Safety and tolerability of deltoid and gluteal injections of paliperidone palmitate in schizophrenia. *Prog Neuropsychopharmacol Biol Psychiatry,* **33**(6), 1022–31.

Huyser BA, Parker JC. (1999). Negative affect and pain in arthritis. *Rheum Dis Clin North Am,* **25**(1), 105–21.

Jann MW, Ereshefsky L, Saklad SR. (1985). Clinical pharmacokinetics of the depot antipsychotics. *Clin Pharmacokinet,* **10**(4), 315–33.

Jones JC, Day JC, Taylor JR, Thomas CS. (1998). Investigation of depot neuroleptic injection site reactions. *Psychiatric Bulletin* **22**, 605–7.

Kane JM, Aguglia E, Altamura AC, Ayuso Gutierrez JL, Brunello N, Fleischhacker WW, et al. (1998). Guidelines for depot antipsychotic treatment in schizophrenia. European Neuropsychopharmacology Consensus Conference in Siena, Italy. *Eur Neuropsychopharmacol,* **8**(1), 55–66.

Kane JM, Detke HC, Naber D, Sethuraman G, Lin DY, Bergstrom RF, et al. (2010). Olanzapine long-acting injection: a 24-week, randomized, double-blind trial of maintenance treatment in patients with schizophrenia. *Am J Psychiatry*, **167**(2),181-9.

Kane JM, Eerdekens M, Lindenmayer JP, Keith SJ, Lesem M, Karcher K. (2003). Long-acting injectable risperidone: efficacy and safety of the first long-acting atypical antipsychotic. *Am J Psychiatry* **160**(6), 1125–32.

Kurtz D, Bergstrom R, McDonnell D, Michell M. (2008). Pharmacokinetics (PK) of multiple doses of olanzapine long-acting injection (OLAI), an intramuscular (IM) depot formulation of olanzapine (OLZ), in stabilised patients with schizophrenia. *Biol Psychiatry,* **63** (Suppl 1), 228S.

Lambert, TJ. (2007). Switching antipsychotic therapy: what to expect and clinical strategies for improving therapeutic outcomes. *J Clin Psychiatry*, **68** (Suppl 6), 10–13.

Lancet. (1979). Tardive dyskinesia. *Lancet* **2**(8140), 447–8.

Lauriello J, Lambert T, Andersen S, Lin D, Taylor CC, McDonnell D. (2008). An 8-week, double-blind, randomized, placebo-controlled study of olanzapine long-acting injection in acutely ill patients with schizophrenia. *J Clin Psychiatry*, **69**(5), 790–9.

Leucht S, Corves C, Arbter D, Engel RR, Li C, Davis JM. (2009). Second-generation versus first-generation antipsychotic drugs for schizophrenia: a meta-analysis. *Lancet* **373**(9657), 31–41.

Mamo D, Kapur S, Keshavan M, Laruelle M, Taylor CC, Kothare PA, et al. (2008). D2 receptor occupancy of olanzapine pamoate depot using positron emission tomography: an open-label study in patients with schizophrenia. *Neuropsychopharmacology,* **33**, 298–304.

Mannaert E, Vermeulen A, Remmerie B, Bouhours P, Levron JC. (2005). Pharmacokinetic profile of long-acting injectable risperidone at steady-state: comparison with oral administration. *Encephale,* **31**, 609–15.

Maudsley Prescribing Guidelines. (2009). Tenth Edition. D Taylor, C Paton, S Kapur. (eds). Informa Healthcare.

Montoya A, Ocampo M, Torres-Ruiz A. (2003). Neuroleptic malignant syndrome in Mexico. *Can J Clin Pharmacol,* **10**(3), 111–13.

Nayak RK, Doose DR, Nair NP. (1987). The bioavailability and pharmacokinetics of oral and depot intramuscular haloperidol in schizophrenic patients. *J Clin Pharmacol,* **27**(2), 144–50.

Nisbet AC. (2006). Intramuscular gluteal injections in the increasingly obese population: retrospective study. *BMJ* **332**(7542), 637–8.

Nyberg S, Farde L, Halldin C. (1997). Delayed normalization of central D2 dopamine receptor availability after discontinuation of haloperidol decanoate. Preliminary findings. *Arch Gen Psychiatry,* **54**(10), 953–8.

Patel, MX, Haddad, PM, Chaudhry, IB, McLoughlin, S, Husain, N, David, AS. (2009). Psychiatrists' use, knowledge and attitudes to first and second generation antipsychotic long-acting injections: comparisons over five years. *J Psychopharmacol*, In Press (published online ahead of print 28 May 2009, doi: 10.1177/0269881109104882).

Patel MX, Nikolaou V, David AS. (2003). Psychiatrists' attitudes to maintenance medication for patients with schizophrenia. *Psychol Med,* **33**(1), 83–9.

Patel MX, Yeung FK, Haddad PM, David AS. (2008). Psychiatric nurses' attitudes to antipsychotic depots in Hong Kong and comparison with London. *J Psychiatr Ment Health Nurs,* **15**(9), 758–66.

Patel MX, DE Zoysa N, Baker D, David AS. (2005). Antipsychotic depot medication and attitudes of community psychiatric nurses. *J Psychiatr Ment Health Nurs,* **12**(2), 237–44.

Reeves S, Howard R. (2002). Depot injections and nut allergy. *Br J Psychiatry* **180**, 188.

Reeves RR, Mack JE. (2005). Allergic reaction to depot risperidone but not to oral risperidone. J *Clin Psychiatry*, **66**(7), 949.

Remington G, Mamo D, Labelle A, Reiss J, Shammi C, Mannaert E, et al. (2006). A PET study evaluating dopamine D2 receptor occupancy for long-acting injectable risperidone. *Am J Psychiatry* **163**, 396–401.

Rubio G, Martínez I, Ponce G, Jiménez-Arriero MA, López-Muñoz F, Alamo C. (2006). Long-acting injectable risperidone compared with zuclopenthixol in the treatment of schizophrenia with substance abuse comorbidity. *Can J Psychiatry*, **51**(8), 531–9.

Saxena A, Grace J, Olympia JL, Trigoboff E, Watson T, Cushman S, et al. (2008). Risperidone long-acting injections: successful alternative deltoid muscle injections for refractory schizophrenia. *Psychiatry (Edgmont)*, **5**(9), 40–2.

Shiovitz TM, Welke TL, Tigel PD, Anand R, Hartman RD, Sramek JJ, et al. (1996). Cholinergic rebound and rapid onset psychosis following abrupt clozapine withdrawal. *Schizophr Bull*, **22**(4), 591–5.

Starmark JE, Forsman A, Wahlström. (1980). Abscesses following prolonged intramuscular administration of perphenazine enantate. *Acta Psychiatr Scand*, **62**(2), 154–7.

Svendsen O, Blom L. (1984). Intramuscular injections and muscle damage: effects of concentration, volume, injection speed and vehicle. *Arch Toxicol Suppl*, **7**, 472–5.

Tavcar R, Dernovsek MZ, Zvan V. (2000). Choosing antipsychotic maintenance therapy—a naturalistic study. *Pharmacopsychiatry*, **33**(2), 66–71.

Thyssen A, Rusch S, Herben V, Quiroz J, Mannaert E. (2010). Risperidone long-acting injection: pharmacokinetics following administration in deltoid versus gluteal muscle in schizophrenic patients. *J Clin Pharmacol*, doi:10.1177/0091270009355156.

Tuninger E, Levander S. (1996). Large variations of plasma levels during maintenance treatment with depot neuroleptics. *Br J Psychiatry*, **169**(5), 618–21.

UKPPG. (2009). *Guidance on the administration to adults of oil-based depots and other long-acting intramuscular antipsychotic injections*. United Kingdom Psychiatric Pharmacy Group. June 2009. Available at: www.ukppg.org.uk/long-acting-injections-guidelines-sops. pdf (accessed on 14 May 2010).

van Harten PN, Hoek HW, Matroos GE, Koeter M, Kahn RS. (1998). Intermittent neuroleptic treatment and risk for tardive dyskinesia: Curaçao Extrapyramidal Syndromes Study III. *Am J Psychiatry*, **155**(4), 565–7.

Wiles DG, Gelder MG. (1979). Plasma fluphenazine levels by radioimmunoassay in schizophrenic patients treated with depot injections of fluphenaz ine decanoate. *Br J Clin Pharmacol*, **8**, 565–70.

Wilson RN. (1998). Iatrogenic complications of depot antipsychotics given to unfamiliar patients. *J R Soc Med*, **91**(1), 38–40.

ZypAdhera®: Summary of Product Characteristics. Eli Lilly and Company Limited. http://www.emc.medicines.org.uk/emc/assets/c/html/DisplayDoc.asp?DocumentID=21361 (accessed 16 March 2010).

Chapter 4

First-generation antipsychotic long-acting injections

Mark Taylor and Polash Shajahan

Correspondence: marktaylor2@nhs.net

Introduction

In this chapter we provide an up to date review of the evidence base surrounding the use of first-generation antipsychotic long-acting injections (FGA-LAIs) in schizophrenia and bipolar disorder. We start by considering the historical background to long-acting antipsychotic medications and the current patterns of use within the United Kingdom, before systematically reviewing the randomized controlled studies (RCTs) and observational studies concerning FGA-LAIs (both placebo and active comparator) in the treatment of schizophrenia and bipolar disorder. It is important to consider all study designs because different studies assess different outcomes i.e. RCTs assess efficacy—does a drug lead to benefit in ideal circumstances? Whereas observational studies assess effectiveness—does a drug have benefit in the real world where dose, patient characteristics, and follow-up may be far more variable than in an RCT? A summary section attempts to synthesize these results. We then consider the implications for future research and clinical practice.

Historical background

The first long-acting injection of antipsychotic medication introduced was fluphenazine enantate in 1966 and the second, fluphenazine decanoate, arrived some 18 months later, largely owing to the influence of GR Daniels, the medical director of Squibb & Sons Pharmaceuticals (Johnson 2009). Early evidence of the effectiveness of long-acting antipsychotic medications came from two mirror-image studies (Denham & Adamson 1971; Johnson & Freeman 1973). Both studies showed a decrease in the number of admissions to hospital and a reduction in morbidity. Lundbeck then developed flupentixol decanoate, and a Swedish mirror-image study (Gottfries & Green 1974) also showed reduced hospitalization rates for long-acting injections of flupentixol compared to the previous treatment. These mirror-image studies catalysed the use of FGA-LAIs in routine clinical practice and are summarized in greater detail in this chapter.

Another early influential study (Hogarty et al. 1979) compared fluphenazine in oral and LAI forms, with or without social therapy. It is important to note that the study duration was 2 years, and the authors found that a lower relapse rate (measured by hospitalization rate) on the LAI formulation was not apparent until after one year of treatment, although the result was not statistically significant (owing to small sample size). It is of interest that it was the interaction between social therapy and the LAI (rather than the LAI alone) that accounted for the reduced relapse rate in the second year compared to the oral form. A later but similar study (Schooler et al. 1997) over 2 years confirmed that intermittent or a very low dose of fluphenazine decanoate was worse in preventing relapse and rehospitalization than continuous moderate dosing (12.5–50 mg each fortnight) regardless of family therapy.

Subsequently, the use of LAI antipsychotic maintenance treatment has become established in chronic schizophrenia but has had a differential uptake around the world. The patterns of use of LAIs in different countries are discussed further in Chapter 10. In terms of the trends in individual LAI usage, comparative data on individual LAI prescriptions in Scotland over a 5-year period is depicted in Figure 4.1. It can be seen that the introduction of risperidone LAI in Scotland in 2003 was followed by an increasing use of this drug accompanied by a decrease in prescription rate of FGA-LAIs, notably flupentixol. The total rate of LAI use however has remained largely unchanged in that 5-year period. Despite the introduction and increasing use of SGA-LAIs it is clear that FGA-LAIs are still widely used in routine clinical practice.

Review of FGA-LAIs in schizophrenia

This review is based on a systematic literature search and extends a previous review that one of the authors (MT) was involved in (Haddad et al. 2009). We review data that compares FGA-LAIs to placebo, other LAIs (FGA or SGA), and oral antipsychotics as well as studies that have investigated the dose–response relationship for different FGA-LAIs. The Medline, Embase, and PsycInfo databases were searched in late 2009

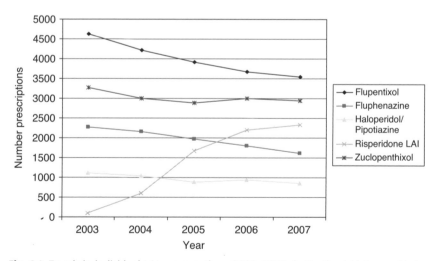

Fig. 4.1 Trends in individual LAI use over time, 2003–2007, in Scotland (data provided by the Information and Statistics Division (ISD) of the Scottish Government).

using the terms 'antipsychotic', 'depot', and 'long-acting injection' with mapping to MESH terms, and with the limits: Humans, Adults, Clinical Trial, Meta-Analysis, Randomized Controlled Trial, Comparative Study, English. There were no limitations by study date. Included studies were then reviewed for additional relevant cited articles, and a citation search facility was used to identify any further potentially relevant original studies. For inclusion, studies were required to include a group of patients treated with an FGA-LAI and provide original quantitative data on efficacy or effectiveness. No specific quality threshold was set for inclusion of studies. Studies were excluded if there were less than 20 patients in the LAI arm or if no original patient data were reported (e.g. 'modelling' studies).

A total of 252 potentially relevant study abstracts were individually scrutinized against the inclusion criteria. Seven further possible studies were identified via citation search. After inclusion/exclusion criteria were applied, remaining studies were divided into the four broad categories: (i) randomized controlled clinical trials (RCTs) which were then subsumed into the nine relevant Cochrane Database Systematic reviews for individual FGA-LAIs, one meta-analytic review (Adams et al. 2001) that considered FGA-LAIs as a group, and two subsequent RCTs; (ii) prospective observational studies (4 studies); (iii) mirror-image studies(11 studies); and (iv) retrospective observational studies (4 studies).

Cochrane systematic reviews for individual FGA-LAIs

1. *Zuclopenthixol decanoate for schizophrenia and other serious mental illnesses.* Da Silva Freire Coutinho et al. (1999) found four studies allowing comparison of zuclopenthixol decanoate with other long-acting (depot) formulations of antipsychotic medication and concluded that zuclopenthixol decanoate prevented or postponed relapse when compared against other long-acting injections of antipsychotic (NNT = 8, CI = 5–53). However, they also showed that zuclopenthixol decanoate may induce more adverse effects than the other LAIs (NNH = 5, CI = 3–31) despite a decreased need for anticholinergic medication (NNT = 9, CI = 5–38). Thus, in summary, the authors felt there was '*a real difference*' between zuclopenthixol decanoate and other FGA-LAIs, despite the limited trial data.

2. *Depot flupentixol decanoate for schizophrenia or other similar psychotic disorders.* David et al. (1999) noted there were no placebo trials and not many studies in total but concluded there was '*nothing to choose between flupentixol decanoate and other depots*'. Furthermore, they observed that no benefit accrued from dosing higher than a 'standard' dose of 40 mg per fortnight.

3. *Depot haloperidol decanoate for schizophrenia* (Quraishi et al. 1999). A variety of trial data were available for haloperidol decanoate. Two small studies confirmed its superiority over placebo as fewer individuals on haloperidol decanoate left the trials early or failed to improve. One study (*n* = 22) showed no difference in a variety of clinical outcomes (including the Clinical Global Impression scale) when haloperidol decanoate was compared to oral haloperidol, and eight separate studies revealed no difference between haloperidol decanoate and other FGA-LAIs in terms of clinical outcomes and tolerability.

4. *Depot fluphenazine decanoate and enantate for schizophrenia* (David et al. 2004). Here, the authors noted there were 70 relevant randomized studies in total available for review thus making this the most widely studied FGA-LAI, although generally the individual trials were small in size. Both fluphenazine decanoate and enantate were effective when compared to placebo as depicted in Figure 4.2. The trials of fluphenazine against both oral antipsychotics and other FGA-LAIs revealed that the '*outcomes were similar*' but the available data even for this widely studied FGA-LAI were limited.

5. *Depot pipotiazine palmitate and undecylenate for schizophrenia.* Dinesh et al. (2004) found that there was no difference between pipotiazine and oral antipsychotic medications in the relevant studies in terms of clinical global impression, relapse, study attrition, or side-effects. The review also included 16 studies ($n = 1123$) of pipotiazine compared to other FGA-LAIs and concluded that pipotiazine was '*consistently equivalent*' to the other FGA-LAIs on the outcomes of clinical global impression, relapse rate, and adverse event occurrence.

6. *Depot bromperidol decanoate for schizophrenia* (Adams et al. 2004). Four controlled studies ($n = 117$) which were described as 'poorly reported' showed that bromperidol was better than placebo but that individuals randomized to fluphenazine decanoate or haloperidol decanoate had less relapses than those given bromperidol decanoate ($n = 77$, RR = 3.95, CI = 1.05–14.6).

7. *Depot perphenazine decanoate and enantate for schizophrenia.* David et al. (2005) reviewed four studies ($n = 313$) which were described as having 'limited data', and compared perphenazine LAI to other FGA-LAIs. They concluded that perphenazine LAI was '*no better or worse*' than the other FGA-LAIs in the outcomes reported.

8. *Penfluridol for schizophrenia* (Soares & Silva de Lima 2005). Penfluridol is perhaps anomalously included here as it is a long-acting oral antipsychotic medication, being usually prescribed once a week. Nevertheless, there are six studies ($n = 274$) comparing penfluridol with FGA-LAIs, and the review concluded that there was no difference between the different medications except perhaps counter-intuitively for the outcome of 'leaving the study early', which favoured penfluridol (NNT = 6, CI = 3.4–50). Also of interest were 11 studies ($n = 449$) of penfluridol against other FGA orals including chlorpromazine and trifluoperazine. No important differences were observed in global state improvement, leaving the trial early, or need for anti-Parkinsonian medication.

9. *Depot fluspirilene for schizophrenia* (Abhijnhan et al. 2007). Here there were 12 suitable studies available for systematic review, and the authors concluded that there was '*no clear difference*' between fluspirilene and the other FGA oral medications and FGA-LAIs involved.

In summary, the Cochrane reviews of FGA-LAIs provide unequivocal evidence of superiority over placebo in the maintenance treatment of schizophrenia, even though the number and size of the available studies are surprisingly low. Moreover, no dramatic difference between individual FGA-LAIs emerges from these Cochrane reviews, both in terms of efficacy and tolerability, except for perhaps a modest superior efficacy for zuclopenthixol decanoate.

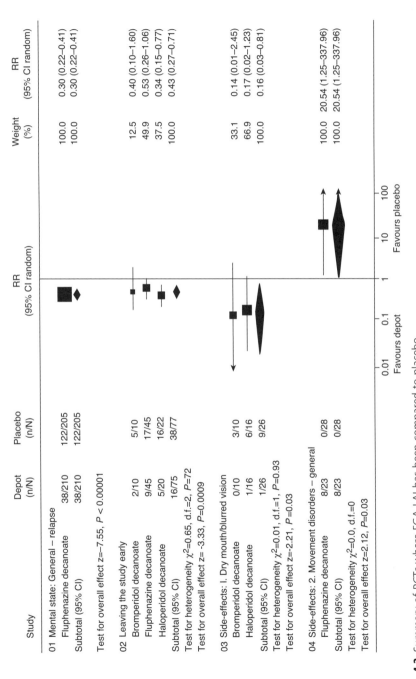

Fig. 4.2 Summary of RCTs where FGA-LAI has been compared to placebo (from Adams et al. 2001, with permission).

The comprehensive systematic meta-review of LAIs by Adams et al. (2001) was based on a synthesis of data from existing Cochrane reviews on individual FGA-LAIs in patients with schizophrenia or schizophrenia-like illnesses. Adams et al. (2001) noted that there were surprisingly few LAI versus placebo studies. A review of fluphenazine decanoate over placebo favoured the active drug in terms of relapse rates ($n = 415$, NNT = 2, CI = 1.8–2.6). The combined (Cochrane style) results from all placebo studies are depicted in Figure 4.2.

Three of the LAI reviews summarized above showed that individuals on LAIs stayed on treatment longer than those on placebo ($n = 152$, RR = 0.43, CI = 0.27–0.71). In terms of tolerability, more people on placebo (curiously) suffered blurred vision or dry mouth, but more individuals in the active LAI group had movement disorders ($n = 51$, NNH = 3, CI = 6.5–1.9).

The relapse data on FGA-LAIs versus oral antipsychotics are based on a total sample of 848 patients randomized to an FGA-LAI (fluphenazine decanoate, fluspirilene decanoate, pipotiazine palmitate) or an FGA-oral medication (including chlorpromazine, haloperidol, penfluridol, and trifluoperazine). The risk of relapse did not differ between the two groups (RR = 0.96, CI = 0.8–1.1) which is perhaps not surprising given the typical study duration, but global improvement was more likely with FGA-LAI than FGA-oral medication with a number needed to treat being 4 (NNT = 4, CI = 2–9). The FGA-LAI and FGA-oral groups were also similar in terms of study attrition, and anticholinergic medication (a proxy marker for the presence of extrapyramidal symptoms (EPS)) was prescribed to approximately two-thirds of both the FGA-LAI and FGA-oral cohorts. The prevalence of tardive dyskinesia (TD) in the FGA-LAI cohort was 9.0%, and in the FGA-oral cohort it was 14.1% supporting the notion that FGA-LAIs are unlikely to cause more TD than their oral counterparts.

When Adams et al. (2001) reviewed the data comparing specific FGA-LAIs with each other, they reached the conclusion that 'there were few convincing data that any real differences exist between depots'. Only the outcome of mental state relapse showed that zuclopenthixol decanoate was statistically superior to the control LAIs (largely fluphenazine: $n = 296$, NNT = 8, CI = 5–53). However, publication bias could not be excluded as an explanation for this finding.

Adams et al. (2001) provided some data regarding the relative efficacy of high, standard, and low doses of certain FGA-LAIs. They found no difference between high dose (e.g. 250 mg fluphenazine per week or flupentixol 200 mg per fortnight) versus standard dose (12.5–50 mg fluphenazine every fortnight and 40 mg flupentixol per fortnight) on a variety of outcomes including mental state, global state, or study attrition. Adams et al. (2001) noted that the data comparing standard to low-dose FGA-LAIs were limited (Adams et al. 2001) but for three preparations (flupentixol, fluphenazine decanoate, and enanthate) relapse rate was improved at the standard dose ($n = 638$, NNT = 7, CI = 5–12) compared to the low dose. These conclusions regarding dose are similar to those reached in an earlier review by Kane (1995) who concluded that low doses of FGA-LAIs were less effective than moderate or standard doses of maintenance treatment. For example, 50 mg and 200 mg per month of haloperidol decanoate had similar relapse rates (25% and 16%, respectively), whereas the relapse rate in those randomly allocated to 25 mg per month was higher (60%).

However, Kane (1995) also observed that the lowest efficacious dose was associated with better psychosocial and vocational adjustment.

More recent RCTs

Our search revealed two RCTs that were not included in the original or updated Cochrane reviews of FGA-LAIs. The first one, by Arango et al. (2006), was a small RCT comparing oral zuclopenthixol (n = 20) and zuclopenthixol decanoate (n = 26) over 1 year in patients with schizophrenia and a history of violence. A lower frequency of violent acts was seen in the LAI group but end-point scores of the Positive and Negative Symptoms Scale (PANSS) did not differ.

The only RCT published at the time of writing that compares an FGA-LAI with an SGA-LAI is that by Rubio et al. (2006), which compared risperidone long-acting injection (RLAI) to zuclopenthixol decanoate in patients with schizophrenia and co-morbid substance use (cannabis, cocaine, opiates, and ecstasy). This study randomized patients who had been admitted to hospital with worsening psychosis. After stabilizing their illness in hospital, 115 of 183 patients interviewed agreed to participate and were alternately allocated to RLAI (n = 57) or zuclopenthixol decanoate (n = 58) and followed up for 6 months as outpatients. The clinical assessors were blind to the treatment. The primary outcome measure was number of positive urine drug tests during the 6 months. Secondary outcome measures were PANSS subscales and compliance with the weekly psychotherapeutic programme. In terms of the primary outcome measures there was a statistically significant advantage with RLAI for number of positive urine drug tests (8.7 for RLAI vs. 10.3 for zuclopenthixol, p = .005). However, relapse rate and survival time to first positive urine drug test did not differ. PANSS scores, particularly for negative symptoms and measures of EPS showed an advantage for RLAI. The RLAI group also demonstrated better adherence to the psychotherapeutic programme.

The Rubio et al. (2006) study involved an important group of patients seen in routine psychiatric practice (and not just in addiction specialties) but caution should be exercised in generalizing these results to all patients with schizophrenia as patients with co-morbid substance use may differ in terms of aetiology, clinical presentation, and treatment response compared with those with no substance misuse disorder.

Prospective observational studies

Four prospective observational studies compared an FGA-LAI to one or more oral antipsychotic cohorts, and they adopted various pragmatic outcome measures including risk of readmission and time to all-cause discontinuation of medication. The results were mixed; two studies found a better outcome for FGA-LAI compared to an FGA-oral (Tiihonen et al. 2006; Zhu et al. 2008). The Schizophrenia Health Outcomes Study (SOHO) found poorer outcomes for FGA-LAI than oral olanzapine (Haro et al. 2006, 2007) and a fourth study (Conley et al. 2003) found oral antipsychotics to be superior to haloperidol decanoate but equivalent to fluphenazine decanoate.

Tiihonen et al. (2006) assessed the outcome of patients after their first admission with schizophrenia or schizoaffective disorder in relation to the antipsychotic they were taking on discharge. Initial use of perphenazine LAI was associated with a significantly lower adjusted risk for all-cause medication discontinuation than haloperidol and the second lowest discontinuation rate of the 10 drugs studied. An analysis of rehospitalization rates, calculated according to the ongoing antipsychotic, showed that perphenazine LAI had the lowest risk of rehospitalization (68% reduction in fully adjusted relative risk compared to haloperidol). It is interesting to note that perphenazine LAI performed better than oral perphenazine on both measures.

The study by Zhu et al. (2008) used data from the US-SCAP (Schizophrenia Care and Assessment Program) study to assess the time to all-cause medication discontinuation in the first year after initiation of an FGA-LAI or oral antipsychotic. The same two antipsychotics—haloperidol and fluphenazine—in oral or LAI form were assessed, being the only two FGA-LAIs available in the United States. The LAI-group had a significantly longer mean time to all-cause medication discontinuation and patients receiving an LAI were twice as likely to stay on treatment than the oral group.

The SOHO study was a 3-year observational study of patients with schizophrenia. The likelihood of not achieving remission, the risk of relapse, and the all-cause discontinuation rate of medication were all higher for those treated with FGA-LAI compared to oral olanzapine (Haro et al. 2006). By 3 years the baseline medication had been discontinued by 36.4% of those who initiated treatment with olanzapine, 50.2% for those who initiated an FGA-LAI and 53.1% for those who initiated an FGA-oral drug. The hazard ratio (risk) for discontinuation relative to olanzapine for FGA-LAIs was 1.43 (95% CI 1.19–1.70).

Conley et al. (2003) assessed readmission rates in patients discharged on fluphenazine decanoate and haloperidol decanoate and compared this with cohorts discharged on one of three SGA-orals. The one-year readmission risk (with adjustment for baseline variables) for each of the three SGA-oral groups was lower than for haloperidol decanoate but similar to that seen with fluphenazine decanoate.

Only the SOHO study presented tolerability data and this was limited to descriptive data without statistical analysis. The period prevalence for EPS was 42.8% for the FGA-LAI cohort, 31.4% for FGA-oral cohort, and for the various SGA-orals values ranged from 13.4% (quetiapine) to 32.2% (risperidone). Assessment of both EPS and TD was based on clinical judgement and not objective rating scales. The proportion of patients who gained more than 7% weight from baseline to medication-discontinuation was higher for FGA-LAI than FGA-oral (21.8% vs. 15.7%) as was mean weight gain (2.6 kg vs. 1.5 kg).

Mirror-image studies

Our search identified 11 mirror-image FGA-LAI studies (see Figure 4.3). These studies have been previously reviewed and analysed in detail (Haddad et al. 2009). In each of the 11 studies, total inpatient days and number of admissions were lower on FGA-LAI than during the preceding treatment period, as indicated in Figure 4.3. Furthermore where *p* values were available, or could be calculated, the differences were statistically significant. Ten studies provided the mean number of inpatient days for the LAI-treatment period and preceding treatment period. Based on these 10 studies, the mean number of inpatient days per patient fell from 114.9 in the pre-FGA-LAI period to 28.6 during FGA-LAI treatment (Haddad et al. 2009). Thus Haddad et al. (2009)

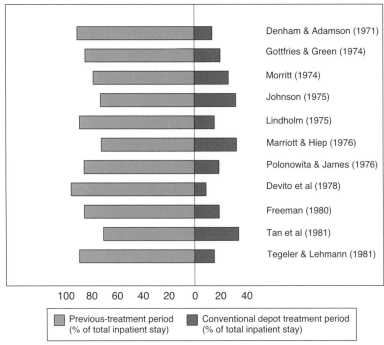

Fig. 4.3 Summary of all mirror-image studies examining time in hospital, comparing FGA-LAIs with oral antipsychotic medications (with permission, from Haddad et al. 2009). Distribution (%) of total inpatient stay between previous-treatment and FGA-LAI treatment periods for each mirror image study (*n* = 11), Each horizontal bar is equivalent to 100%.

confirmed the conclusions of an earlier important review (Davis et al. 1994) regarding the utility of LAIs in maintenance treatment of schizophrenia.

Other retrospective observational studies

We identified four retrospective observational studies. Shajahan et al. (2010) examined patients with schizophrenia or related psychosis who had been commenced on any long-acting antipsychotic injection in a discreet Scottish population of approximately 500,000 within a defined period (2002 to 2008). They utilized an electronic chart review of patients' medical records and assigned retrospective Clinical Global Impression ratings as well as recording discontinuation and rehospitalization events as putative markers of treatment failure. The advantage of this study was that all new medication starts after the electronic record initiation were included, so patients were more representative of real clinical populations requiring treatment rather than those seen in controlled trials. Shajahan et al. (2010) found that RLAI were the most popular choice of new start long-acting injection outnumbering all the other conventional long-acting injections; however, when compared with RLAI and flupentixol, patients

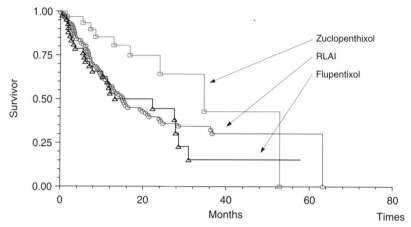

Fig. 4.4 All cause discontinuation (unadjusted) from LAIs (from Shajahan et al. 2010, with permission).

on zuclopenthixol decanoate showed significantly better outcomes in terms of time to discontinuation (see Figure 4.4) and hospitalization rates. However, fewer of those on zuclopenthixol decanoate were considered 'much improved' or 'very much improved' in terms of CGI compared with flupentixol decanoate or RLAI.

Olfson et al. (2007) used the California Medicaid database to analyse the use of fluphenazine decanoate ($n = 948$), haloperidol decanoate ($n = 1631$), and RLAI ($n = 116$) for 180 days before and 180 days after initiating treatment. This study was not included in the 'mirror-image' section above as patients who were admitted for 14 days or more were excluded. They found few clinical or demographic differences between the three treatment groups and recent oral non-adherence was frequently seen. Only a small minority of patients continued on the three long-acting injections for the full 180 days post-initiation (5%, 10%, and 3% respectively), this represents a much lower continuation rate for LAI treatment than reported in several European studies. The authors also noted a high rate of co-prescribing of antidepressants, mood stabilizers, and benzodiazepines in their LAI cohort.

In the two remaining studies, the readmission rate was lower in the FGA-LAI group compared with oral medication in one study (Devito et al. 1978) but did not differ between LAI and oral medication in another (Marchiaro et al. 2005). In the Marchiaro et al. (2005) study the two groups had similar rates of baseline anticholinergic drug use but during the study anticholinergic drugs were prescribed more frequently to the patients prescribed an LAI than those prescribed an oral drug (47 % vs. 13 %; $p = .01$).

Review of FGA-LAIs in bipolar disorder

The use of LAIs in bipolar disorder has been reviewed by El Mallakh in 2007. LAIs are widely used in bipolar disorder as well as schizophrenia as illustrated by the following (unpublished) data from the city of Glasgow in Scotland (population ~1 million). Here, a case register of all cases of psychosis (i.e. 'broad' schizophrenia and bipolar disorder)

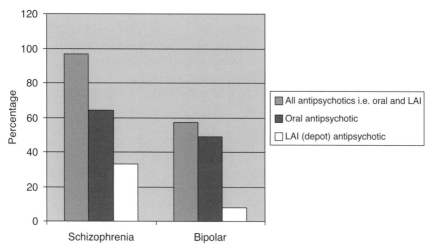

Fig. 4.5 Psycis cases (*n* = 5221) showing use of maintenance antipsychotic medication (%) by diagnosis.

followed up in secondary care has been developed from 2002. This 'Psycis' (Psychosis clinical information system) register comprises (at the time of analysis) 5221 individuals and contains demographic and clinical details. The large and comprehensive nature of the Psycis case register, albeit from secondary care, suggests that the findings are generalizable to the rest of the United Kingdom if not to other government-based health care systems. Figure 4.5 provides percentage figures for use of antipsychotic medication in both schizophrenia (2323 individuals) and bipolar disorder (1048 individuals) from this case register, broken down by total, oral only, and LAI or depot antipsychotic.

Figure 4.5 reveals that the LAI usage rate in maintenance treatment in this large UK cohort is 33% for broad schizophrenia (one-third of the total antipsychotic prescriptions) and 8% in bipolar disorder (14% of the total antipsychotics prescribed). A total of 23% of men and 18% of women received LAI maintenance treatment in the total psychosis cohort. Co-prescription of regular oral antipsychotic medication, in combination with a regular long-acting injection of antipsychotic medication, occured in a significant minority of cases namely 24.5% of individuals with schizophrenia and 28% of those with bipolar disorder. In addition, within the Psycis sample described above that includes both community- and hospital-based patients (as of January 2010), 15% of those individuals receiving regular LAI or depot antipsychotic were currently under long-term treatment orders under the Mental Health Act, compared to 12% of the total sample, i.e. a negligible difference, suggesting that at the current time in Glasgow the use of LAIs is not strongly linked to compulsory treatment under the Mental Health Act.

To date, no RCTs of FGA-LAI use in bipolar disorder are available, although there are a number of switching and retrospective observational studies that are summarized in Table 4.1. The largest switching study was that by Ahlfors et al. (1981) that followed up 93 patients, of whom 85 were bipolar. The study involved switching from lithium

Table 4.1 Summary of studies in bipolar affective disorder with an FGA-LAI cohort

Study	Participants/type of study	Follow-up period	LAI group (number of participants)	Comparator group(s)	Outcomes
Ahlfors et al. (1981)	◆ Patients switched from lithium carbonate to flupentixol decanoate ◆ 85% had bipolar disorder, remainder had unipolar depression	14 months	Flupentixol decanoate (n = 93)	Lithium carbonate (n = 93)	◆ No difference in terms of illness episodes per year ◆ Non-significant increase in illness time ◆ Reduction in manic episodes ◆ Increase in depressive episodes
Fernando et al. (1984)	◆ Retrospective chart review of patients with schizoaffective disorder (n = 9) and bipolar disorder (n = 6) treated with LAI	23 months	Haloperidol decanoate		◆ All patients described as 'improved in clinical state, discharged from hospital and improved social function'
Lowe and Batchelor (1986)	◆ Patients switched from lithium carbonate plus FGA oral antipsychotic to lithium plus LAI	23 months	Haloperidol decanoate plus lithium carbonate (n = 12)	FGA oral antipsychotic plus lithium carbonate (n = 12)	◆ Reduction in rapid cycling episodes (n = 4) ◆ Less extrapyramidal side effects with LAI

Study	Design	Duration	Treatment	Comparator	Findings
Esparon et al. (1986)	◆ Blinded cross-over design, 1 year on then 1 year off LAI.	2 years	Flupentixol decanoate plus lithium carbonate (n = 15)	Lithium carbonate alone (n = 15)	◆ Both groups spent less time in hospital (reduced by half) than in the 2 years prior to entry into study ◆ No differences in hospitalization rates or time spent in hospital on flupenthixol decanoate plus lithium carbonate
White et al. (1993)	◆ Patients switched from either lithium carbonate or carbamazepine due to inadequate response. ◆ Mirror design study	44 months	Haloperidol decanoate (n = 16)	Lithium carbonate or carbamazepine	◆ Reduction in manic episodes and time spent manic ◆ Non-significant increase in depressive episodes and time spent depressed
Littlejohn et al (1994)	◆ Retrospective chart review of patients treated with various LAIs	23 months	Haloperidol decanoate plus lithium carbonate (n = 12)	FGA oral antipsychotic plus lithium carbonate (n = 12)	◆ Reduction in hospitalization rates and time spent in hospital ◆ Reduction in manic, depressive and mixed episodes

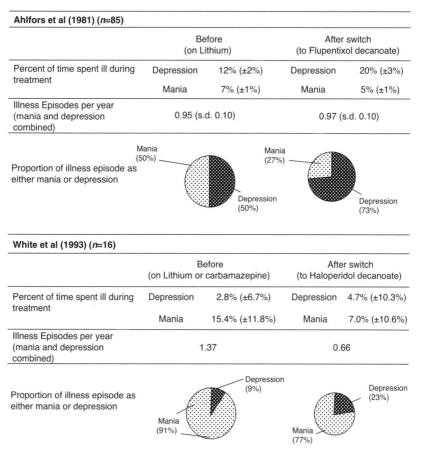

Fig. 4.6 Outcomes of switching from a mood stabiliser to a FGA-LAI in bipolar disorder.

carbonate to flupentixol decanoate. Reasons for switching were side-effects and poor adherence. Patients were observed prospectively in terms of percentage of time spent ill, number of illness episodes, and these were subcategorized into mania or depression. Similar data are available from the smaller study ($n = 16$) by White et al. (1993) that involved switching patients on lithium carbonate or carbamazepine to haloperidol decanoate. Prospectively collected data were compared with retrospective data for the equivalent period. The results from these two studies (Ahlfors et al. 1981; White et al. 1993) are summarized in Figure 4.6. Switching to the LAI in both studies was not associated with worsening in terms of number of illness episodes per year, indeed the smaller study of White et al. (1993) showed a statistically significant reduction in half of the number of episodes, perhaps related to improved adherence with the LAI formulation. However, the cost of switching to either LAI formulation from a mood stabilizer was a relative increase in the proportion of illness time spent in a depressive phase.

That is, the FGA-LAI appeared to be protecting against recurrence of mania but increased the burden from depression. The three other studies available (Fernando et al. 1984; Littlejohn et al. 1994; Lowe & Batchelor 1986) reported findings following treatment with haloperidol decanoate. Generally, these studies showed no worsening in terms of illness episodes and favourable reduction in hospitalization rates.

In summary, the limited data available support the hypothesis that FGA-LAIs such as flupentixol and haloperidol decanoate are associated with some clinical improvements in bipolar disorder. More specifically they are effective in preventing manic relapse and days spent suffering from mania. However, FGA-LAIs do not necessarily prevent depressive relapse or days spent in a depressive phase of bipolar disorder. This is of interest in light of previous reports supporting the hypothesis that flupentixol has anti-depressant effects in unipolar depressive disorder (Gruber & Cole 1991). The Psycis data indicate that the use of LAIs in bipolar disorder is not unusual, whereas the evidence base outlined here for FGA-LAIs is thin, being restricted to observational studies. Thus there is a need for further research into the use of LAIs in bipolar disorder.

Summary of evidence

There is an extensive evidence base concerning FGA-LAIs in schizophrenia, comprising both RCTs and observational studies although most studies date from the 1970s and 1980s. In terms of relapse prevention, the Adams et al. (2001) meta-analysis shows that FGA-LAIs are superior to placebo and equally effective as oral antipsychotics. Adams et al. (2001) found that global clinical improvement was twice as likely in the FGA-LAI compared to the FGA-oral group, although it is worth noting that this analysis was based on a relatively small sample. This increased likelihood of clinical improvement may reflect LAIs overcoming the problem of partial adherence with oral medication. At first sight the equivalent effect of LAIs and oral antipsychotics in relapse prevention in Adams et al.'s (2001) review may seem surprising, but it may reflect an important weakness of RCTs namely that they tend to recruit a highly selected population, and the same factors that influence a patient to adhere to prescribed medication are precisely the factors that will influence willingness to cooperate with research or volunteer for a RCT. Adams et al. acknowledged this bias commenting, 'those for whom depots (LAIs) are most indicated may not be represented.'

Adams et al. (2001) also found that high dosing of LAIs conferred no therapeutic advantage and thus should be avoided owing to dose-related adverse events. Low dosing (e.g. less than 12.5 mg fluphenazine decanoate per fortnight) cannot be recommended either as it is less effective compared to standard LAI dosing. Finally, there is a modest signal from Adams et al. (2001) that zuclopenthixol decanoate may be the most effective single FGA-LAI—consistent with the findings of the retrospective study of Shajahan et al. (2010).

To date the only randomized comparison of an FGA-LAI and SGA-LAI is that of Rubio et al. (2006) that compared zuclopenthixol decanoate with RLAI. This was a relatively small study and was conducted in a specific population, namely patients with schizophrenia and co-morbid substance misuse. This study found that most outcome measures were superior in the RLAI group.

We identified four prospective observational studies showing mixed results. In two studies the FGA-LAI was superior to an FGA-oral comparator, whereas the two studies that showed a worse outcome for FGA-LAIs used an SGA-oral comparator(s). These conflicting results may reflect greater selection bias when simultaneously comparing between formulation (oral or LAI) and between class (FGA or SGA). Consistent with this, outcomes in SOHO appeared similar for FGA-LAI and FGA-oral cohorts although statistical analysis was not provided.

The 11 mirror-image studies (see Figure 4.3) of FGA-LAIs showed that a switch to an LAI was associated with a reduced number of inpatient days and number of admissions compared to previous treatment (Haddad et al. 2009). This is a striking finding but must be interpreted in light of the methodological weaknesses of mirror-image designs. Nevertheless, the combined weight of the mirror-image studies illustrated in Figure 4.3 provides strong evidence for the use of FGA-LAIs in the maintenance treatment of schizophrenia.

We identified four retrospective studies that were not mirror-image studies. Two compared an FGA-LAI to an oral comparator group and the other two made comparison to another LAI. Of the two studies with an oral comparator, one found a lower readmission rate with the FGA-LAI compared oral medication, whereas the other found comparable readmission rates for oral medication and LAI. The two studies that made comparison to another LAI (Olfson et al. 2007; Shajahan et al. 2010) are of particular interest as they both included a cohort of patients receiving RLAI. The most striking finding of the Olfson et al. study from the United States was the extremely low continuation rate of all three LAIs over six months, coupled with supplementary oral psychotropic polypharmacy. Shajahan et al. (2010) found that zuclopenthixol decanoate was superior to RLAI and flupentixol decanoate in terms of discontinuation and hospitalization rate over the long (up to 5 years) study period, although the global improvement scores did not favour any particular LAI. This advantage of zuclopenthixol decanoate over other FGA-LAIs is consistent with the conclusion of Adams et al. (2001) and the Cochrane review of zuclopenthixol decanoate, which suggested it may have (a modest) superiority over other FGA-LAIs. This finding that zuclopenthixol decanoate was superior to RLAI is contrary to the findings of Rubio et al. (2006). Both studies have their weaknesses, and at present it would probably be reasonable to assume that the comparative effectiveness of these two drugs is unclear. Further research is warranted especially given the cost differential of SGA-LAIs compared to FGA-LAIs.

In bipolar disorder, first choice maintenance pharmacotherapy remains a traditional mood stabilizer such as lithium or valproic acid, or one of the second-generation oral antipsychotics that are licensed for this indication. Where adherence is an issue, there is a place for an LAI. The data for FGA-LAIs in the maintenance phase of bipolar disorder are limited by a lack of randomized controlled trials. The 'switching' studies that are available are limited by small numbers of subjects and variation in end-point measures. In clinical practice, LAIs are used in a significant minority of patients with bipolar disorder (8%; see Figure 4.5). This represents an important subgroup of patients and the relative risks and benefits need to be considered. The data available are sparse but suggest that FGA-LAIs appear to be effective in preventing manic relapse and days spent suffering from mania. However, they do not necessarily prevent depressive relapse or days spent in a depressive phase of bipolar disorder. From a clinical perspective, particularly where manic phases owing to non-adherence can lead to catastrophic decision-making, LAIs may have an important role.

In terms of safety and tolerability, several studies have calculated prevalence rates for EPS in patients on FGA-LAI, including 42.8% in the SOHO prospective study, 47.0% in a retrospective case note study (Marchiaro et al. 2005), and 69.5% in a meta-analysis (Adams et al. 2001). Rates for TD emergence in FGA-LAIs range between 9.0% and 12.9%. The only study to make a statistical comparison between rates of EPS and TD in patients prescribed for FGA-LAI and FGA-oral drugs is the meta-analysis by Adams et al. (2001) and the rates were comparable. These results demonstrate that EPS and TD are common in many patients prescribed certain FGA-LAIs.

Future research

An RCT comparing oral antipsychotic medication with an FGA-LAI and an SGA-LAI would be of value. This is of particular relevance given the higher aquisition cost of SGA-LAIs and recent RCTs of oral medication, including CATIE (Lieberman et al. 2005) and CUtLASS (Jones et al 2006), which showed no striking differences between specific oral FGAs and oral SGAs in either efficacy or tolerability, although it is worth bearing in mind that CATIE found high rates of medication discontinuation (its primary outcome) for all the oral antipsychotic medications studied. Future studies involving LAIs should be of adequate duration to assess relapse e.g. 18 months or more, and outcome measures should include relapse, symptomatic improvement, and a range of adverse effects including EPS, TD, weight gain, and metabolic parameters. Patient satisfaction and cost-effectiveness also need to be examined. To reduce the problem of selective recruitment such a trial should be pragmatic and have minimal exclusion criteria.

Currently the only head-to-head studies of an FGA-LAI and an SGA-LAI are an RCT (Rubio et al. 2006) and a retrospective observational study (Shajahan et al. 2010). Both compared zuclopenthixol decanoate and RLAI, both had methodological weaknesses, and the results of the two studies were contradictory. Clearly more work in this important area is required.

Implications for clinical practice

RCTs and observational studies have their individual strengths and weaknesses, and reviewing all these study designs together provides the most comprehensive analysis of the data. The four designs we considered (RCTs, prospective observational studies, mirror-image studies, other retrospective studies) all provided at least some evidence that FGA-LAIs can result in superior outcome than oral antipsychotic medication in the treatment of schizophrenia. The reduced readmission rates found in the prospective study by Tiihonen et al. and in mirror-image studies (Figure 4.3) suggest that FGA-LAIs have the potential to reduce treatment costs because inpatient admission is one of the largest contributors to the direct costs of schizophrenia.

In the 1970s and 1980s there were claims that there were differences in the actions of various FGA-LAIs e.g. that flupentixol was said to be more effective in patients with depressive symptoms, fluphenazine could make depressive symptoms worse, pipotiazine was less likely to cause EPS, and zuclopenthixol was more useful in aggressive or agitated patients. These supposed differences appear to have originated from marketing strategies when these compounds were initially presented to clinicians, as our review found little evidence of differences among FGA-LAIs. The only exception is some limited data (Adams et al. 2001; Shajahan et al. 2010) that suggest that a moderate dose of zuclopenthixol decanoate may be more effective than certain other FGA-LAIs. Figure 4.1 illustrates that zuclopenthixol decanoate remains a popular prescribing choice of LAI for clinicians, at least in Scotland.

The rates of EPS and TD seen with FGA-LAIs (e.g. in the meta-review of Adams et al. 2001) are no higher than those seen with oral FGA-LAIs but remain a concern and emphasize the need to screen patients regularly for EPS. Screening for adverse medication effects should cover a full range of potential adverse effects including weight gain and metabolic abnormalities and ideally occur in a systematic manner using a practical but valid scale (Waddell & Taylor 2008). The finding that higher doses of FGA-LAIs are no more effective than moderate doses (Adams et al. 2001) highlights the importance of avoiding inappropriately high doses of these drugs given that most adverse effects, including EPS and TD, are dose related.

Our findings support the view that LAIs should be considered in patients with schizophrenia at risk of relapse who adhere poorly with oral medication. This is consistently recommended in various authorial guidelines (e.g. Kane & Garcia-Ribera 2009) Furthermore, there is some tentative evidence that suggests that FGA-LAIs may be beneficial in bipolar disorder maintenance treatment, particularly where manic relapse owing to limited treatment adherence is a concern. However, it seems that clinicians often regard LAIs as a treatment of last resort (Waddell & Taylor 2009) and use them only when the risk of relapse is perceived as very high. We argue that the evidence suggests that a broader range of patients could benefit. For example, the Tiihonen et al. (2006) study demonstrates that FGA-LAIs can be of benefit early in the course of schizophrenia. The Adams et al. (2001) meta-review finding of a higher likelihood of clinical improvement on FGA-LAI than oral medication, even though relapse rates did not differ, suggests that LAIs can be of benefit in partial adherence, which is a common and underestimated problem. Good clinical practice suggests that the decision to use an LAI should be made at an individual level, reflecting the evidence base and being an informed decision jointly made by the clinician and patient.

References

Abhijnhan A, Adams CE, David A, Ozbilen M. (2007). Depot fluspirilene for schizophrenia. *Cochrane Database Syst Rev,* (1), CD001718.

Adams CE, David A, Quraishi SN. (2004). Depot bromperidol decanoate for schizophrenia. *Cochrane Database Syst Rev,* (3), CD001719.

Adams CE, Fenton MKP, Quraishi S, David AS. (2001). Systematic meta-review of depot antipsychotic drugs for people with schizophrenia. *Br J Psych,* **179**, 290–9.

Ahlfors UG, Baastrup PC, Dencker SJ, Elgen Ket al. (1981). Flupenthixol decanoate in recurrent manic depressive illness. A comparison with lithium. *Acta Psych Scand,* **64**, (3) 226–37.

Arango C, Bombin I, Gonzalez-Salvador T, Garcia-Cabeza I, Bobes J. (2006). Randomised clinical trial comparing oral versus depot formulations of zuclopenthixol in patients with schizophrenia and previous violence. *European Psychiatry*, **21**(1), 34–40.

Conley RR, Kelly DL, Love RC, McMahon RP. (2003). Rehospitalization risk with second-generation and depot antipsychotics. *Ann Clin Psychiatry*, 15 23–31.

da Silva Freire Coutinho E, Fenton M, Quraishi, SN. (2009). Zuclopenthixol decanoate for schizophrenia and other serious mental illnesses. *Cochrane Database Syst Rev*, (3), CD001164.

David A, Adams CE, Eisenbruch M, Quraishi S, Rathbone J. (2004). Depot fluphenazine decanoate and enanthate for schizophrenia. *Cochrane Database Syst Rev*, (2), CD000307.

David A, Adams CE, Quraishi SN. (1999). Depot flupenthixol decanoate for schizophrenia or other similar psychotic disorders. *Cochrane Database Syst Rev*, CD001470.

David A, Quraishi S, Rathbone J. (2005). Depot perphenazine decanoate and enanthate for schizophrenia. *Cochrane Database Syst Rev*, (3), CD001717.

Davis JM, Matalon L, Watanabe MD, Blake L. (1994). Depot antipsychotic drugs. Place in therapy. *Drugs*, **47**(5), 741–73.

Denham J, Adamson L. (1971). The contribution of fluphenazine enanthate and decanoate in the prevention of readmission of schizophrenic patients. *Acta Psychiatr Scand*, **47**(4), 420–30.

Devito RA, Brink L, Sloan C, Jolliff F. (1978). Fluphenazine decanoate vs oral antipsychotics: a comparison of their effectiveness in the treatment of schizophrenia as measured by a reduction in hospital readmissions. *J Clin Psychiatry*, **39**(1), 26–34.

Dinesh M, David A, Quraishi SN. (2004). Depot pipotiazine palmitate and undecylenate for schizophrenia. *Cochrane Database Syst Rev*, (3), CD001720.

El Mallakh Rif S. (2007).Medication adherence and the use of long-acting antipsychotics in bipolar disorder. *J Psychiatr Practice*, **13**(2), 79–85.

Esparon J, Kolloori J, Naylor GJ, McHarg AM, Smith AH, Hopwood SE. (1986). Comparison of the prophylactic action of flupenthixol with placebo in lithium treated manic-depressive patients. *Br J Psychiatry*, **148**, 723–5.

Fernando J, Krishna Raju R, Jones GG, Stanley RO. (1984). The use of depot neuroleptic haloperidol decanoate. *Acta Psychiatr Scand*, **69**(2), 175–6.

Freeman H. (1980). Twelve years' experience with the total use of depot neuroleptics in a defined population. *Adv Biochem Psychopharmacol*, **24**, 559–64.

Gottfries CG, Green L. (1974). Flupenthixol decanoate–in treatment of out-patients. *Acta Psychiatr Scand Suppl*, **255**, 15–24.

Gruber AJ, Cole JO. (1991). Antidepressant effects of flupenthixol. *Pharmacotherapy*, **11**, 450–9.

Haddad PM, Taylor M, Niaz OS. (2009). First-generation antipsychotic long-acting injections v. oral antipsychotics in schizophrenia: systematic review of randomised controlled trials and observational studies. *Br J Psychiatry*, **195**, S20–8.

Haro JM, Novick D, Suarez D, Alonso J, Le´ pine JP, Ratcliffe M. (2006). Remission and relapse in the outpatient care of schizophrenia: three-year results from the Schizophrenia Outpatient Health Outcomes study. *J Clin Psychopharmacol*, **26**, 571–8.

Haro JM, Suarez D, Novick D, Brown J, Usall J, Naber D. (2007). Three-year antipsychotic effectiveness in the outpatient care of schizophrenia: observational versus randomized studies results. *Eur Neuropsychopharmacol*, **17**, 235–44.

Hogarty GE, Schooler NR, Ulrich R, Mussare F, Ferro P, Herron E. (1979). Fluphenazine and social therapy in the aftercare of schizophrenic patients. Relapse analyses of a two-year controlled study of fluphenazine decanoate and fluphenazine hydrochloride. *Arch Gen Psychiatry*, **36**, 1283–94.

Johnson DAW, and Freeman HL, . (1973). Drug Defaulting by Patients on Long-Acting Phenothiazines. Psychol Med. *Arch Gen Psychiatry*, **3**(1), 115–119.

Johnson DAW. (1975). Observations on the dose regime of fluphenazine decanoate in maintenance therapy of schizophrenia. *Br J Psychiatry*, **126**, 457–61.

Johnson DAW. (2009). Historical perspective on antipsychotic long-acting injections. *Br J Psychiatry* **195**, S7–S12.

Jones PB, Barnes TR, Davies L, Dunn G, Lloyd H, Hayhurst KP, et al. (2006). Randomized controlled trial of the effect on Quality of Life of second- vs first-generation antipsychotic drugs in schizophrenia: Cost Utility of the Latest Antipsychotic Drugs in Schizophrenia Study (CUtLASS 1). *Arch Gen Psychiatry*, **63**(10), 1079–87.

Kane JM. (1995). Dosing issues and depot medication in the maintenance treatment of schizophrenia. *Int Clin Psychopharmacol,* **10**(Suppl 3), 65–71.

Kane JM, Garcia-Ribera C. (2009). Clinical guideline recommendations for antipsychotic long-acting injections. *Br J Psychiatry,* **195**, S63–7.

Lieberman JA, Stroup TS, McEvoy JP, Swartz MS, Rosenheck RA, Perkins DO, et al. (2005). Clinical Antipsychotic Trials of Intervention Effectiveness (CATIE) Investigators. Effectiveness of antipsychotic drugs in patients with chronic schizophrenia. *N Engl J Med*, **353**, 1209–23.

Lindholm H. (1975). The consumption of inpatient psychiatric resources prior to and during treatment with a depot neuroleptic, perphenazine enanthate. A mirror study. *Nord Psykiatr Tidsskr,* **29**(6), 513–20.

Littlejohn R, Leslie F, Cookson J. (1994). Depot antipsychotics in the prophylaxis of bipolar affective disorder. *Br J Psychiatry,***165**, 827–9.

Lowe MR, Batchelor DH. (1986). Depot neuroleptics and manic depressive psychosis. *Int Clin Psychopharmacol,* **1**(Suppl 1), 53–62.

Marchiaro L, Rocca P, LeNoci F, Longo P, Montemagni C, Rigazzi C, et al. (2005). Naturalistic, retrospective comparison between second-generation antipsychotics and depot neuroleptics in patients affected by schizophrenia. *J Clin Psychiatry*, **66**(11), 1423–31.

Marriott P, Hiep A. (1976). A mirror image out-patient study at a depot phenothiazine clinic. *Aust N Z J Psychiatry*, **10**(2), 163–7.

Morritt C. (1974). Long-acting phenothiazines and schizophrenia. *Nurs Mirror Midwives J*, **138**(4), 57–9.

Olfson M, Marcus SC, Ascher-Svanum H. (2007). Treatment of schizophrenia with long-acting fluphenazine, haloperidol, or risperidone. *Schiz Bulletin,* **33**(6), 1379–87.

Polonowita A, James NM. (1976). Fluphenazine decanoate maintenance in schizophrenia: a retrospective study. *N Z Med J*, **83**(563), 316–18.

Quraishi SN, David A, Brasil MA, Alheira FV. (1999). Depot haloperidol decanoate for schizophrenia. *Cochrane Database Syst Rev*, (3), CD001361.

Rubio G, Martinez I, Ponce G, Jimenez-Arriero MA, Lopez-Munoz F, Alamo C. (2006). Long-acting injectable risperidone compared with zuclopenthixol in the treatment of schizophrenia with substance abuse comorbidity *Can J Psychiatry/La Revue canadienne de psychiatrie*, **51**, 531–9.

Schooler NR, Keith SJ, Severe JB, Matthews SM, Bellack AS, Glick ID, et al. (1997). Relapse and rehospitalisation during maintenance treatment of schizophrenia. The effects of dose reduction and family treatment. *Arch Gen Psychiatry*, **54**(5), 453–63.

Shajahan P, Spence E, Taylor M, Darlington D, Pelosi A. (in press). A long term 'real world' head-to-head comparison of the effectiveness of risperidone consta and first generation depot antipsychotics. *The Psychiatrist*.

Soares B, Silva de Lima M. (2005). Penfluridol for schizophrenia. *Cochrane Database Sys Rev*, CD002923.

Tan CT, Ong TC, Chee KT. (1981). The use of fluphenazine decanoate (Modecate) depot therapy in outpatient schizophrenics—a retrospective study. *Singapore Med J*, **22**(4), 214–8.

Tegeler J, Lehmann E. (1981). A follow-up study of schizophrenic outpatients treated with depot-neuroleptics. *Prog Neuropsychopharmacol*, **5**(1), 79–90.

Tiihonen J, Walhbeck K, Lönnqvist J, Klaukka T, Ioannidis JP, Volavka J, et al. (2006). Effectiveness of antipsychotic treatments in a nationwide cohort of patients in community care after first hospitalisation due to schizophrenia and schizoaffective disorder: observational follow-up study. *BMJ*, **333**(7561), 224–7.

Waddell L, Taylor M. (2008). A new self-rating scale for detecting atypical or second-generation antipsychotic side effects. *J Psychopharmacol*, **22**, 238–43.

Waddell L, Taylor M. (2009). Attitudes of patients and mental health staff to antipsychotic long-acting injections: systematic review. *Br J Psychiatry* **195**, S43–S50.

White E, Cheung P, Silverstone T. (1993). Depot antipsychotics in bipolar affective disorder. *Int Clin Psychopharmacol*, **8**, 119–22.

Zhu B, Ascher-Svanum H, Shi L, Faries D, Montgomery W, Marder SR. (2008). Time to discontinuation of depot and oral first-generation antipsychotics in the usual care of schizophrenia. *Psychiatr Serv*, **59**(3), 315–17.

Chapter 5

Risperidone long-acting injection

Pierre Chue

Correspondence: pchue@ualberta.ca

Introduction

Risperidone is a second-generation (SGA) or atypical (novel) antipsychotic first marketed worldwide in the 1990s as an oral preparation. In 2003, the US Federal Drugs Administration (FDA) approved risperidone long-acting injection (RLAI), the first SGA to be available commercially in an injectable sustained-action formulation (Chue 2003; Ereschefsky & Mascarenas 2003). This chapter describes the development of RLAI, reviews aspects of the pharmacokinetics, summarizes the pivotal trials and clinical data including pharmacoeconomic, and discusses the potential future directions for this novel formulation.

Oral risperidone

Risperidone, a benzisoxazole derivative, possesses a high affinity for serotoninergic 5-HT_{2A} and dopaminergic D_2 receptors. It binds to dopaminergic D_2 receptors with a slightly lower affinity than haloperidol and also binds to α_1-adrenergic receptors as well as to H_1-histaminergic and α_2-adrenergic receptors with a lower affinity but has no affinity for cholinergic receptors (Chue 2003). Although risperidone is a potent D_2 antagonist (considered to improve the positive symptoms of schizophrenia), it causes less suppression of motor activity and induction of catalepsy than haloperidol (Grant & Fitton 1994). It is therefore postulated that balanced central serotonin and dopamine antagonism may reduce extrapyramidal side-effects (EPS) liability and contribute to efficacy in the treatment of negative and affective symptoms of schizophrenia (Keegan 1994). In pivotal trials risperidone showed comparable efficacy for positive symptoms, greater efficacy for negative symptoms and less EPS when compared to haloperidol (Gupta et al. 1994). Subsequent studies and meta-analyses demonstrated higher response rates, less use of anticholinergic medications, lower treatment dropout rates, and greater prevention of relapse, but more weight gain versus oral first-generation or typical (conventional) antipsychotics (FGAs) (Davies et al. 1998; Hunter et al. 2003; Kennedy et al. 2000). Other reviews of risperidone versus other SGAs indicated comparable efficacy but differential side-effect profile with risperidone being associated with more sexual dysfunction but less weight gain than olanzapine (Gilbody et al. 2000; Jayaram & Hosalli 2006).

Pharmacokinetics of risperidone long-acting injection

The pharmacokinetics of RLAI are discussed in detail in Chapter 2 but are briefly reviewed here given the unique release profile characteristics of the formulation. In contrast to first-generation long-acting injectables (FGA-LAIs) or conventional depots that are composed of a prodrug dissolved in an oil vehicle, RLAI is a reconstituted injection of *microspheres* comprising risperidone encapsulated in a biodegradable polymer of glycolic and lactic acids (Poly D, L-Lactide-co-glycolide or PLG) (Ramstack et al. 2003). The microspheres progressively and completely degrade through a process of hydrolysis catalysed by risperidone, the end-products being risperidone, carbon dioxide, and water.

The RLAI is unique in terms of administration and possesses differences in pharmacokinetic profile when compared to FGA-LAIs (Ereshefsky & Mannaert 2005). After a single intramuscular (IM) injection there is a very small initial release of drug (<1% of the dose), principally from the surface of the microspheres, followed by a lag time of at least 3 weeks until the main release of the drug begins. Therapeutic serum drug levels are achieved between weeks 4 and 6, subsiding by week 7 (Figure 5.1; Eerdekens et al. 2004).

Antipsychotic supplementation is therefore recommended at least during the first 3 weeks of RLAI treatment (either in the form of oral antipsychotic supplementation or coverage from previous FGA-LAI). With IM injections repeated every 2 weeks, steady-state plasma concentrations of RLAI are reached after four injections. Data from PET studies with [11C] raclopride confimed that RLAI at steady state doses, of 25, 50, and 75 mg every 2 weeks, resulted in peak dopamine D_2 receptor occupancy levels above the 65% threshold associated with optimal clinical response, although the 75-mg dose reached the 80% threshold associated with the potential of extrapyramidal symptoms (Gefvert et al. 2005; Medori et al. 2006; Remington et al. 2006).

Theoretical models and human studies have demonstrated that with RLAI, the peak-to-trough fluctuations in plasma levels of the active moiety (risperidone and 9-hydroxyrisperidone) and C_{max} are reduced by comparison with orally administered risperidone (Eerdekens et al. 2004; Mannaert et al. 2005) although there can be

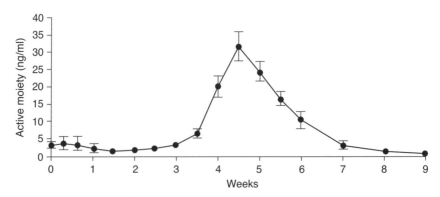

Fig. 5.1 RLAI single dose pharmacokinetic profile (Chue 2003).
Reproduced from Expert Rev. Neurotherapeutics 3(4), 435–446 (2003) with permission from Expert Reviews Ltd.

some individual variation (Castberg & Spigset 2005). Other pharmacokinetic studies have shown that patients receiving RLAI not only had significantly lower serum concentrations of the active moiety than patients taking oral risperidone but that the 9-hydroxyrisperidone/risperidone ratio was also significantly lower (Nesvåg et al. 2006). In fact, data from therapeutic drug monitoring (TDM) of 46 patients on RLAI and 50 patients on oral risperidone demonstrated that approximately 25% of patients on RLAI had total serum drug levels below the established reference range compared to 6% of patients on oral risperidone (Nesvåg & Tanum 2005). Although it is postulated that this may account for the differences in side-effect profile for RLAI when compared with an equivalent oral risperidone dose, this does raise the question of the equivalency of recommended switching doses (Bai et al. 2007a). The bioequivalence and tolerability of RLAI were evaluated in a multicentre, prospective, open-label, 15-week study ($n = 86$) (Eerdekens et al. 2004). Maintenance of effect was demonstrated from oral risperidone to RLAI despite mean C_{Max} of the active moiety being 25% to 32% lower than with oral risperidone, although PANSS total and subscale scores showed the most robust improvement with the 75 mg dose; the ESRS scores decreased for all treatment groups. Reduction in mean PANSS total scores was also noted in a pharmacokinetic and D_2 receptor occupancy study ($n = 13$) (Gefvert et al. 2005). Neither race nor CYP2D6 metabolizer status appears to affect the efficacy and tolerability of RLAI (Ciliberto et al. 2005; Ereshefsky & Mannaert 2005), although one recent study found differences in concentrations of active moiety and 9-hydroxyrisperidone/risperidone ratio correlated with metabolizer status in patients receiving RLAI or oral risperidone (Hendset et al. 2009).

Dosing of RLAI

According to the product monograph the recommended dose of RLAI is 25 mg/ 2 weeks with the maximum dose not exceeding 50 mg/2 weeks (Janssen-Ortho Inc 2009). Dose increments from 25 mg to 37.5 mg or from 37.5 mg to 50 mg should be considered after a minimum of 4 weeks after the previous dose adjustment. The effect of this dosage adjustment on the patient's clinical status should not be anticipated earlier than 3 weeks after the first injection with the higher dose. A lower initial dose of RLAI may be appropriate when clinical factors warrant dose adjustment, such as in patients with renal or hepatic impairment, for certain drug interactions that increase risperidone plasma concentrations, or in patients sensitive to psychotropic medications. A 12.5-mg dose is available in the United States but not in Europe but there are no published studies evaluating the efficacy of this dose. The only recommended dose for the elderly (>65 years) age group is 25 mg/2 weeks. Of note, RLAI has not been studied in children and adolescents younger than 18 years of age.

Supplementation with oral risperidone (at the previous dose) should be provided for at least the first 3 weeks after the first RLAI, after which the oral risperidone should be discontinued. For hepatically or renally impaired patients a lower starting dose of oral risperidone e.g. 0.5 mg b.i.d. is recommended during the first week and for the second week, 1 mg b.i.d. or 2 mg o.d. can be given. However, if clinically appropriate, oral risperidone up to 4 mg/day can be temporarily added to the treatment with RLAI while establishing an individual patient's optimal dose. The clinical value of adding oral risperidone should be routinely reassessed and, if there is continuing need for oral supplementation, consideration should be given to increasing the dose of RLAI. However, if sedation is required, an additional drug (such as a benzodiazepine) should be considered rather than increasing the dose of RLAI. Patients without any previous history of risperidone exposure should be pre-treated with oral risperidone for several days as clinically feasible, to assess tolerability before the first injection of RLAI.

The product monograph (Janssen-Ortho Inc 2009) recommends that for patients stabilized on a fixed dose of oral risperidone (for 2 weeks or more) the following con-version scheme should be considered: patients treated with a dosage of 4 mg or less oral risperidone should receive 25 mg RLAI, whereas for patients receiving higher oral doses a dose of 37.5 mg of RLAI should be considered. These recommended dosing strategies and conversions have been subject to some discussion (Keith et al. 2004a; Mauri et al. 2009; Taylor et al. 2006; Viner et al. 2006). In a study of 50 patients with schizophrenia converted to 25 mg and 37.5 mg/2 weeks of RLAI from a doses of 4 mg/ day or less and 4 to 6 mg/day of oral risperidone, respectively, an increase in PANSS scores and risk of relapse were observed (Bai et al. 2007a). The authors suggested that based on these findings the equivalent switching dose should in fact be as follows: patients on an oral risperidone dose of 3 mg/day or less should receive 25 mg of RLAI, patients taking an oral dose of more than 3 mg/day but of 5 mg/day or less should receive 37.5 mg/2 weeks, and patients taking an oral dose of more than 5 mg/day should receive 50 mg of RLAI/2 weeks. An RCT comparing treatment with 25 mg (n = 163) or 50 mg (n = 161) doses of RLAI over 52 weeks found time to relapse was comparable (p =.131) for both groups, but projected median time to relapse was 161.8 weeks (95%CI = 103.0–254.2) with 25 mg and 259.0 weeks (95% CI = 153.6–436.8) with 50 mg and one-year incidences of relapse were 21.6% and 14.9%, respectively (p = .059) (Simpson et al. 2006). These findings together with the phar-macokinetic data (Nesvåg et al. 2006; Nesvåg & Tanum 2005) suggest that the recom-mended dose of 25 mg of RLAI may require some adjustment in real world populations. However, data from a sub-analysis of a 6-month open-label study, the Switch to Risperidone Microspheres (SToRMi) (n = 1849) conducted in 22 European countries, found that patients treated with lower RLAI doses were more likely to be female, have shorter illness duration, milder symptoms, and on less polypharmacy (Mauri et al. 2009), although the strongest predictors that a patient would remain on a 25 mg dose were baseline PANSS hallucinatory scores (OR = 0.78), baseline Clinical Global Impression-Severity (CGI-S) scores (OR = 1.56), and intriguingly, the country of residence but the latter did not correlate with baseline disease severity.

It is the degradation characteristics of the microspheres that determine the injection frequency of RLAI to maintain stable serum levels. Unlike FGA-LAIs that allow considerable variation in dosing frequency as oil-based vehicles tend to persist in the body for much longer periods, RLAI is recommended to be given every 2 weeks. This frequency of dosing does pose some limitations in clinical practice and case reports of attempts at longer dosing intervals have described limited success (Singh & O'Connor 2007). However, a pilot study of 50 mg RLAI (n = 87) administered every 4 weeks over 52 weeks concluded that most symptomatically stable patients could be safely and effectively managed with an alternate dosing interval (Gharabawi et al. 2007b). The relapse rate in this study was 17.9% (Kaplan-Meier estimate of the risk of relapse was 22.4%), which is comparable to other long-term data for RLAI (Simpson et al. 2006), even though at this dosing frequency the mean ±SD dopamine D_2 receptor occupancy is 56% ±24% (range, 29%–82%; Uchida et al. 2008).

Efficacy of RLAI

The initial efficacy and safety of RLAI was evaluated in three pivotal trials, two short-term (12 and 24 weeks) studies comparing RLAI to placebo and RLAI to oral risperidone respectively, and one long-term (52 weeks) study involving a switch of stable patients to RLAI. All 3 pivotal studies generated subsequent analyses that are further discussed in the relevant sections of this chapter. A summary of these studies is presented in Table 5.1 (Chue et al. 2005a; Fleischhacker et al. 2003; Kane et al. 2003a). It should be noted that although RLAI is available in doses of 12.5, 25, 37.5, or 50 mg, the pivotal trials investigated the use of a 75-mg dose that was not marketed because this dose did not appear to offer greater efficacy than the 50 mg dose and was associated with more side-effects particularly EPS.

Given the pharmacokinetic differences of RLAI compared to FGA-LAI and thus, potential issues in initiating and switching in clinical practice, a number of early studies looked at different strategies for switching, one such large scale study was the SToRMi study, in which 1876 symptomatically stable patients with schizophrenia or other psychoses were transitioned directly to RLAI from their previous antipsychotic medication without an oral risperidone run-in (Möller 2005). There was a significant reduction from baseline to end point in mean total PANSS and subscale scores and symptom factors ($p < .001$) and CGI-S score improved significantly ($p < .001$). Data are also been presented from a 12-month extension ($n = 508$) of StoRMi showing significant reductions in mean PANSS total score from baseline to end point ($p = .001$) and with 47% of patients having a 20% or more improvement in PANSS total score (Kissling et al. 2005). Although an 18-month follow-up ($n = 529$) also showed significant reductions in total PANSS and all subscale scores ($p = .0001$) compared to baseline, 47% of patients showing a 20% decrease or more in total PANSS score (Llorca et al. 2008b). Similar observations were made in a 12-week, open-label study of patients ($n = 141$) transitioned directly to RLAI without an intervening period of oral risperidone but with continuation of their previous oral medication (haloperidol, $n = 46$; quetiapine, $n = 45$; olanzapine, $n = 50$) (Lindenmayer et al. 2004). Improvements in symptoms of schizophrenia were observed with RLAI at week 4 and continued through the 12-week treatment with significant reductions in total PANSS scores at week 8 ($p < .01$) and week 12 (p < .001). At end point, 37% of these stable patients were rated as clinically improved (≥20% decrease in PANSS total scores). Lindemayer et al. (2007) reported on the long-term efficacy of the 12-month extension of this study as well the extension of the 12-week pivotal trial describing maintenance of efficacy with CGI-S ratings of 'not ill' and 'mild' increasing from 42% to 65% at baseline and from 14% to 54%, respectively at end point for the two studies. Parellada (2007) in a review of the use of RLAI in the treatment of schizophrenia in

Table 5.1 Overview of pivotal studies evaluating the efficacy and safety of RLAI

Study details	Treatment groups	Efficacy	Adverse events
Short-term studies			
Kane et al. 2003a ◆ 12-week, double-blind, placebo controlled study in patients with schizophrenia ◆ Run-in with oral risperidone	Placebo (n = 98) RLAI doses included: 25 mg (n =99) 50 mg (n = 103) 75 mg (n = 100)	◆ 68% of placebo patients and 51%–52% of RLAI patients discontinued the study ◆ Withdrawals owing to insufficient response: RLAI 25 mg, 22%; RLAI 50 mg, 15%; RLAI 75 mg, 12%; placebo, 30% ◆ Withdrawals owing to non-compliance: RLAI 25 mg 0%; RLAI 50 mg, 3%; RLAI 75 mg, 3%; placebo 4% ◆ Mean (±SD) improvement in PANSS scores at end point: RLAI 25 mg, −6.2±16.9; RLAI 50 mg, −8.5±16.9; RLAI 75 mg, −7.4±16.9; placebo, 2.6±16.9 ◆ Clinical improvement (≥20% reduction in PANSS) occurred in 47%, 48%, 39%, and 17% of patients in the RLAI 25 mg, 50 mg, 75 mg, and placebo groups, respectively, p < .001	◆ Incidence of AEs: RLAI 25 mg, 80%; RLAI 50 mg, 83%; RLAI 75 mg 82%; placebo, 83% ◆ Incidence of serious AEs in respective groups: RLAI 25 mg, 13%; RLAI 50 mg, 14%; RLAI 75 mg, 15%; placebo, 24% ◆ AEs occurring in ≥5% of patients: RLAI: headache (20%), agitation (15%), insomnia (15%), psychosis (12%), anxiety (9%); placebo: agitation (25%), psychosis (23%), anxiety (15%), insomnia (14%), headache (12%) ◆ Withdrawals owing to AEs: RLAI 25 mg, 11%; RLAI 50 mg, 12%; RLAI 75 mg, 14%; placebo, 12% ◆ Incidence of EPS: RLAI 25 mg, 10%; RLAI 50 mg, 24%; RLAI 75 mg, 29%; placebo, 13% ◆ Mean change in total ESRS at endpoint: RLAI 25 mg, −1.5±4.0; RLAI 50 mg, 0.1±3.6; RLAI 75 mg 0.0±5.3; placebo, −0.1± 4.8 ◆ Change in mean body weight: RLAI 25 mg, +0.5 kg; RLAI 50 mg, +1.2 kg; RLAI 75 mg, +1.9 kg; placebo −1.4 kg ◆ 80%, 81%, 84%, 90% of patients in the RLAI 25 mg, 50 mg, 75 mg and placebo groups rated injection site pain as absent after the sixth injection

Chue et al. 2005a

◆ 12-week, double-blind study in symptomatically patients with schizophrenia taking oral risperidone who either continued oral risperidone or switched to RLAI

Oral risperidone 2, 4 and 6 mg/day (n = 321)

RLAI 25, 50 and 75 mg (n = 319)

◆ Patients completing the study: oral risperidone, 84%; RLAI, 80%

◆ Withdrawals owing to insufficient response: oral risperidone, 2.5%; RLAI, 3.8%

◆ Mean (±SE) improvement in PANSS scores at endpoint: oral risperidone, −6.3±0.7; RLAI, −5.4± 0.7, p<0.001 for each

Percentage of patients rated as 'not ill' or with 'mild illness' increased from 46.9% in the oral risperidone group and 49.2% in the RLAI group at baseline to 57.8% and 57.9%, respectively, at end point

◆ Incidence of AEs: oral risperidone 60%, RLAI 61%

◆ AEs occurring in ≥5% of patients— oral risperidone: insomnia (9%), anxiety (7%), headache (7%), psychosis (5%); RLAI: anxiety (10%), insomnia (10%), headache (8%), psychosis (5%)

◆ Withdrawals owing to AEs: oral risperidone, 4.7%; RLAI, 5.6%

◆ Incidence of EPS: oral risperidone, 6%; RLAI, 7%

◆ Change in mean bodyweight: oral risperidone, +0.3 kg; RLAI, +0.5 kg

◆ AEs potentially related to prolactin: oral risperidone, 2.5%; RLAI, 1.3%

◆ Decrease in prolactin levels from baseline to endpoint: oral risperidone group, 38.9±1.6 ng/mL to 38.0±1.8 ng/mL; RLAI group, 37.4±1.7 ng/mL to 32.6±1.6 ng/mL

Pain at injection site was low (mean scores of 18–20 on a 100 point VAS)

(Continued)

Table 5.1 (continued) Overview of pivotal studies evaluating the efficacy and safety of RLAI

Study details	Treatment groups	Efficacy	Adverse events
Long-term studies			
Fleischhacker et al. 2003	RLAI 25 mg (n = 120)	◆ 65% completed the study	◆ Incidence of AEs in respective treatment groups: 82%, 84%, 87%
◆ 1-year, open label study in symptomatically stable patients with schizophrenia switched from other oral or long-acting antipsychotics	RLAI 50 mg (n = 228) RLAI 75 mg (n = 267)	◆ 7.8% withdrew due to insufficient response ◆ 1.8% withdrew due to noncompliance ◆ Mean (±SE) improvement in PANSS scores at endpoint (all doses): −6.1±0.7, $p<0.01$ ◆ Clinical improvement (≥20% reduction in PANSS) was seen in 49% of patients: 55% of the 25 mg group, 56% of the 50 mg group and 40% of the 75 mg group	◆ Withdrawals due to AEs in respective treatment groups: 4%, 6%, 5% ◆ Most commonly reported AEs: anxiety (24%), insomnia (21%), psychosis (17%), depression (15%), headache (12%) ◆ Incidence of EPS: RLAI 25 mg, 21%; RLAI 50 mg, 27%; RLAI 75 mg, 25%
◆ Run-in with oral risperidone		◆ CGI-S ratings of 'not ill', 'very mildly ill' or 'mildly ill' increased from 58% at baseline to 78% at endpoint in the 25 mg group, from 40% to 65% in the 50 mg group and from 33% to 44% in the 75 mg group ◆ 18% of patients were rehospitalized during the study	◆ Incidence of tardive dyskinesia: 0.7% ◆ Mean (SE) change in total ESRS at endpoint (all doses): −2.5±0.2 ◆ Change in mean body weight: RLAI 25 mg, +1.7 kg; RLAI 50 mg, +2.6 kg; RLAI 75 mg, +1.9 kg ◆ Patients with no injection site pain (all doses): 68% at first injection; 80% at last injection

Note. AE = adverse event; CGI-S = Clinical Global Impression-Severity; ESRS = Extrapyramidal Symptoms Rating Scale; PANNS = Positive and Negative Syndrome Scale; RLAI= long-acting risperidone; SD = Standard deviation; SE = Standard error; VAS = Visual Analogue Scale.

patients of different ethnicity as well as elderly, early psychosis (EP) (≤ 3 years of illness) and schizoaffective disorder patients concluded that RLAI was efficacious in all
patient groups.

Other open-label studies have described the use of RLAI in diverse patient populations
in terms of ethnicity, severity including difficult-to-treat patient and non-adherent
populations (Camacho et al. 2008; Giradi et al. 2010; Lee et al. 2006; Lindenmayer
et al. 2006; Martin et al. 2003; Raignoux et al. 2007). For outpatients ($n = 50$) of mainly
Hispanic origin switched to RLAI, a retrospective chart review reported a significant
improvement in patient adherence with appointments and functioning as measured
by the GAF (Camacho et al. 2008). Inpatients tend to reflect a more difficult to treat
population thus, an initial post hoc analysis of patients who were inpatients ($n = 214$)
from the 12-week pivotal trial showed that RLAI versus placebo was associated with a
significant reduction in total PANSS score at end point ($p < .001$), a significantly
higher rate of treatment response defined as a 20% reduction or more in total PANSS
score (50% vs. 27%, $p < .05$), and CGI assessments of 'not ill, very mild or mild' (32%
vs. 5%, $p < .01$) (Lauriello et al. 2005). There were no significant differences in ESRS
scores between RLAI and placebo groups but mean increase in body weight, although
small in magnitude (2.3 kg vs. 0.43 kg) was greater with RLAI ($p = .0003$) Similarly, an
open-label study of inpatients who were unstable or non-compliant with their previous treatment reported that 40.5% of the patients experienced more than a 20%
decrease of their initial PANSS score accompanied by global improvement in CGI
ratings (Raignoux et al. 2007). Lee et al. (2006) in a study of Korean outpatients treated
for 48 weeks found significant improvement in mean PANSS total and subscale and
CGI scores (both $p = .0001$). A cohort of chronically psychotic patients ($n = 88$; initial
BPRS = 93±5) was treated for 6 months with oral medication and then converted to
RLAI for 6 months in a matched mirror comparison design, with further follow-up
over 18 months (Giradi et al. 2010). With RLAI (at a mean dose of 47 mg/2 weeks at
6 and up to 23.1±3.3 months) there were improvements in all outcome measures
(BPRS, CGI-S and SF-36) ($p < .001$) and initial BPRS scores fell by an average of 50%
within 6 months; hospitalizations declined from 19.8% to 0% and clinical benefit was
maintained over the 18 months. Finally, data from 100 subjects (79% inpatients)
switched to RLAI from oral atypical (58%) or FG-LAI (28%) antipsychotics primarily
because of poor patient acceptability demonstrated an improvement in CGI scores
and a reduction in antipsychotic coprescriptions from 71% of subjects to 8% (Taylor
et al. 2004). Overall, 51% of the subjects discontinued RLAI; of the completers, 61%
beginning RLAI as inpatients were discharged.

Although the majority of open-label studies have reported on the efficacy of RLAI, a
Cochrane review did not find a substantial benefit for RLAI based on 2 RCTs (Hosalli
& Davis 2003). The authors commented on the high discontinuation rate in an RCT
of RLAI compared to placebo (52%) which limited generalizability; however it should
be noted that both the rates of discontinuation ($n = 400$, RR = 0.74, CI = 0.63–0.88;
NNT = 6, CI = 4–12) and adverse events (AEs) were greater in the placebo group ($n = 400$, RR = 0.59 CI = 0.38–0.93; NNT = 11, CI = 7–70). The discontinuation rate was
comparable to that reported for other placebo-controlled studies with antipsychotics
(Lindemayer 2005). Furthermore, although no clear difference in the RCT of RLAI

versus oral risperidone was observed, this was in fact a non-inferiority study designed to show the comparability of RLAI with its oral equivalent. It is clear that there are numerous additional methodological problems when evaluating effectiveness of long-acting treatments; in particular, RCTs are difficult to conduct when comparing oral versus injectable treatments, may not recruit the very patients who are likely to do best on LAIs, and may be of insufficient duration to demonstrate effectiveness. Thus, not only is it the more severe and less adherent patients who are likely to be selected for injectable treatments, but it is often the more difficult patients again who are selected for RLAI. Consistent with this are the findings of a study of pharmacy dispensing data from the Netherlands that found predictors for switching to FGA-LAI versus oral antipsychotics included male sex, previous use of FGA-LAI, recent anticholinergic drug use, and poor adherence, whereas predictors for switching to RLAI versus FGA-LAI included previous use of FGA-LAI and specialist recommendation (Vehof et al. 2008). The authors concluded that compared with oral antipsychotics, patients receiving an FGA-LAI were less adherent and with more extrapyramidal side-effects but compared with FGA -LAI, patients receiving RLAI tended to be more severely ill patients.

Given the limited relevance of short-term RCT data in real world populations the National Institute of Health and Clinical Excellence has recommended well-designed observational studies in schizophrenia that reflect usual clinical practice. One such large-scale naturalistic study is the electronic Schizophrenia Treatment Adherence Registry (e-STAR) which is an ongoing, international (Europe and Canada), multicentre, prospective, observational registry assessing use of RLAI in patients with schizophrenia or schizoaffective disorder in a normal clinical practice setting. Clinical and demographic information were collected at baseline with treatment-related data, including RLAI discontinuation, psychiatric hospitalization, and medication utilization, collected prospectively every 3 months and continued for 24 months, even for patients who discontinued RLAI. Hospitalization and medication utilization were collected retrospectively by chart review for the 12-month period prior to RLAI initiation. Early results from six European countries ($n = 1649$) demonstrated a high retention rate of 85% at 24 months, with the main reasons for discontinuation being insufficient response (28.5%), patient/family choice (26.1%), adverse events (9.6%), and unacceptable tolerability (6.0%) (Peuskens et al. 2010). At baseline, compared to completers, discontinuers were younger (37.4 vs. 39.6 years, $p = .01$), had shorter duration of schizophrenia (10.2 vs. 11.9 years, $p = .02$), lower GAF scores (43.5 vs. 48.0, $p = .0001$), higher utilization of benzodiazepines (56.5 vs. 43.3%), and were more likely to be inpatients at baseline (30 vs. 16%). Early data reported significant improvement in GAF scores ($p < .001$) for all groups with greater improvements in the completers and compared to pre-RLAI, completers had greater reductions than discontinuers in the percentage of patients hospitalized (66.2% reduction vs. 29.2%) and in the length (68% reduction vs. 0%) and number (80.0 vs. 14.3%) of hospital stays at 12 months—differences that persisted at 24 months.

Risperidone long-acting injection and remission

The concept of remission in schizophrenia has been proposed as a clinical relevant end point that represents an important step towards functional recovery. Operational definitions of remission based on core symptom ratings have been ventured by the

Remission in Schizophrenia Working Group (RSWG) and applied to treatment outcomes in schizophrenia (Andreasen et al. 2005; van Os et al. 2006). A post hoc analysis of the 1-year pivotal trial found that although considered clinically 'stable', 68.2% of patients (*n* = 578) did not meet the symptom-severity component of remission criteria at baseline (Lasser et al. 2005b). Following RLAI treatment, 20.8% of non-remitted patients achieved symptom remission for at least 6 months, with significant decreases in mean PANSS total and cluster scores (*p* < .0001) and CGI-S scores (*p* < .05). Among 31.8% of patients meeting the symptom-severity component of remission criteria at baseline, 84.8% maintained these criteria at end point. Remitted patients had a higher study completion rate and lower use of concomitant medications compared to non-remitted patients together with significant improvements in SF36 factors (social functioning and vitality, *p* < .05). Kissling et al. (2005) reported that of patients from the StoRMi study (*n* = 506) who did not meet severity remission criteria at baseline, 31% achieved remission after 12 months. Among those patients meeting severity criteria for remission at baseline, 84% were in remission at end point. A similar analysis conducted of 579 patients from the StoRMi study but followed for up to 18 months found that among those patients not meeting severity remission criteria at baseline, 44.8% achieved remission by end point (Llorca et al. 2008b). A total of 93.7% of the patients who achieved or maintained remission at 6 months were in remission at endpoint. In a post hoc analysis of an extension phase of StoRMi, the proportion of patients meeting severity criteria for remission increased from 29% at baseline to 60% at end point, and the proportion of patients who met these criteria for 6 months or less increased from 24% at month 6 to 45% at end point (Kissling et al. 2005). Similar findings were reported by Lambert et al. (2010) in a futher analysis of the StoRMi extension (*n* = 529; symptomatic remission (≥6 months) was obtained in 33% of patients with 21% achieving global remission as defined by symptomatic remission, functional level, and mental-health HRQoL. Symptomatic remission was predicted by better baseline symptom severity and country of origin, whereas global remission was predicted by RLAI dose, additional use of psychoactive medications, and country of origin. These data suggest that even 'stable' patients can further benefit from appropriate treatment review and switching of therapies. Remission criteria have also been applied to special populations including first-episode (FE) patients (Emsley 2008b) and elderly patients (Tadger 2008). In 50 FE patients treated with RLAI over 12 months, 64% achieved remission and 97% maintained this status until study completion (Emsley 2008b). Remission was associated with greater improvements in multiple symptom domains, insight, and social and occupational functioning. Predictors of remission included female sex and early treatment response. Although use of oral risperidone in FE patients resulted in remission rates of 70%, only 24% were able to maintain remission duration or severity criteria, which suggests that the improved adherence with RLAI plays a major role in maintaining clinical response (Emsley et al. 2007).

Side-effects of RLAI

In general, RLAI is well tolerated and side-effects are consistent with those associated with oral risperidone (Möller 2006). A marker of tolerability is the percentage of patients discontinuing owing to AEs which was low with RLAI even with long-term studies; ranging from 5% in the 1-year study to 12.3% (vs. placebo 12%) in the 12-week study, and 13% in an 18-month switch study (Fleischhacker et al. 2003; Kane et al. 2003a; Llorca et al. 2008b). Lindenmayer et al. (2007) reviewed the long-term safety of patients over 12 months of completing extension phases of 12-week studies and concluded that treatment with RLAI was well tolerated. Finally, Bai et al. (2007a) reported that the overall side-effect burden as measured with the UKU scale was reduced in patients switched to RLAI compared to oral risperidone.

According to the product monograph, common (>1%) adverse effects reported with RLAI have included weight gain, depression, fatigue, and EPS. In the 1-year study, mean weight changes in the 25-, 50-, and 75-mg risperidone groups were 1.7, 2.6, and 1.9 kg, respectively (Fleischhacker et al. 2003), whereas in the 12-week study mean weight changes in the 25-, 50-, and 75-mg risperidone groups were 0.5, 1.2, and 1.9 kg, respectively (Kane et al. 2003a). Most switch studies, short- and long-term are within this range (Lasser et al. 2004a; Lindenmayer et al. 2004; Marinis 2007; Turner et al. 2004) with a few demonstrating either slightly greater weight gain or statistically significant weight gain possibly reflective of more real world scenarios (Kissling et al. 2005; Möller et al. 2005; Paralleda et al. 2005). In the 18-month follow-up of the StoRMi study, body weight increased from (mean±SD) 77.7± 15.5 kg at baseline to 78.7± 15.6 kg at end point with weight observed predominantly in patients whose BMI was less than 25 kg/m^2 (Llorca et al. 2008b). From the metabolic perspective, glucose and lipid parameters do not appear adversely affected, with some studies reporting reduction in these values (Lindenmayer et al. 2004) and overall, a low level of treatment emergent glucose-related abnormalities, in the range 0.3% to 0.8% (Llorca et al. 2008b). As a class, the SGAs are associated with a lower risk for tardive dyskinesia (TD) than FGAs, and it is suggested that an LAI, given more consistent blood levels and lower peak serum levels, may be associated with less liability for movement disorder compared with an oral formulation. The incidence of EPS in patients receiving 25 mg of RLAI in the 12-week study (10%) was comparable with that for patients receiving placebo (13%), with higher rates in the 50- and 75-mg groups (Kane et al. 2003a). In general, studies with RLAI have demonstrated a reduction in EPS compared to prior treatment (Bai et al. 2007a; Fleischhacker et al. 2003; Lauriello et al. 2005; Lindenmayer et al. 2004; Llorca et al. 2008a; Kane et al. 2003a; Möller et al. 2005; Nick et al. 2006; Simpson et al. 2006; van Os et al. 2004), whether receiving FGA-LAI (Lai et al. 2009; Lasser et al. 2004b; Marinis et al. 2007), oral SGAs (Gastpar et al. 2005) including risperidone (Eerdekens et al. 2004; Lasser et al. 2005a; Schmauss et al. 2007), or oral FGAs (Lindemayer et al. 2004; Marinis 2007). However, one study found that EPS was the most common AE (29.7%) (Raignoux et al. 2007) and Lindemayer et al. (2007) reported EPS-related AEs in 33% and 22% of patients in two 1-year extension phase studies. A retrospective analysis of TD by defined research criteria in patients treated with RLAI in the 1-year study (Fleischhacker et al. 2003) found that 0.94% of subjects (n = 530), without dyskinesia at baseline, met the predefined criteria for emergent persistent TD during therapy. The overall 1-year rate based on either exposure to study medication or Kaplan–Meier analysis was 1.19% (Gharabawi et al. 2005). Furthermore, for subjects with dyskinesia at baseline (n = 132), the mean dyskinesia score on the ESRS improved significantly at end point (−2.77; p <.0001), regardless of anticholinergic drug use (p = .243 for patients with or without anticholinergic drug use). Finally, improvement in movement disorder has been reported with RLAI in susceptible populations including EP (Emsley 2008b; Lasser et al. 2007; Paralleda et al. 2005), elderly (Lasser et al. 2004c), schizoaffective (Mohl et al. 2005), and bipolar patients (Han et al. 2007).

According to the product monograph, uncommon (>0.1%) adverse effects reported with RLAI have included weight decrease, nervousness, sleep disorder, apathy, impaired concentration, abnormal vision, hypotension, syncope, rash, pruritus, peripheral oedema, injection-site reaction, and symptoms potentially related to hyper-prolactinemia such as nonpuerperal lactation, amenorrhoea, abnormal sexual function, ejaculation failure, decreased libido, and impotence. Increases in white blood cell counts and in hepatic enzymes have occasionally been reported. Prolactin level increases (Kim et al. 2009; Lai 2009; Lindenmayer et al. 2004; Peng et al. 2008; Raignoux et al. 2007) as well as decreases (Bai et al. 2007b; Chue et al. 2005a; Docherty et al. 2007; Turner et al. 2004) have been described following switches to RLAI. Although the decreases relative to oral risperidone likely reflect lower steady state concentrations of active moiety, overall prolactin levels remain elevated compared to the normal range. Bai et al. (2007b) followed a cohort of 24 patients switched to RLAI from oral risperidone and found a significant decrease in prolactin levels from 68.44±39.63 ng/mL at baseline to 50.57±30.73 ng/mL at 12 weeks (p <.001). In contrast, Peng et al. (2008) following a cohort of 18 patients dosed very similarly reported a non-significant increase in prolactin levels from 72.7±58.8 ng/mL to 76.3±60.6 ng/mL. An RCT comparison between RLAI and oral risperidone treated patients reported prolactin–related AEs occurring in 1.3% and 2.5%, respectively (Chue et al. 2005a) but in an FE study no differences were seen between the two groups (Kim et al. 2008).

Unlike FGA-LAIs, RLAI must be reconstituted prior to IM injection by mixing with the supplied diluent and then administered using a specific wide-bore and thin-walled, 20-gauge, 2-inch needle as a 2 mL volume (for all doses). In the pivotal clinical trials, patients rated injection-site pain using a 100-mm Visual Analogue Scale (VAS) and investigators rated injection-site pain, redness, swelling and induration. VAS pain ratings were low at all visits across all doses and decreased from first to final injection (significantly for all doses in the 1-year trial and the 75 mg dose in the 12-week trial) (Fleischhacker et al. 2003; Lindenmayer et al. 2005; Kane et al. 2003a). Other studies have reported similar low rates of injection-site pain with a decrease in ratings and concerns about pain over study period as well as low rates of skin reactions (Chue et al. 2005a; Docherty et al. 2007; Eerdekens et al. 2004; Gefvert et al. 2005; Kissling et al. 2005; Lasser et al. 2004a, c, 2005a, 2007; Lauriello 2005; Raignoux et al. 2007). However, it should be noted that in some of these studies subjects experiencing pain or injection complications were more likely to discontinue RLAI treatment by dropping out of the study.

It is suggested that RLAI administered by gluteal injection may be less painful in comparison to traditional oil-based injections (Bloch et al. 2001) because of its aqueous composition. In both the United States and the European Union the deltoid site has been approved as an alternate injection site using a specifically developed administration kit with a shorter and narrower needle. This allows use in patients who may be reluctant to accept a gluteal injection because of paranoid or other beliefs. Deltoid injections may be a further advantage in obese individuals (of which there is a high prevalence in patients with schizophrenia) who may be at greater risk of skin reactions such as fat necrosis and in whom IM injections are difficult because of the needle length required to penetrate the muscle layer. In fact, FGA-LAIs have been utilized in this way despite an absence of specific data or indication. For RLAI, two recent studies support the use of the deltoid muscle as an alternative injection site. The first study being a bioequivalence study ($n = 170$) of deltoid versus gluteal administration with two-way, crossover design (Thyssen et al. 2010). Both sites were shown to be bioequivalent at equal doses with respect to peak and total plasma exposure and exhibited dose-proportional pharmacokinetics, independent of injection site. Overall, 64% of patients experienced approximately one adverse event of swelling or redness (48% for gluteal injection and 49% for deltoid injection). No patient withdrew owing to injection-site tolerability issues, and there were no nodule formations. In the second study, patients ($n = 53$) who previously received gluteal injections and required higher doses received RLAI 37.5 mg or 50 mg/2 weeks into the deltoid muscle over 8 weeks (Ning et al. 2008). No patients withdrew owing to injection-site tolerability issues, there were no nodule formations, and 83% completed the study. Investigator-rated mild injection-site reactions were observed in 19% of patients after injection but returned to normal prior to the next injection. Patients receiving the higher dose of medication reported higher pain than those receiving the lower dose.

In the CATIE study, 74% of patients ($n = 1432$) discontinued their first assigned study medication before 18 months, providing a real world demonstration of discontinuation rates for oral antipsychotics, atypical or conventional (Lieberman et al. 2005). In contrast, with RLAI studies, discontinuation rates, with the exception of several studies of specific populations, have been lower—as low as 18.1% over 24 months (Olivares et al. 2008). This suggests a possible benefit conferred in terms of long-term persistence with the injectable formulation, which together with improved adherence, may well contribute to better outcome. In terms of prognostic factors for discontinuation of RLAI, a British group has evaluated the data in three analyses (Patel et al. 2004; Taylor & Cornelius 2009; Taylor et al. 2009c). In a 6-month follow-up of 88 patients (35.8% had treatment refractoriness), 37.0% discontinued within 6 months (Patel et al. 2004). Preceding antipsychotic type (FGA-LAI vs. oral) (OR = 2.68, 95% CI 0.95–7.53, $p = .061$) was a stronger prognostic indicator than treatment refractoriness (OR =1.55, 95% CI 0.59–4.11, $p = .376$) for RLAI discontinuation, whereas sociodemographic factors and other clinical factors were non-predictive of discontinuation. Of 250 patients starting RLAI, 47.2% were still receiving it at 6 months. Patients were more likely to continue treatment with RLAI to 6 months if older than 55 years (OR = 3.13, 95% CI = 1.32–7.40, $p= .0060$) and if receiving a dose of more than 25 mg/2 week RLAI (OR = 2.37, 95% CI = 1.40–3.99, $p < .001$). Greater improvement was more likely in those prescribed RLAI because of poor prior adherence (OR = 2.28, 95%

CI = 1.35–3.86, p = .002) and less likely in those who had previously been prescribed clozapine (OR = 0.29, 95% CI=0.14–0.61, p = .001) (Taylor et al. 2006). Finally a longer-term evaluation over 3 years determined that factors predictive of a greater probability of discontinuation including younger age (p = .001), longer duration of illness (p = .001), inpatient status at initiation (p = .002), and a RLAI dose of 25 mg/2 weeks (p < .001) (Taylor & Cornelius 2009).

RLAI versus oral antipsychotics

RLAI demonstrated non-inferiority to oral SGAs in two RCTs of outpatients, the first versus oral risperidone in a double-blind, double-dummy design over 12 weeks with 8 week run-in period (Chue et al. 2005a) and the second versus oral olanzapine (Keks et al. 2007), the latter divided into a 13-week initial phase followed by a 12-month phase (n = 318 RLAI, n = 300 olanzapine). There was a trend to more positive long-term responses with RLAI than with olanzapine at months 9 to 12, but significant benefits of RLAI over olanzapine were noted on just two outcomes: clinical improvement (at least 20% reduction in PANSS total score) at month 12 and at end point (p < .001), and improvement on a PANSS factor at month 12 (disorganized thoughts); significantly greater improvement in anxiety/depression was seen in the olanzapine group at end point. The incidence of EPS-related AEs was greater at baseline in the RLAI group but comparable to the olanzapine group by months 9 to 12; weight gain was significantly greater in the olanzapine group (4.0 kg vs. 1.7 kg, p < .05). Of particular interest is a recently completed large-scale (n = 710), 2-year, open-label trial that compared time to relapse for patients randomized to receive RLAI or oral quetiapine. At the time of writing this study is in press (Gaebel et al 2010) but previous conference presentations of the data (Medori et al 2008) indicate that not only did RLAI significantly extend time to relapse versus quetiapine (Kaplan-Meier estimate, p < .0001), but also fewer RLAI patients relapsed compared with quetiapine (16.5% and 31.3% respectively) and more patients on RLAI completed the study than on quetiapine. Overall both drugs appeared well tolerated.

An open-label, 2-year, prospective, naturalistic, controlled study of early psychosis (EP) patients found that the RLAI cohort (n = 22) showed significantly lower relapse rates and higher medication adherence than the oral risperidone cohort (n = 28) (Kim et al. 2008). Although there was no significant difference between groups in terms of PANSS, GAF, and CGI scales when time versus treatment interactions were considered (assesses comparative change over time), the RLAI cohort showed significant differences on all of these scales. There were no differences in overall adverse effect profile between the two groups. A study of hospitalized patients (n = 50), maintained on oral risperidone for more than 3 months, randomized to RLAI or oral risperidone showed no greater efficacy of RLAI over oral risperidone except for PANSS positive subscale scores (0.72±3.52 vs. −1.24±3.81, p = .022) but with advantages of improved side-effect profiles on the UKU (p = .037), short form 36 (SF-36) social life domain (p = .011), and reduced prolactin levels (p = .001) (Bai et al. 2007b).

Sub-analyses of early pivotal trials and subsequent switch studies have been conducted examining the antipsychotic prior to switch. From the StoRMi study, 568 patients were identified and grouped according to pre-trial oral risperidone dosage (56% ≤4 mg; 30% >4 to ≤6 mg; 14% >6 mg) (Schmauss et al. 2007). Efficacy significantly improved from baseline to end point in all groups with total PANSS scores of 20% or more in 39% of patients switched to RLAI over 6 months as well as improvements in CGI, GAF, and SF-36 mental component summary scores. Even longer-term data from the 1-year pivotal trial focusing on stable patients on oral risperidone ($n = 336$) switched to RLAI found that PANSS total scores significantly improved from baseline at end point ($p < .001$) and by 20% or more in 50% of patients, with the greatest improvement in negative symptoms, whereas the proportion with CGI-S scores representing the lowest levels of illness severity increased 2.4-fold ($p < .0001$) (Lasser et al. 2005a). Retention was high at 66.4% at 12 months and ESRS improved significantly ($p < .0001$). Similarly, patients previously symptomatically stable on olanzapine treatment ($n = 192$) switched to RLAI showed a significant improvement in PANSS total and subscale scores and CGI-S scores (all $p = .0001$), patient satisfaction with treatment ($p = 0.0001$), and SF-36 domains, (all $p = .0001$ except for role physical, bodily pain, and physical component summary, and $p < .05$ for vitality) (Gastpar et al. 2005). Body weight did not change but ESRS scores decreased significantly. Finally, data from e-STAR for patients initiated on RLAI ($n = 1345$) or an oral antipsychotic ($n = 277$; 35.7% and 36.5% on risperidone and olanzapine, respectively) indicated that at 24 months, RLAI was associated with better treatment retention with 81.8% for RLAI and 63.4% for oral antipsychotic ($p < .0001$), and greater improvement in CGI-S scores ($p = .0165$) (Olivares et al. 2009b).

Similar data are published concerning switches from oral FGAs with significant improvements in PANSS total scores ($p = .0006$) reported in stable patients receiving oral FGAs ($n = 46$) switched to RLAI as part of the 1-year pivotal trial (van Os et al. 2004). Improvement of 20% or more PANSS was achieved by 49% of patients. Movement disorder symptom severity according to the ESRS improved significantly and use of anti-Parkinsonian medications decreased throughout the study; patients rated their injection-site pain as low with a significant decrease from baseline to end point ($p = .0042$). A 12-week, prospective study of symptomatically stable patients previously taking haloperidol ($n = 46$), quetiapine ($n = 45$), or olanzapine ($n = 50$) switched to RLAI (25, 50, and 75 mg) reported significant reductions in PANSS scores ($p < .001$) with 37% showing a decrease of 20% or more in PANSS total scores; mean CGI-S scores were also reduced, significantly for the haloperidol and quetiapine groups ($p < .05$) (Lindenmayer et al. 2004). Glucose and triglyceride levels were reduced in all groups, and ESRS scores decreased for all groups, particularly for the haloperidol group. Mean serum prolactin levels increased from 23.5±2.4 ng/mL to 52.2±3.7 ng/mL, and mean body weight increase was 0.4 kg; the olanzapine group experienced a mean weight loss of 0.5 kg. A 12-week study ($n = 206$) reported clinical benefit in stable inpatients or outpatients switched from risperidone, olanzapine, quetiapine, amisulpride, and ziprasidone with greater changes noted in patient satisfaction and health-related quality of life (HRQoL) for patients previously on the other SGAs compared to prior treatment with risperidone (Schmauß et al. 2010).

It is interesting to learn that one small study that focused on cognition using brain imaging (functional MRI) compared 16 patients on RLAI, 16 patients on conventional antipsychotics (matched for clinical symptoms and other illness variables), and 8 healthy controls concluded that RLAI may contribute to normalization of brain activation in regions involved in working memory functioning in chronic schizophrenia (Surguladze et al. 2007). Although a recent open-label, 26-week, study ($n = 36$) involving a switch from oral SGAs to RLAI reported significant improvements in cognitive function, scores on the PANSS, SOFAS, Scale to Assess Unawareness of Mental Disorder (SUMD), and the Simpson-Angus Rating Scale (SARS) also improved significantly with most improvements in neurocognitive function not being correlated with clinical measures (Kim et al. 2009).

RLAI versus FGA-LAIs

There are very few studies that have prospectively compared RLAI to an FGA-LAI. Such studies are difficult to do for a number of reasons; in many countries particularly North America the use of FGA-LAIs has seen a significant reduction outside of special populations (secure, refractory, non-adherent, public payor source) and thus, FGA-LAIs are not considered a standard of treatment for most patients with schizophrenia, which limits likelihood of approval by many research ethics boards. There is one published study in which patients fulfilling DSM-IV criteria for schizophrenia and substance abuse disorder were allocated to receive either RLAI ($n = 57$) or zuclopenthixol decanoate ($n = 58$) over 6 months (Rubio et al. 2006). Overall, RLAI was shown to be more effective than zuclopenthixol decanoate in improving the symptoms of schizophrenia with PANSS total scores (mean ±SD) improving from 93.79±22.9 at baseline to 64.39±19.9 at end point for RLAI in comparison to 93.69±22.5 at baseline to 74.03±20.9 for zuclopenthixol decanoate and was more effective in treating substance abuse (mean [±SD] number of total positive tests for substance abuse: for RLAI 8.67±3.0 vs. 10.36±3.1 for zuclopenthixol decanoate, $p = .005$). More patients receiving RLAI attended more than 75% of addiction counselling sessions compared to patients receiving zuclopenthixol decanoate (92.9% vs. 67.8%, $p = .001$). Of note, an RCT study examining the effect of RLAI in cocaine addicts did not find any benefit compared to placebo; in fact RLAI was associated with worsening of depressive symptoms and weight gain (Loebl et al. 2008).

A study comparing three 3 cohorts of patients with schizophrenia before, during, and after initiating treatment with fluphenazine decanoate, haloperidol decanoate, or RLAI did not find any substantial differences in terms of treatment duration but reported that patients treated with LAIs tended to have complex pharmacological regimens and recent medication non-adherence (Olfson et al. 2007). Other studies have examined switches from FGA-LAI to RLAI. An open-label, 12-week study of Chinese patients switched from FGA-LAI to RLAI ($n = 25$) found PANSS total, negative and general psychopathology scores ($p = .002, p = .006, p = .001$, respectively), and mean ESRS scores ($p < .001$) improved significantly (Lai et al. 2009). Another open-label, 12-week study involving a switch from flupentixol decanoate, fluphenazine decanoate, haloperidol decanoate, or zuclopenthixol decanoate to RLAI demonstrated significant reductions in PANSS total and factor scores and CGI-S scores with 48% of these stable patients showed further symptom improvement ($\geq$20% decrease in PANSS score at end point). Severity of movement disorders decreased significantly with movement disorder-related AEs reported in 3% (Turner et al. 2004). A sub-analysis of the 1-year pivotal trial of patients receiving FGA-LAI at entry (n = 188), showed significant improvement in PANSS total scores with RLAI (p < .001); clinical improvement of 20% or more, 40%, or 60% reduction in PANSS-total score occurred in 52%, 34%, and 16% of patients, respectively, whereas ESRS subjective ratings and objective physician ratings decreased significantly (p < .001) (Lasser et al. 2004b)). A sub-analysis of StoRMi focusing on patients switching from oral antipsychotic (n = 100) or FGA-LAI (n = 565) reported improvements for PANSS total and subscale scores, GAF, HRQoL, treatment satisfaction, and hospitalizations (Marinis 2007). Treatment emergent AEs occurring in >5% were: anxiety (11.0%), insomnia (9.0%), weight increase (6.0%) for patients switching from oral, and weight increase (6.0%) and disease exacerbation (5.3%) for patients switching from FGA-LAI.

RLAI in early psychosis

Early psychosis (EP) patients are particularly sensitive to side-effects of medication and often lack insight into their illness, all of which likely contributes to poor adherence and high treatment-discontinuation rates. However, the use of a long-acting injectable medication has been somewhat controversial in EP patients (Chue & Emsley 2007; Pinninti & Mago 2005). Early and subsequent post hoc analyses of pivotal and switch studies with RLAI reported significant improvements in efficacy, patient satisfaction, and movement disorder ratings for young adults with schizophrenia or schizoaffective disorder (Lasser et al. 2007; Paralleda et al. 2005) and specifically in patients diagnosed with schizophrenia for 3 years or less compared with those diagnosed more than 3 years (MacFadden et al. 2010). Recently published data from e-STAR assessed the outcome of patients treated with RLAI who had a recent diagnosis (<2 years) in comparison to a longer-term diagnosis (>2 years) (Olivares et al. 2009a). The recent diagnosis group had a better outcome than the longer-term diagnosis group in terms of improvement in CGI-S scores and reduction in hospitalization (proportion of patients hospitalized, number of hospital stays, and length of stay) compared to pre-RLAI treatment.

An interesting prospective study examined non-adherence behaviour in FP patients randomly assigned to continuing on oral therapy (n = 11) or switching to RLAI (n = 37) (Weiden et al. 2009). Although there were no differences in adherence behaviour at 12 weeks with 76% (95% CI 35%–90%) adherent for RLAI versus 72% (95% CI 55%–89%) for oral ITT population (log-rank p = .78), patients accepting RLAI were significantly more likely to be adherent than patients staying on oral, with 89% (95% CI 64%–97%) adherent for RLAI vs. 59% (95% CI 32%–78%) for oral for the per protocol population (log-rank p = .035).

Several prospective, open-label studies of RLAI have been conducted specifically in EP patients with encouraging results (Emsley et al. 2008a, b; Kim et al. 2008). For example, in a 2-year study (n=50) reported by Emsley et al. (2008a) there was a high trial completion rate (72%), a high clinical response rate (78%) and most patients achieving RSWG-defined remission (64%) (Emsley et al. 2008b). A post hoc comparison of this study with a randomized controlled trial of flexible doses of oral risperidone or haloperidol found that compared with patients treated with oral risperidone or haloperidol (n = 47), RLAI-treated patients had significantly fewer all-cause discontinuations (26.0% vs. 70.2% at 24 months, p < .005), greater reduction on the PANSS total scores (p = .009), higher remission rates (64.0% vs. 40.4%, p = .028), and lower relapse rates (9.3% vs. 42.1%, p = .001) (Emsley 2008c). Clearly further RCTs of LAIs are needed in early phase schizophrenia compared to oral SGAs in particular, but these results suggest that this group can benefit from an SGA-LAI. The literature relating to the use of LAIs in EP patients is examined in detail in Chapter 7.

RLAI in the elderly

Numerous factors contribute to increased risk of psychosis in the elderly including age-related brain deterioration, co-morbid physical illnesses and social isolation (Masand & Gupta 2003). Cognitive and sensory deficits coupled with polypharmacy further contribute to difficulties with adherence. The elderly are at risk of adverse effects particularly movement disorder, which influences choice and dosing of medications. Reviews of RLAI use in the elderly have been generally positive but limited by paucity of data (Singh & O'Connor 2009). Early data from the 1-year pivotal trial of patients aged 65 years or more (n = 57) demonstrated significant improvement in PANSS total and factor scores (positive symptoms, negative symptoms, disorganized thoughts, uncontrolled hostility/excitement, and anxiety/depression) (p < .01), accompanied by improvement in CGI-S scores (Lasser et al. 2004c). Overall, treatment was well tolerated and associated with improvements in HRQoL SF36 scores, and ESRS scores were reduced significantly. A sub-group analysis of the StoRMi study evaluated long-term safety and efficacy of a direct conversion to RLAI in patients (≥65 years) with psychosis stabilized on oral or FG-LAI antipsychotic (n = 52) (Kissling et al. 2007). Modal dose at end point was 25 mg/2 weeks (60%), and the trial was completed by 81% of patients. Six patients discontinued treatment owing to an AE. Mean PANSS total decreased significantly by 15.8 at end point with significant reductions in every subscale and symptom factor at every assessment (p = .001). A total of 46.9% of patients experienced an improvement of 20% or more, with significant improvements in GAF scores, SF36 sub-domains, and patient satisfaction. The severity of movement disorder according to ESRS scores improved significantly from baseline with significant changes in patients switched from FGA-LAI. There were no cerebrovascular events. A higher rate of EPS side-effects was reported in one case series (3/6) (Hudson-Jessop et al. 2007), whereas in another sample of 18 patients 2 discontinued because of EPS AEs and in fact 6 patients with a history of EPS improved on RLAI (Singh & Connor 2007). A retrospective chart review of elderly patients (n > 60) treated with RLAI (n = 25) using the RSWG remission criteria found that symptomatic remission was achieved in 60%, with 76% continuing treatment for at least 6 months with a mean dose of 36 mg/2 weeks (Tadger 2008). Although in all of these studies, the lowest dose of RLAI was 25mg/2 weeks, a dose of 12.5 mg/2 weeks was introduced in the United States with the goal of increasing the treatment options for subjects sensitive to adverse effects such as the elderly. However, this dose has not been studied in clinical trials and is not available in Europe.

RLAI in schizoaffective and bipolar disorder

Early sub-analyses with respect to the efficacy of RLAI in schizoaffective disorder coupled with the approved indications for most of the atypical antipsychotics in the treatment of bipolar disorder led logically to research in this domain in which adherence is also problematic and there exists no 'long-acting' mood stabiliser (Savas et al. 2006). Two *post hoc* analyses of stable patients with schizoaffective disorder found significant improvement in symptomatically stable patients with schizoaffective disorder following a switch to RLAI (Lasser et al. 2004a, Mohl et al. 2005). Although no specific mood symptom scales were administered patients demonstrated reductions in symptoms (particularly the mood symptom domains) and a reduction in movement disorders. In an analysis of the 1-year study ($n = 110$), mean PANSS total scores improved significantly ($p < .001$) at each measured time point, including end point, compared with baseline with 57.7% achieving an improvement of 20% or more in total PANSS scores (Lasser et al. 2004a). Significant reductions were observed on mean PANSS cluster scores for both anxiety/depression ($p < .001$) and uncontrolled hostility/excitement ($p < .05$). In addition, scores improved significantly for positive symptoms ($p < .001$), negative symptoms ($p < .001$), and disorganized thoughts ($0.4, p < .001$). The overall subjective score of movement disorders was low at baseline and significantly decreased at endpoint ($p < .05$). Mean weight (±SE) was 80.3±1.7 kg at baseline and 82.8±0.4 kg at end point ($p < .001$). An analysis from the StoRMi study ($n = 249$) found mean scores for the total PANSS and all three subscales were significantly reduced from baseline to week 4 ($p < .001$), with further improvements until end point accompanied by significant reductions in CGI-S scores ($p < .001$) (Mohl et al. 2005). Significant improvements from baseline to end point were seen in the mood symptom domains of anxiety/depression and uncontrolled hostility/excitement. A total of 74% of patients completed the 6-month study and of 87 patients hospitalized at baseline, 67% were discharged at end point. Total ESRS scores decreased significantly from 4 weeks ($p < .001$) although small but statistically significant ($p < .001$) mean shifts of 1.8% were noted in body weight and BMI.

Since the introduction of RLAI, a number of studies have been conducted of its use in bipolar disorder mostly in maintenance therapy but including two in acute mania. The first, a small, 6-month study of 12 bipolar patients switched to RLAI reported significant improvements in mean Bech-Rafaelsen Mania Rating Scale (BRMAS) and CGI-S scores beginning at month 1 and through to end point (both $p = .02$) (Savas et al. 2006). Response, defined as a decrease of 50% more in BRMAS score from baseline was achived in 100% of patients at month 6. A long-term (2 years) observational study of mirror design of acutely manic bipolar inpatients ($n = 29$) with a history of poor or partial adherence to medication receiving treatment as usual and RLAI showed a significant decrease in the number ($p < .006$) and average length of hospitalizations ($p < .001$) per patient, in the number of manic or mixed episodes leading to hospitalisation ($p < .007$) (but not in the hospitalizations owing to depressive episodes), a significant increase in the time to any new episode (first relapse) ($p <.001$), and significant improvements in treatment adherence ($p < .0001$) and hetero-aggressive episodes ($p <.0001$), but not suicide attempts ($p =$ ns) (Vieta 2008). At study end point, 48% patients were very much improved according to the CGI. Three studies have been published concerning maintenance therapy including a 6-month, open-label, randomized trial of bipolar outpatients ($n = 49$) taking a mood stabilizer and an atypical antipsychotic and randomized to continuation of their current antipsychotic ($n = 23$) or switched to RLAI ($n = 26$) (Yatham et al. 2007). The RLAI group had significant reductions in symptoms as measured by changes in CGI-S scores and YMRS at end point relative to baseline and oral antipsychotic group had reductions in HAM-A scale scores relative to baseline but no significant differences were noted between the groups on any of the efficacy measures. The authors concluded that RLAI demonstrated similar effectiveness, safety, and tolerability compared to oral antipsychotics. A small, 12-month, prospective study ($n = 11$) of stable patients on antipsychotic maintenance monotherapy who switched to RLAI did not observe any significant changes in the YMRS, HAM-D, and BPRS scores but CGI-S and ESRS scores were significantly decreased at end point ($p < 0.05$), and patients and caregivers reported high levels of satisfaction with no significant weight change (Han et al. 2007). There were no relapses and the majority of patients (90.9%) completed the 12 months of evaluation. A slightly larger study of poorly adherent inpatients with bipolar disorder or schizoaffective disorder found a significant reduction in YMRS and CGI-S scores (both $p < .001$) but scores on HAM-D and UKU scales did not reach a statistically significant reduction (Benabarre et al. 2009).

Finally, two randomized controlled studies have confirmed the efficacy of RLAI in the maintenance treatment of bipolar disorder (Macfadden et al 2009; Quiroz et al 2010). The first study evaluated whether adjunctive maintenance treatment with RLAI, added to treatment-as-usual (TAU) medications, delayed relapse in patients with frequently relapsing (≥ 4 mood episodes in the 12 months prior to study entry) bipolar I disorder (Macfadden et al. 2009). Following a 16-week, open-label stabilization phase with RLAI plus TAU, remitted patients entered a 52-week, double-blind, phase in which randomized patients continued treatment with adjunctive RLAI plus TAU ($n = 65$) or switched to adjunctive placebo injection plus TAU ($n = 59$). Time to relapse was longer in patients receiving adjunctive RLAI ($p = .010$) and relative relapse risk was 2.3-fold higher with adjunctive placebo ($p = .011$). Completion rates were higher for adjunctive RLAI compared to adjunctive placebo (60.0% vs. 42.4%; $p = .050$) and adverse event-related discontinuations were 4.6% and 1.7%, respectively. In the second study (Quiroz et al 2010), patients with bipolar 1 disorder stabilized on RLAI were randomized to either RLAI ($n = 154$) or placebo injections ($n = 149$). Time to recurrence for any mood episode (primary outcome variable) was significantly longer for RLAI-treated patients versus placebo-treated patients ($p < .001$); the difference was significant for time to recurrence of elevated-mood episode ($p < .001$) but not time to recurrence of depressive episode ($p = .805$). Of note, use of RLAI to support treatment adherence and mood stabilization has also been described in pediatric bipolar patients (Fu-I et al. 2009).

Given the increasing data with respect to RLAI use in bipolar disorder, the Canadian Network for Mood and Anxiety Treatments (CANMAT) has recently published updated guidelines for the management of bipolar disorder supporting the use of RLAI for the prevention of mood events (Yatham et al. 2009). Furthermore, the FDA granted approval for use of RLAI both as a monotherapy and adjunctive therapy in the maintenance treatment of Bipolar I Disorder in May 2009 in the United States.

Relationship of RLAI with functionality, patient satisfaction, insight, and health-related quality of life

The concept of effectiveness encompassing the domains of efficacy, tolerability, functionality, and patient satisfaction with treatment may be regarded as a measure of a drug's worth in real-world settings (Lalonde 2003; Streiner 2002). These domains significantly influence the acceptability of a treatment to a patient and hence adherence as well as HRQoL but are difficult to measure reliably in this population (Lee et al. 2006; Lenert et al. 2005,). In a 3-month naturalistic study of RLAI in 10 US community mental health centres ($n = 60$), patients reported RLAI as being more convenient and easier to use than previous medication with the number of patients being 'very' to 'extremely' satisfied increasing from baseline to end point and patient concern about injection-site pain decreasing significantly over time (p<.06; Docherty et al. 2007). Although the majority of patients (72.6%) felt that taking RLAI was 'better' or 'much better' than taking oral risperidone, HRQoL scores were numerically but not significantly improved.

A post hoc analysis of the 12-week pivotal trial found that the HRQoL of patients receiving RLAI ($n = 93$) improved significantly ($p < .05$) in five domains of the SF-36 (bodily pain, general health, social functioning, role-emotional, and mental health) compared with patients receiving placebo ($n = 92$; Nasrallah et al. 2004). The effect was greatest for the 25-mg group, with significant improvement compared with placebo in six domains ($p < .05$) and at end point, scores in seven domains were not statistically different from normal values after 12 weeks. A similar post hoc analysis of the 1-year pivotal trial ($n = 615$) found significant improvements were found on the SF-36 mental component summary score ($p < .05$) and vitality and social functioning scales ($p < .05$; Fleischhacker et al. 2005). In this study, mean Drug Attitude Inventory (DAI) ratings indicated high patient satisfaction from baseline throughout the trial idependent of sex or diagnostic group ($p < .0001$; Lindenmayer et al. 2005). Another post hoc analysis from this trial ($n = 323$) explored the role of insight as a mediator of functioning and found that insight scores correlated significantly with changes in efficacy outcome measures (CGI-S, PANSS), functionality measures (PSP, LOF), and several cognitive measures (Gharabawi et al. 2007a). Even the elderly cohort ($n = 57$) in this trial showed improvement in SF-36 mean scores with significant improvements in mental component ($p < .05$), vitality ($p < .05$), social functioning ($p < .01$), and role-emotional ($p < .05$) subscales (Lasser et al. 2004a).

Primary analysis of the StoRMi trial reported significant improvements in GAF, ($p < 0.001$), all SF-36 domains ($p < .001$ for role physical, bodily pain, general health, social functioning, role emotional, and mental health) and patient satisfaction with treatment ($p < .001$; Möller 2005), with 31% rating the treatment as 'very good' at end point, compared with 6% at baseline. Similar findings were reported by Lorca et al. (2008b) with 31% rating the treatment as 'very good' at end point, compared with 8% at baseline. Gastpar et al. (2005) reported improvement in multiple SF-36 domains for patients switched directly to RLAI from oral olanzapine. A sub-analysis of schizoaffective patients ($n = 297$) from StoRMi reported that mean GAF scores improved significantly from baseline to end point ($p < .001$; Mohl et al. 2005). There were significant increases in mean scores for all domains of the SF-36 ($p < .01$) with marked improvements in social functioning, role emotional, and mental health (all p < .001), whereas satisfaction with treatment also improved significantly at end point (p < .001) with 78% of patients rating RLAI treatment as 'good' or 'very good'. Nick et al. (2006) reporting on a cohort of Swiss patients from StoRMi (n = 60) described significant improvement in mean PANSS total and subscale score, CGI, GAF, and patient satisfaction (all p < .001) with a study completion rate of 65%. Finally a sub-analysis of EP patients (n = 382) from StoRMi reported that mean GAF scores improved very significantly from baseline to end point (p < .0001; Paralleda et al. 2005). There were significant increases in mean scores for all SF-36 domains ($p \leq$ .001) at end point from baseline except for vitality. Satisfaction with treatment also improved significantly at end point (p < .0001) with 30% expressing their satisfaction as 'very good' at end point compared to 7% at baseline. Two studies did not show any change in HRQoL measures; the first in Korean outpatients over 48 weeks in which despite significant improvements in the primary outcome measures including GAF there were no significant differences in DAI, SWN, or SF-36 scores (Lee et al. 2006), and the second in inpatients in three hospitals treated with RLAI over 6 months again in which there were significant improvements in primary outcome measures but not in HrQoL as measured with the Tableau d'Evaluation Assistée de la Qualité de Vie (TEAQV; Raignoux et al. 2007).

RLAI and hospitalization data

Several studies have demonstrated that treatment with RLAI is associated with a reduction in hospitalization rates. Many of these studies use a mirror image analysis to compare the RLAI treatment period to pre-RLAI treatment in the same cohort of patients. Mirror image studies have various methodological weaknesses that may include regression to the mean, selection bias and interference from independent factors (Haddad et al. 2009). Other studies have a parallel control group but are non-randomized. Despite these methodological weaknesses, these studies do have their strengths including the fact that most are observational and thus, assess real world patients.

A post hoc analysis of the 1-year pivotal study found that the number of patients requiring hospitalization (n = 397) decreased continuously and significantly, from 38% in the 3 months before treatment to 12% during the last 3 months of treatment (p < .001) (Chue et al. 2005c). In this analysis, of baseline inpatients, 71% were discharged during treatment and the overall 1-year re-hospitalization rate was 17.6%, with a rate of 15.9% for baseline outpatients. The rates of psychiatric hospitalizations were 15.4% and 14.3% for all inpatients and outpatients, respectively. A further post hoc analysis reported outpatient consultations also decreased significantly from 70% of patients to 30% in the first 3 months of treatment and remained stable thereafter (p < .0001) with a reduction in ER use particularly for psychiatric consultations (Leal et al. 2004).

Reductions in hospitalization were noted during from baseline to end point in various analyses from the StoRMi study (Llorca et al. 2008b; Mohl et al. 2005; Möller et al. 2005; Paralleda et al. 2005) and the e-STAR study (Olivares et al. 2008, 2009a, b

Peuskens et al. 2009). The primary analysis of StoRMi reported that 16% of patients were hospitalized at endpoint compared to 35% at baseline with 65% of patients hospitalized at end point being discharged (Möller et al. 2005). Llorca et al. (2008b) in an 18-month follow-up of StoRMi (*n* = 529) reported that 18.6% of inpatients at baseline were rehospitalized at end point, whereas 14.2% of outpatients at baseline were hospitalized at end point. Although a sub-analysis of patients with schizoaffective disorder (*n* = 249) reported that of the 87 patients hospitalized at baseline, 66.7% had been discharged at end point (Mohl et al. 2005). Finally, in a subgroup analysis of EP patients from StoRMi (*n* = 382), of 41% hospitalized at baseline, 81% were discharged at end point and the mean number of hospitalizations during the 6 months prior to study entry was higher than during the study (0.7 vs. 0.1) (Paralleda et al. 2005). A retrospective chart review of patients treated with RLAI (*n* = 44) in a community mental health care setting in Canada found that mean (SD) duration of hospitalization and mean (SD) number of hospitalizations decreased significantly from 15.7 (19.7) days before treatment to 2.4 (6.0) days after treatment (*p* < .05) and from 2.0 (1.8) before treatment to 0.5 (1.3) after treatment (*p* < .01) respectively (Ganesan et al. 2007). This was accompanied by significant improvements in CGI-S scale scores (*p* < .001).

A mirror-image analysis of patients treated with RLAI in the United Kingdom (*n* = 100) reported 62 admissions in the 12 months before initiation of RLAI, falling to 22 admissions in the first 12 months of treatment with RLAI (Taylor et al. 2008). Another UK mirror-image study (*n* = 74) showed that RLAI, prescribed for varying periods of up to 35 months, was associated with a reduction in the number of admissions (65 vs. 33, *p* < .005) and in total inpatient days (4550 vs. 2188 days, *p* < .005) (Niaz & Haddad 2007). A 6-month pre- and post-RLAI mirror-image study (*n* = 253) conducted in Taiwan reported that compared to the 6-month pre-RLAI period, the total number of admissions was reduced by 35% (*p* = .00070 and total hospital stays by 47% (*p* = .002; Chang et al. 2009). A recently published Swedish retrospective chart review within-subject mirror-image study (*n* = 164) in patients over 2 years reported a significant reduction in mean annual days in hospital from 39 to 21 days per year (45%) and in the number of hospitalizations from 0.86 to 0.63 per year (27%) after switching to RLAI (Willis et al. 2010). Finally, a study in US veterans with schizophrenia (*n* = 106) over 309 days (±196; range, 42–737 days) found that there were fewer psychiatric-related hospitalisations (mean [SD] change, –0.8 [2.0]; *p* < .001), shorter length of stay (–25 [63.6] days; *p* < .001), and fewer inpatient days/month (–3.1 [7.2] days) in the post-RLAI compared to matched pre-RLAI period (Fuller et al. 2009). In fact, less than half experienced hospitalisation after initiation (75% vs. 42%; *p* < .001).

Two studies have been conducted comparing outcomes of patients initiated on RLAI with patients initiated on oral antipsychotics, with hospitalization prior to therapy assessed by a retrospective chart review (Beauclair et al. 2007; Olivares et al. 2009b). In the first, compared to the pre-switch period, RLAI patients had greater reductions in the number (reduction of 0.37 stays per patient vs. 0.2, *p* < .05) and days (18.74 vs. 13.02, *p* < .01) of hospitalizations at 24 months than oral antipsychotic patients (Olivares et al. 2009b). Patients initiated on RLAI were twice as likely to remain on therapy after 24 months (HR = 2.3, 95% CI = 1.79–2.97, *p* < .0001) and demonstrated significant reductions in CGI-S and GAF scores (*p* = .0165 and *p* = .03) compared to oral antipsychotic patients, despite greater duration of illness and higher proportion of prior FGA-LAI and combination antipsychotic therapy. In the second study, during RLAI-treatment (41.5 months) compared with pre-treatment (40.8 months), there were significant decreases in hospitalization (50.7 vs. 4.3%, $p < .0001$) and duration of hospitalization (23.5 vs. 0.3 days per patient, $p < .0001$) and compared with patients receiving oral SGAs for 57.2 months, RLAI patients had a reduced risk of hospitalization (95% CI 1.8–16.5% vs. 54.7–76.4%) and medication switching (95% CI 34.6–58.4% vs. 55.7–76.4%) (Beauclair et al. 2007). The oral SGAs included olanzapine (41.9%), risperidone (43%), and quetiapine (8.6%), with mean daily doses of 12.2, 3.4, and 643.8 mg/day, respectively; the remaining subjects (6.5% of total) were prescribed other oral atypicals.

Two observational studies of cohorts of patients prescribed RLAI in the United Kingdom have not found a reduction in hospitalizations or a low rate of discontinuation. In the first study, resource use data were collected for 3 years before and for 1 year after the initiation of RLAI (Young & Taylor 2006). Of those who started RLAI the days spent in hospital increased from (mean number/patient) 31 in year –3 to 44 in year –2 to 90 in year –1 to 141 in year +1. This result must be interpreted in light of the 'intent to treat' design and the fact that only 32.4% of patients in the analysis were continuing RLAI by the end of year 1. Another analysis of these data with a longer follow-up over 3 years ($n = 211$) found a reduction only in bed days for patients initiating RLAI as outpatients, with significantly greater costs being associated with RLAI treatment and high rates of discontinuation (84%) (Taylor & Cornelius 2009). Taylor et al. (2009c) also reported that while the number of hospital admissions did not increase, the number of hospital bed days increased by a median of 74 days in the 3 years post- compared with the 3 years pre-RLAI initiation ($p < .0001$) for the 211 patients initiated on RLAI. Only subjects starting RLAI as outpatients showed no increase in bed days after RLAI initiation. A greater than expected number of bed days was observed in women (36% increase), patients prescribed more than 25 mg/2 weeks (70% increase) and patients previously treated with clozapine (118% increase). A further analysis of the data examining the 34 patients who continued RLAI for 3 years showed no change in median bed days [64 days (6.5–182) before vs. 64 days (12–180) after] and median number of admissions was decreased (1.5 (1–2.25) before compared to (1.00 (0–1.25)) after ($p = .001$) (Taylor et al. 2009b). Healthcare costs more than doubled for the whole cohort ($p < .001$) and discontinuers ($p < .001$) and increased significantly for continuers ($p = .010$).

The difference in outcomes in the studies above is likely influenced by differences in patient selection particularly proportion of refractory patients or poor prognosis patients and inpatients at study start, study methodology, and how the pre- and post-periods of treatment are selected and compared, dropout rates, and finally adequacy of dosing. It is also postulated that the relative frequency of contact with RLAI given the 2-weekly dosing interval and administration through specialized programmes influences the overall effectiveness of the treatment, both in terms of increased support and closer monitoring.

RLAI and cost-effectiveness

Schizophrenia remains one of the most expensive illnesses to treat with relapse and the consequent necessity for hospitalization contributing significantly to the overall cost.

The potential of RLAI to increase adherence and thus, to improved clinical and economic outcomes for individuals with schizophrenia through reduced relapse and hospitalization has been postulated in a number of pharmacoeconomic models (Annemans 2005; Bartkó & Fehér 2005; Haycox 2005). These models represent the health and economic outcomes of patients or populations under a variety of scenarios and are used to evaluate the economic implications of schizophrenia treatment (Annemans 2005; Haycox 2005). Country-specific models for the United States (Edwards et al. 2005a, b), Canada (Chue et al. 2005b), Germany (Laux et al. 2005), Spain (Baca et al. 2005), France (Llorca et al. 2005), Belgium (De Graeve et al. 2005), Taiwan (Yang et al. 2005), and Portugal (Heeg et al. 2008) were developed to test the hypothesis using discrete event simulation (DES) models or decision (tree) analytical structures. Direct costs included medication, type of physician visits, and treatment location but indirect costs were not included (Laux et al. 2005). Outcomes may be expressed in terms of the number and duration of psychotic episodes, cumulative symptom scores, costs, and quality-adjusted life-years (QALY). Published medical literature, clinical trials reports, consumer health databases, and expert opinion are utilized to populate a decision analytical model comparing possible treatment alternatives and transition probabilities. These models can capture rates of patient adherence, rates, frequency and duration of relapse, incidence of AEs, and health care resource utilization and associated costs. Sensitivity analyses confirmed that the results were robust to a wide variation of different input variables (effectiveness, dosing distribution, patient status according to health care system) and sensitive to changes in the reported relative effectiveness of SGAs and FGAs for preventing symptom recurrence, and in relative adherence with oral and long-acting formulations (De Graeve et al. 2005). In all scenarios, RLAI produced additional clinical benefit and cost savings compared with other treatment strategies (oral risperidone, olanzapine, quetiapine, ziprasidone, aripiprazole, and haloperidol LAI), despite significant variations in heath care systems, cost-effectiveness, and therapeutic approaches. Consistently with RLAI, higher acquisition costs are offset by reduced rates of relapse because of improved adherence thus providing a cost-effective strategy for treating patients with schizophrenia (Bartkó & Fehér 2005). Results for RLAI are even more favourable among patients at high risk of being non-adherent or with more severe disease (Laux et al. 2005).

Real world cost savings with RLAI have been demonstrated in a number of analyses (Beauclair et al. 2007; Olivares et al. 2008). An e-STAR analysis ($n = 757$) found that cost-effectiveness per month per patient was lower for RLAI than previous antipsychotic medication in the three patient scenarios: without hospitalization (€539.82 vs. €982.13), without relapse (€519.67 vs. €1242.03) and without hospitalization and without relapse (€597.22 vs. €1059.39) despite higher medication costs per month compared with previous antipsychotic medication after 12 (€405.80 vs. €128.16) and 24 months (€407.33 vs. €142.77; Olivares 2008). This was attributed to higher percentage of patients who did not require hospitalization (89.1%), did not relapse (85.4%), neither required hospitalization nor relapsed (82.4%) as compared retrospectively with the same period for the previous treatment (67%, 47.8%, and

59.8%) at 12 months and at at 24 months (85.2% vs. 60%, 88.5% vs. 47.4%, and 77% vs. 53.6%).

Future research

RLAI, the first SGA-LAI, represents an important new treatment option for the long-term management of patients with schizophrenia. Overall, it has demonstrated good efficacy and tolerability equal to and possibly superior to oral SGAs. Clearly combining the benefits of an SGA with the advantages of a long-acting formulation addresses the adherence problems that are recognized as being one of the major barriers to the achievement of successful long-term outcomes in chronic mental illness. However, the necessity of refrigerated storage, difficulties of reconstitution, and administration utilizing only the supplied kit, have contributed to the complexity and expense of RLAI administration (Amdur 2004), which together with the greater acquisition costs, particularly compared to oral risperidone or FGA-LAI, have led to less widespread use than perhaps anticipated for the first SGA-LAI. Negative patient and clinician attitudes have also influenced the perception and uptake of an injectable treatment in the current era of oral atypical agents despite recommendations for RLAI use from various working groups (Kane 2003c; Kane et al. 2003b; Keith et al. 2004a). Use of a clinical manual, integrated multidisciplinary team with family participation, psycho-social interventions and motivational enhancement interviewing may be helpful in re-aligning clinician–patient expectations, further decreasing relapse potential, and enhancing long-term maintenance of therapy with RLAI (Bechelli 2003; Docherty et al. 2007; Keith et al. 2004b; Lasser et al. 2009; Lee et al. 2010). In addition, an adequate understanding of the pharmacokinetics of RLAI is important to achieve optimal results when switching and titrating (Marder et al. 2003) and in clinical situations such as dealing with missed or delayed injections (Docherty et al. 2007).

Some older practice guidelines throughout the world do not discuss RLAI as they predate its launch in the respective countries. Recommendations for the use of RLAI, in more recent guidelines, are primarily in the context of poor adherence (Argo et al. 2007; Canadian Psychiatric Association 2005). New agents are frequently used in refractory or difficult patients and particularly with RLAI because of the perceptions and expectations associated with an injectable and novel agent. There has been a tendency to switch complex patients e.g. those on high dose FGA-LAIs, combination treatments, or clozapine, leading to inconsistent results, particularly when coupled with unclear data concerning the most appropriate dosing of RLAI. Nonetheless, the limited improvement in long-term outcomes in schizophrenia despite the advent of atypical antipsychotics begs the question as to whether consistent treatment or the choice of agent is the more relevant determinant. Thus, a pragmatic trial of long duration of RLAI versus an oral SGA would perhaps provide an answer to such a question and such research is under way. However, the benefits of a long-acting treatment over its oral equivalent or an alternate oral comparator are only likely to become apparent over an adequate duration of study, minimum 2 years, and such a trial would not be without its difficulties in terms of patient selection, controlling for frequency of contact and type of intervention, choice and dosing of oral comparator as well as adherence and retention issues. To date only one long-term randomized trial of RLAI versus an oral SGA has been conducted, and the results showed a lower relapse rate for RLAI than quetiapine over a 2-year period (Gaebel et al 2010). Clearly, further studies are needed comparing SGA LAIs to oral SGAs.

References

Amdur MA. (2004). Impractical features of long-acting risperidone. *Psychiatr Serv*, **55**(12), 1443.

Andreasen N, Carpenter WT Jr, Kane J, Lasser RA, Marder SR, Weinberger DR. (2005). Remission in schizophrenia: Proposed criteria and rationale for consensus. *Am J Psychiatry*, **162**, 441–9.

Annemans L. (2005). Cost effectiveness of long-acting risperidone: what can pharmacoeconomic models teach us? *Pharmacoeconomics*, **23**(1), 1–2.

Argo TR, Crismon ML, Miller al., Moore TA, Bendele SD, Suehs B. (2007). *Texas Medication Algorithm Project Procedural Manual: Schizophrenia Treatment algorithms*. The Texas Department of State Health Services.

Baca E, Bobes J, Cañas F, Leal C, Salvador L, Badia X, et al. (2005). Cost-effectiveness analysis of long-acting injectable risperidone v. olanzapine and v. fluphenazine decanoate in treating schizophrenia. *Rev Esp Econ Salud*, **4**(5), 273–85.

Bai YM, Ting Chen T, Chen JY, Chang WH, Wu B, Hung CH, et al. (2007a). Equivalent switching dose from oral risperidone to risperidone long-acting injection: a 48-week randomized, prospective, single-blind pharmacokinetic study. *J Clin Psychiatry*, **68**(8), 1218–25.

Bai YM, Ting Chen T, Kuo Lin W, Chang WH, Wu B, Hung CH, et al. (2007b). Pharmacokinetics study for hyperprolactinemia among schizophrenics switched from risperidone to risperidone long-acting injection. *J Clin Pyschopharmacology*, **27**(3), 306–308.

Bartkó G, Fehér L. (2005). Pharmacoeconomic review of the use of injectable long-acting risperidone. *Neuropsychopharmacol Hung*, **7**(4), 199–207.

Beauclair L, Chue P, McCormick J, Camacho F, Lam A, Luong D. (2007). Impact of risperidone long-acting injectable on hospitalisation and medication use in Canadian patients with schizophrenia. *J Med Econ*, **10**(4), 427–2.

Bechelli LP. (2003). Long-acting antipsychotics in the maintenance treatment of schizophrenia. Part II. Management of medications, integration of the multiprofessional team, and perspectives with the formulation of new a new generation of long-acting antipsychotics. *Rev Lat Am Enfermagem*, **11**(4), 507–15.

Benabarre A, Castro P, Sánchez-Moreno J, Martínez-Arán A, Salamero M, Murru A, et al. (2009). Efficacy and safety of long-acting injectable risperidone in maintenance phase of bipolar and schizoaffective disorder. *Actas Esp Psiquiatr* **37**(3), 143–7.

Bloch Y, Mendlovic S, Strupinsky S, Altshuler A, Fennig S, Ratzoni G. (2001). Injections of depot FG-LAI antipsychotic medications in patients suffering from schizophrenia: do they hurt? *J Clin Psychiatry*, **62**(11), 855–9.

Camacho A, Ng B, Galangue B, David F. (2008). Use of risperidone long-acting injectable in a rural border community clinic in southern california. *Psychiatry (Edgmont)*, **5**(6), 43–9.

Castberg I, Spigset O. (2005). Serum concentrations of risperidone and 9-hydroxyrisperidone after administration of the long-acting injectable form of risperidone: evidence from a routine therapeutic drug monitoring service. *Ther Drug Monit*, **27**(1), 103–6

Chang HC, Tang CH, Tsai SJ, Yen FC, Su KP. (2009). Long-acting injectable risperidone and hospital readmission: a mirror-image study using a national claim-based database in Taiwan. *J Clin Psychiatry*, **70**(1), 141.

Chue P. (2003). Risperidone long-acting injection. *Expert Review of Neurotherapeutics*, 3(1), 435–446.

Chue P, Eerdekens M, Augustyns I, Lachaux B, Molcan P, Eriksson L, et al. (2005a). Comparative efficacy and safety of long-acting risperidone and risperidone oral tablets. *Eur Neuropsychopharmacol*, **15**(91), 111–17.

Chue PS, Heeg B, Buskens E, van Hout BA. (2005b). Modelling the impact of adherence on the costs and effects of long-acting risperidone in Canada. *Pharmacoeconomics*, **23**(1), 62–74.

Chue P, Llorca P, Duchesne I, Leal A, Rosillon D, Mehnert A. (2005c). Hospitalisation rates in patients during long-term treatment with long-acting risperidone injection. *J Appl Res*, 5(2), 266–74.

Chue P, Emsley R. (2007). Long-acting formulations of atypical antipsychotics: time to reconsider when to introduce depot FG-LAI antipsychotics. *CNS Drugs*, **21**(96), 441–8.

Ciliberto N, Bossie CA, Urioste R, Lasser RA. (2005). Lack of impact of race on the efficacy and safety of long-acting risperidone versusvs. placebo in patients with schizophrenia or schizoaffective disorder. *Int Clin Psychopharmacol*, **20**(4), 207–12.

Canadian Psychiatric Association. (2005). Clinical practice guidelines treatment of schizophrenia. *Can J Psych*, **50**, S1–S56.

Davies A, Adena MA, Keks NA, Catts SV, Lambert T, Schweitzer I. (1998). Risperidone versus haloperidol: I. Meta-analysis of efficacy and safety. *Clin Ther* **20**(1), 58–7.

De Graeve D, Smet A, Mehnert A, Caleo S, Miadi-Fargier H, Mosqueda GJ, et al. (2005). Long-acting risperidone compared with oral olanzapine and haloperidol depot in schizophrenia: a Belgian cost-effectiveness analysis. *Pharmacoeconomics*, **23**(Suppl 1), 35–47.

Docherty JP, Jones R, Turkoz I, Lasser RA, Kujawa M. (2007). Evaluation of a treatment manual for risperidone long-acting injectable. *Community Ment Health J*, **43**(3), 267–80.

Edwards NC, Locklear JC, Rupnow MF, Diamond RJ. (2005a). Cost effectiveness of long-acting risperidone injection versusvs. al.ternative antipsychotic agents in patients with schizophrenia in the USA. *Pharmacoeconomics*, **23**(Suppl 1), 75–89.

Edwards NC, Rupnow MF, Pashos CL, Botteman MF, Diamond RJ. (2005b). Cost-effectiveness model of long-acting risperidone in schizophrenia in the US. *Pharmacoeconomics*, **23**(3), 299–314.

Eerdekens M, Van Hove I, Remmerie B, Mannaert E. (2004). Pharmacokinetics and tolerability of long-acting injectable risperidone in schizophrenia. *Schizophr Res*, **70**(1), 91–100.

Emsley R, Medori R, Koen L, Oosthuizen PP, Niehaus DJ, Rabinowitz J. (2008a). Long-acting injectable risperidone in the treatment of subjects with recent-onset psychosis: a preliminary study. *J Clin Psychopharmacol*, **28**(2), 210–13.

Emsley R, Oosthuizen P, Koen L, Niehaus DJ, Medori R, Rabinowitz J. (2008b). Remission in patients with first-episode schizophrenia receiving assured antipsychotic medication: a study with risperidone long-acting injection. *Int Clin Psychopharmacol*, **23**(6), 325–31.

Emsley R, Oosthuizen P, Koen L, Niehaus DJ, Medori R, Rabinowitz J. (2008c). Oral versus injectable antipsychotic treatment in early psychosis: post hoc comparison of two studies. *Clin Ther*, **30**(12), 2378–86.

Emsley R, Rabinowitz J, Medori R; Early PsychosisEP Global Working Group. (2007). Remission in early psychosis: Rates, predictors, and clinical and functional outcome correlates. *Schizophr Res*, **89**(1–3), 129–39.

Ereshefsky L, Mannaert E. (2005). Pharmacokinetic profile and clinical efficacy of long-acting risperidone: potential benefits of combining an atypical antipsychotic and a new delivery system. *Drugs R D*, **6**(3), 129–37.

Ereshefsky L, Mascarenas CA. 2003. Comparison of the effects of different routes of antipsychotic administration on pharmacokinetics and pharmacodynamics. *J Clin Psychiatry*, **64**(Suppl 16), 18–23.

Fleischhacker WW, Eerdekens M, Karcher K, Remington G, Llorca PM, Chrzanowski W, et al. (2003). Treatment of schizophrenia with long-acting injectable risperidone: a 12-month open-label trial of the first long-acting second-generation antipsychotic. *J Clin Psychiatry*, **64**(10), 1250–7.

Fleischhacker WW, Lasser R, Mehnert A. (2005). Perceived functioning and well-being and association with psychiatric symptomatology in clinically stable schizophrenia patients treated with long-acting risperidone for 1 year. *Br J Psychiatry*, **187**, 131–6.

Fu-I L, Boarati MA, Stravogiannis A, Wang YP (2009). Use of risperidone long-acting injection to support treatment adherence and mood stabilization in pediatric bipolar patients: a case series. *J Clin Psychiatry*, **70**(4), 604–6.

Fuller M, Shermock K, Russo P, Secic M, Dirani R, Vallow S, et al. (2009). Hospitalisation and resource utilisation in patients with schizophrenia following initiation of risperidone long-acting therapy in the Veterans Affairs Healthcare System. *J Med Econ*, **12**(4), 317–24.

Gaebel W, Schreiner A, Bergmans P, et al. (2010). Relapse Prevention in Schizophrenia and Schizoaffective Disorder with Risperidone Long-Acting Injectable Versus Quetiapine: Results of a Long-Term, Open-Label, Randomized Clinical Trial. Neuropsychopharmacology. In press.

Ganesan S, McKenna M, Procyshyn R, Zipursky S. (2007). Risperidone long-acting injection in the treatment of schizophrenia spectrum illnesses: A retrospective chart review of 19 patients in the Vancouver Community Mental Health Organization (Vancouver, Canada). *Current Therapeutic Research*, **68**(6), 409–20.

Gastpar M, Masiak M, Latif MA, Frazzingaro S, Medori R, Lombertie ER. (2005). Sustained improvement of clinical outcome with risperidone long-acting injectable in psychotic patients previously treated with olanzapine. *J Psychopharmacology*, **19**(5), 32–8.

Gefvert O, Eriksson B, Persson P, et al. (2005). Pharmacokinetics and D2 receptor occupancy of long-acting injectable risperidone (Risperdal Consta) in patients with schizophrenia. *Int J Neuropsychopharmacol*, **8**(1), 27–36.

Gharabawi GM, Bossie CA, Zhu Y, Lasser RA. (2005). An assessment of emergent tardive dyskinesia and existing dyskinesia in patients receiving long-acting, injectable risperidone: results from a long-term study. *Schizophr Res*, **77**(2–3), 129–39.

Gharabawi G, Bossie C, Turkoz I, Kujawa M, Mahmoud R, Simpson G. (2007a). The impact of insight on functioning in patients with schizophrenia or schizoaffective disorder receiving risperidone long-acting injectable. *J Nerv Ment Dis*, **195**(12), 976–82.

Gharabawi GM, Gearhart NC, Lasser RA, Mahmoud RA, Zhu Y, Mannaert E, Naessens I. (2007b). Maintenance therapy with once-monthly administration of long-acting injectable risperidone in patients with schizophrenia or schizoaffective disorder: a pilot study of an extended dosing interval. *Ann Gen Psychiatry*, **6**, 3.

Gilbody SM, Bagnall AM, Duggan L, Tuunainen A. Risperidone versus. other atypical antipsychotic medication for schizophrenia. (2000). *Cochrane Database Syst Rev*, (3), CD002306.

Girardi P, Serafini G, Pompili M, Innamorati M, Tatarelli R, Baldessarini RJ. (2010). Prospective, open study of long-acting injected risperidone versus oral antipsychotics in 88 chronically psychotic patients. *Pharmacopsychiatry*, **43**(2), 66–72.

Grant S, Fitton A. (1994). Risperidone. A review of its pharmacology and therapeutic potential in the treatment of schizophrenia. *Drugs*, **48**(2), 253–73.

Gupta S, Black DW, Smith DA. (1994). Risperidone: review of its pharmacology and therapeutic use in schizophrenia. *Ann Clin Psychiatry*, **6**(3), 173–80.

Haddad PM, Taylor M, Niaz O. (2009). First generation antipsychotic long-acting injections versus oral antipsychotics in schizophrenia: systematic review of randomised controlled trials and observational studies. *Br J Psych*, **52**, S20–8.

Han C, Lee MS, Pae CU, Ko YH, Patkar AA, Jung IK. (2007). Usefulness of long-acting injectable risperidone during 12-month maintenance therapy of bipolar disorder. *Prog Neuropsychopharmacol Biol Psychiatry*, **31**(6), 1219–23.

Haycox A. (2005). Pharmacoeconomics of long-acting risperidone: results and validity of cost-effectiveness models. *Pharmacoeconomics*, **23**(1), 3–16.

Heeg BM, Antunes J, Figueira ML, Jara JM, Marques Teixeira J, Palha AP, et al. (2008). Cost-effectiveness and budget impact of long-acting risperidone in Portugal: a modeling exercise. *Curr Med Res Opinion*, **24**(2), 349–58.

Hendset M, Molden E, Refsum H, Hermann M. (2009). Impact of CYP2D6 genotype on steady-state serum concentrations of risperidone and 9-hydroxyrisperidone in patients using long-acting injectable risperidone. *J Clin Psychopharmacol*, **29**(6), 537–41.

Hosalli P, Davis JM. (2003). Depot risperidone for schizophrenia. *Cochrane Database Syst Rev*, (4), CD004161.

Hudson-Jessop P, Hughes B, Brinkley N. (2007). New for old? Risperidone long-acting injection in older patients. *Australas Psychiatry*, **15**(6), 461–4.

Hunter RH, Joy CB, Kennedy E, Gilbody SM, Song F. (2003). Risperidone versus typical antipsychotic medication for schizophrenia. *Cochrane Database Syst Review*, (2), CD000440.

Janssen-Ortho Inc. (2009). Risperdal Consta Product Monograph-.

Jayaram MB, Hosalli P. (2005). Risperidone versus olanzapine for schizophrenia. *Cochrane Database Syst Rev*, (18), CD005237.

Kane JM, Eerdekens M, Lindenmayer JP, Keith SJ, Lesem M, Karcher K. (2003a). Long-acting injectable risperidone: efficacy and safety of the first long-acting atypical antipsychotics. *Am J Psychiatry*, **160**(6), 1125–32.

Kane JM, Leucht S, Carpenter D, Docherty JP; Expert Consensus Panel for Optimizing Pharmacologic Treatment of Psychotic Disorders. (2003b). The expert consensus guideline series. Optimizing pharmacologic treatment of psychotic disorders. Introduction: methods, commentary, and summary. *J Clin Psychiatry*, **64**(12), 5–19.

Kane JM. (2003c). Strategies for improving adherence in treatment of schizophrenia by using a long-acting formulation of an antipsychotic: clinical studies. *J Clin Psychiatry*, **64**(Suppl 16), 34–40.

Keegan D. (1994). Risperidone: neurochemical, pharmacologic and clinical properties of a new antipsychotic drug. *Can J Psychiatry*, **39**(9), 46–52.

Keith SJ, Kane JM, Turner M, Conley RR, Nasrallah HA. (2004a). Academic highlights: guidelines for the use of long-acting injectable atypical antipsychotics. *J Clin Psychiatry*, **65**(1), 120–31.

Keith SJ, Pani L, Nick B, Emsley R, San L, Turner M, et al. (2004b). Practical application of pharmacotherapy with long-acting risperidone for patients with schizophrenia. *Psychiatr Serv*, **55**(9), 997–1005.

Keks NA, Ingham M, Khan A, Karcher K. (2007). Long-acting injectable risperidone vs. olanzapine tablets for schizophrenia or schizoaffective disorder. Randomised, controlled, open-label study. *Br J Psychiatry*, **191**, 131–9.

Kennedy E, Song F, Hunter R, Clarke A, Gilbody S. (2000). Risperidone versus. typical antipsychotic medication for schizophrenia. *Cochrane Database Syst Rev*, (2), CD000440.

Kim B, Lee SH, Choi TK, Suh S, Kim YW, Lee E, et al. (2008). Effectiveness of risperidone long-acting injection in first-episode schizophrenia: in naturalistic setting. *Prog Neuropsychopharmacol Biol Psychiatry*, **32**(5), 1231–5.

Kim SW, Shin Il-S, Kim JM, Lee SH, Lee YH, Ynag SJ, et al. (2009). Effects of switching to long-acting injectable risperidone from oral atypical antipsychoticsoral second generation antipsychotics on cognitive function in patients with schizophrenia. *Human Psychopharmacology: Clinical and Experimental*, **24**(7), 565–73.

Kissling W, Glue P, Medori R, Simpson S. (2007). Long-term safety and efficacy of long-acting risperidone in elderly psychotic patients. *Hum Psychopharmacology*, **22**(8), 505–13.

Kissling W, Heres S, Lloyd K, Sacchetti E, Bouhours P, Medori R, et al. (2005). Direct transition to long-acting risperidone—analysis of long-term efficacy. *J Psychopharmacology*, **19**(5), 15–21.

Lai YC, Huang MC, Chen CH, Tsai CJ, Pan CH, Chiu CC. (2009). Pharmacokinetics and efficacy of a direct switch from conventional depotFG-LAI to risperidone long-acting injection in Chinese patients with schizophrenic and schizoaffective disorders. *Psychiatry Clin Neurosci*, **63**(4), 440–8.

Lalonde P. (2003). Evaluating antipsychotic medications: predictors of clinical effectiveness. Report of an expert review panel on efficacy and effectiveness. *Can J Psychiatry*, **48**(3), 3S–12S.

Lambert M, De Marinis T, Pfeil J, et al. (2010). Establishing remission and good clinical functioning in schizophrenia: Predictors of best outcome with long-term risperidone long-acting injectable treatment. *Eur Psychiatry*, **25**(4), 220–9.

Lasser R, Bossie C, Gharabawi G, Baldessarini RJ. (2005a). Clinical improvement in 336 stable chronically psychotic patients changed from oral to long-acting risperidone: a 12-month open trial. *Int J Neuropsychopharmacol*, **8**(3), 427–38.

Lasser R, Bossie CA, Gharabawi G, Eerdekens M, Nasrallah HA. (2004a). Efficacy and safety of long-acting risperidone in stable patients with schizoaffective disorder. *J Affect Disord*, **83**(2-3), 263–75.

Lasser R, Bossie CA, Gharabawi GM, Kane JM. (2005b). Remission in schizophrenia: Results from a 1-year study of long-acting risperidone injection. *Schizophr Res*, **77**(2–3), 215–27.

Lasser R, Bossie C, Gharabawi G, Turner M. (2004b). Patients with schizophrenia previously stabilized on conventional depot antipsychotics experience significant clinical improvements following treatment with long-acting risperidone. *Eur Psychiatry*, **19**(4), 219–25.

Lasser R, Bossie CA, Zhu Y, Gharabawi G, Eerdekens M, Davidson M. (2004c). Efficacy and safety of long-acting risperidone in elderly patients with schizophrenia and schizoaffective disorder. *Int J Geriatr Psychiatry*, **19**(9), 898–905.

Lasser RA, Bossie CA, Zhu Y, Locklear JC, Kane JM. (2007). Long-acting risperidone in young adults with early schizophrenia or schizoaffective illness. *Ann Clin Psychiatry*, **19**(2), 65–71.

Lasser RA, Schooler NR, Kujawa M, Docherty J, Weiden P. (2009). A new psychosocial tool for gaining patient understanding and acceptance of long-acting injectable antipsychotic therapy. *Psychiatry (Edgmont)*, **6**(4), 22–7.

Lauriello J, McEvoy JP, Rodriquez S, Bossie CA, Lasser RA. (2005). Long-acting risperidone vs. placebo in the treatment of hospital inpatients with schizophrenia. *Schizophr Res*, **72**(2–3), 249–58.

Laux G, Heeg B, van Hout B, Mehnert A. (2005). Costs and effects of long-acting risperidone compared with oral atypical and conventional depotconventional depot formulations in Germany. *Pharmacoeconomics*, **23**(Suppl 1), 49–61.

Leal A, Rosillon D, Mehnert A, Jarema M, Remington G. 2004. Healthcare resource utilization during 1-year treatment with long-acting, injectable risperidone. *Pharmacoepidemiol Drug Safety*, **13**(11), 811–6.

Lee MS, Ko YH, Lee SH, Seo YJ, Kim SH, Joe SH, et al. (2006). Long-term treatment with long-acting risperidone in Korean patients with schizophrenia. *Hum Psychopharmaco*, **21**(6), 399–407.

Lee SH, Choi TK, Suh S, Kim YW, Kim B, Lee E, et al. (2010). Effectiveness of a psychosocial intervention for relapse prevention in patients with schizophrenia receiving risperidone via long-acting injection. *Psychiatry Res*, **175**(3), 195–9.

Lenert LA, Rupnow MF, Elnitsky C. (2005).Application of a disease-specific mapping function to estimate utility gains with effective treatment of schizophrenia. *Health Quality Life Outcomes*, **11**(3),57.

Lieberman JA, Stroup TS, McEvoy JP, Swartz MS, Rosenheck RA, Perkins DO, et al. (2005). Clinical Antipsychotic Trials of Intervention Effectiveness (CATIE) Investigators. Effectiveness of antipsychotic drugs in patients with chronic schizophrenia. *N Engl J Med*, **353**(12), 1209–23.

Lindenmayer JP, Eerdekens E, Berry SA, Eerdekens M. (2004). Safety and efficacy of long-acting risperidone in schizophrenia: a 12-week, multicenter, open-label study in stable patients switched from typical and atypical oral antipsychotics. *J Clin Psychiatry*, **65**(8), 1084–9.

Lindenmayer JP, Jarboe K, Bossie CA, Zhu Y, Mehnert A, Lasser R. (2005). Minimal injection site pain and high patient satisfaction during treatment with long-acting risperidone. *Int Clin Psychopharmacol*, **20**(4), 213–21.

Lindenmayer JP, Khan A, Eerdekens M, Van Hove I, Kushner S. (2007). Long-term safety and tolerability of long-acting injectable risperidone in patients with schizophrenia or schizoaffective disorder. *Eur Neuropsychopharmacol*, **17**(2), 138–44.

Lindenmayer JP, Parak M, Gorman JM. (2006). Improved long-term outcome with long-acting risperidone treatment of chronic schizophrenia with prior partial response. *J Psychiatr Pract*, **12**(1), 55–7.

Llorca PM, Bouhours P, Moreau-Mallet V, et al. (2008a) Improved symptom control, functioning and satisfaction in French patients treated with long-acting injectable risperidone. *Encephale*, **34**(2), 170–8.

Llorca PM, Miadi-Fargier H, Lançon C, Jasso Mosqueda G, Casadebaig F, Philippe A, et al. (2005). Cost-effectiveness analysis of schizophrenic patient care settings: impact of an atypical antipsychotic under long-acting injection formulation. *Encephale*, **31**(2), 235–46.

Llorca PM, Sacchetti E, Lloyd K, Kissling W, Medori R. (2008b). Long-term remission in schizophrenia and related psychoses with long-acting risperidone: results obtained in an open-label study with an observation period of 18 months. *Int J Clin Pharmacol Ther*, **46**(1), 14–22.

Loebl T, Angarita GA, Pachas GN, Lee SH, Nino J, Logvinenko T, et al. (2008). A randomized, double-blind, placebo-controlled trial of long-acting risperidone in cocaine-dependent men. *J Clin Psychiatry*, **69**(3), 480–6.

Macfadden W, Alphs L, Haskins JT, Turner N, Turkoz I, Bossie C, et al. (2009). A randomized, double-blind, placebo-controlled study of maintenance treatment with adjunctive risperidone long-acting therapy in patients with bipolar I disorder who relapse frequently. *Bipolar Disord*, **11**(8),827–39.

Macfadden W, Bossie CA, Turkoz I, Haskins JT. (2010). Risperidone long-acting therapy in stable patients with recently diagnosed schizophrenia. *Int Clin Psychopharmacol*, **25**(2), 75–82.

Mannaert E, Vermeulen A, Remmerie B, Bouhours P, Levron JC. (2005). Pharmacokinetic profile of long-acting injectable risperidone at steady-state: comparison with oral administration. *Encephale*, **31**(5 Pt 1), 609–15.

Marder SR, Conley R, Ereshefsky L, Kane JM, Turner MS. (2003). Clinical guidelines: Dosing and switching strategies for long-acting risperidone. *J Clin Psychiatry*, **64**(Suppl 16), 41–6.

Marinis TD, Saleem PT, Glue P, Arnoldussen WJ, Teijeiro R, Lex A, et al. (2007). Switching to long-acting injectable risperidone is beneficial with regard to clinical outcomes, regardless of previous conventional medication in patients with schizophrenia. *Pharmacopsychiatry*, **40**(6), 257–63.

Martin SD, Libretto SE, Pratt DJ, Brewin JS, Huq ZU, Saleh BT. (2003). Clinical experience with the long-acting injectable formulation of the atypical antipsychotic, risperidone. *Curr Med Res Opin*, **19**(4), 298–305.

Masand PS, Gupta S. (2003). Long-acting injectable antipsychotics in the elderly: guidelines for effective use. *Drugs Aging*, **20**(15), 1099–110.

Mauri MC, Turner M, Volonteri LS, Medori R, Maier W. (2009). Dosing patterns in Europe: Efficacy and safety of risperidone long-acting injectable in doses of 25, 37.5 and 50 mg. *Int J Psychiatry in Clinical Practice,* **13**(1), 36–47.

Medori R, Mannaert E, Gründer G. (2006). Plasma antipsychotic concentration and receptor occupancy, with special focus on risperidone long-acting injectable. *Eur Neuropsychopharmacol*, **16**(4), 233–40.

Medori R, Wapenaar R, de Arce R, Rouillon F, Gaebel W, Cordes J, et al. (2008). *Relapse Prevention and Effectiveness in Schizophrenia with Risperidone Long-acting Injectable (RLAI) versus Quetiapine.* Poster presented at 161st Annual American Psychiatric Association Meeting, 2008, Washington, USA.

Mohl A, Westlye K, Opjordsmoen S, Lex A, Schreiner A, Benoit M, et al. (2005). Long-acting risperidone in stable patients with schizoaffective disorder. *J Psychopharmacol*, **19**(Suppl 6), 22–31.

Möller H, Llorca PM, Sacchetti E, Martin SD, Medori R, Parellada E; StoRMi Study Group. (2005). Efficacy and safety of direct transition to risperidone long-acting injectable in patients treated with various antipsychotic therapies. *Int Clin Psychopharmacol*, **20**(3), 121–30.

Möller HJ. (2006). Long-acting risperidone: focus on safety. *Clin Ther*, **28**(5), 633–51.

Nasrallah H, Duchesne I, Mehnert A, Janagap C, Eerdekens M. (2004). Health-related quality of life with schizophrenia during treatment with long-acting risperidone injection. *J Clin Psychiatry*, **65**(8), 531–6.

Nesvåg R, Hendset M, Refsum H, Tanum L. (2006). Serum concentrations of risperidone and 9-OH risperidone following intramuscular injection of long-acting risperidone compared with oral risperidone medication. *Acta Psychiatrica Scandinavica*, **114**(1), 21–6.

Nesvåg R, Tanum L. (2005). Therapeutic drug monitoring of patients on risperidone depot. *Nord J Psychiatry*, **59**(1), 51–5.

Niaz OS, Haddad PM. (2007). Thirty-five months experience of risperidone long-acting injection in a UK psychiatric service including a mirror-image analysis of in-patient care. *Acta Psychiatr Scand*, **116**(1), 36–46.

Nick B, Vauth R, Braendle D et al. (2006) Symptom control, functioning and satisfaction among Swiss patients treated with risperidone long-acting injectable. *Int J Psychiatry in Clinical Practice*, **10**(3), 174–81.

Ning X, Thyssen A, Quiroz J, et al. (2008). Tolerability and safety of long-acting injectable risperidone in chronic schizophrenia subjects using deltoid muscle as an alternative injection site. Poster presented at the 161st Annual American Psychiatric Association Annual Meeting; 3–8 May 2008; Washington, DC.

Olfson M, Marcus SC, Ascher-Svanum H. (2007). Treatment of schizophrenia with long-acting fluphenazine, haloperidol, or risperidone. *Schizophr Bull*, **33**(6), 1379–87.

Olivares JM, Peuskens J, Pecenak J, Resseler S, Jacobs A, Akhras KS; e-STAR Study Group. (2009a). Clinical and resource-use outcomes of risperidone long-acting injection in recent and long-term diagnosed schizophrenia patients: results from a multinational electronic registry. *Curr Med Res Opin*, **25**(9), 2197–206.

Olivares JM, Rodriguez-Morales A, Burón JA, Alonso-Escolano D, Rodriguez-Morales A; e-STAR Study Group. (2008). Cost-effectiveness analysis of switching antipsychotic medication to long-acting injectable risperidone in patients with schizophrenia: a 12- and 24-month follow-up from the e-STAR database in Spain. *Appl Health Econ Health Policy*, **6**(1), 41–53.

Olivares JM, Rodriguez-Morales A, Diels J, Povey M, Jacobs A, Zhao Z, et al.; e-STAR Spanish Study Group . (2009b). Long-term outcomes in patients with schizophrenia treated with risperidone long-acting injection or oral antipsychotics in Spain: results from the electronic Schizophrenia Treatment Adherence Registry (e-STAR). *Eur Psychiatry*, **24**(5), 287–96.

Parellada E. (2007). Long-acting injectable risperidone in the treatment of schizophrenia in special patient populations. *Psychopharmacol Bull*, **40**(2), 82–100.

Parellada E, Andrezina R, Milanova V, Glue P, Masiak M, Turner MS, et al. (2005). Patients in the early phases of schizophrenia and schizoaffective disorders effectively treated with risperidone long-acting injectable. *J Psychopharmacol*, **19**(Suppl 5), 5–14.

Patel MX, Young C, Samele C, Taylor DM, David AS. (2004). Prognostic indicators for early discontinuation of risperidone long-acting injection. *Int Clin Psychopharmacol*, **19**(4), 233–9.

Peng PW, Huang MC, Tsai CJ, Pan CH, Chen CC, Chiu CC. (2008). The disparity of pharmacokinetics and prolactin study for risperidone long-acting injection.The disparity of pharmacokinetics and prolactin study for risperidone long-acting injection. *J Clin Psychopharmacology*, **28**(8), 726–7.

Peuskens J, Olivares JM, Pecenak J, Tuma I, Bij de Weg H, Eriksson L, et al. (2010). Treatment retention with risperidone long-acting injection: 24-month results from the Electronic

Schizophrenia Treatment Adherence Registry (e-STAR) in six countries. *Curr Med Res Opin*, **26**(3), 501–9.

Pinninti NR, Mago R. (2005). Use of long-acting risperidone. *Psychiatr Serv*, **56**(1), 105.

Quiroz JA, Yatham LN, Palumbo JM, Karcher K, Kushner S, Kusumakar V, et al. (2010). Risperidone long-acting injectable monotherapy in the maintenance treatment of bipolar I disorder. *Biol Psychiatry*, **68**(2), 156–62.

Raignoux C, Dusouchet T, Bret P, Queuille E, Biscay ML, Caron J, et al. (2007). Long-acting injectable risperidone: naturalistic study in three hospitals in Aquitaine. *Encephale*, **33**(6), 973–81.

Ramstack J, Grandolfi G, Mannaert E, D'Hoore P, Lasser RA. (2003). Long-acting risperidone: prolonged-release injectable delivery of risperidone using Medisorb® microsphere technology. *Schizophr Research*, **60**, 314.

Remington G, Mamo D, Labelle A, Reiss J, Shammi C, Mannaert E, et al. 2006. A PET study evaluating dopamine D2 receptor occupancy for long-acting injectable risperidone. *Am J Psychiatry*, **163**(3), 396–401.

Rubio G, Martinez I, Ponce G, Jiménez-Arriero MA, López-Muñoz F, Alamo C. (2006). Long-acting injectable risperidone versus zuclopenthixol in the treatment of schizophrenia with substance abuse comorbidity. *Can J Psychiatry*, **51**(8), 531–9.

Savas HA, Yumru M, Ozen ME. (2006). Use of long-acting risperidone in the treatment of bipolar patients. *J Clin Psychopharmacol*, **26**(5), 530–1.

Schmauß M, Diekamp B, Gerwe M, Schreiner A, Ibach B. (2010). Does oral antipsychotic pre-treatment influence outcome of a switch to long-acting injectable risperidone. *Pharmacopsychiatry*, **43**(2), 73–80.

Schmauss M, Sacchetti E, Kahn JP, Medori R. (2007). Efficacy and safety of risperidone long-acting injectable in stable psychotic patients previously treated with oral risperidone. *Int Clin Psychopharmacol*, **22**(2), 85–92.

Simpson GM, Mahmoud RA, Lasser RA, Kujawa M, Bossie CA, Turkoz I, et al. (2006). A 1-year double-blind study of 2 doses of long-acting risperidone in stable patients with schizophrenia or schizoaffective disorder. *J Clin Psychiatry*, **67**(8), 1194–203.

Singh D, O'Connor DW. (2007). Depot risperidone in elderly patients: the experience of an Australian aged psychiatry service. *Int Psychogeriatr*, **19**, 789–92.

Singh D, O'Connor DW. (2009). Efficacy and safety of risperidone long-acting injection in elderly people with schizophrenia. *Clin Interv Aging*, **4**, 351–5.

Streiner DL. (2002). The 2 'Es' of research: efficacy and effectiveness trials. *Can J Psychiatry*, **47**(6), 552–6.

Surguladze SA, Chu EM, Evans A, et al. (2007). The effect of long-acting risperidone on working memory in schizophrenia: a functional magnetic resonance imaging study. *J Clin Psychopharmacol*, **27**, 560–70.

Tadger S, Baruch Y, Barak Y. (2008).Symptomatic remission in elderly schizophrenia patients treated with long-acting risperidone. *Int Psychogeriatr*, **20**, 1245–50.

Taylor D, Cornelius V. (2010) Risperidone long-acting injection: factors associated with changes in bed stay and hospitalisation in a 3-year naturalistic follow-up. *J Psychopharmacol*, **24**(7),995–9.

Taylor DM, Fischetti C, Sparshatt A, Thomas A, Bishara D, Cornelius V. (2009a). Risperidone long-acting injection: a prospective 3-year analysis of its use in clinical practice. *J Clin Psychiatry*, **70**(2), 196–200.

Taylor DM, Fischetti C, Sparshatt A, Thomas A, Bishara D, Cornelius V. (2009b). Risperidone long-acting injection: a 6-year mirror-image study of healthcare resource use. *Acta Psychiatr Scand*, **120**(2), 97–101.

Taylor DM, Young CL, Mace S, Patel MX. (2004). Early clinical experience with risperidone long-acting injection: a prospective, 6-month follow-up of 100 patients. *J Clin Psychiatry*, **65**(8), 1076–83.

Taylor DM, Young C, Patel MX. (2006). Prospective 6-month follow-up of patients prescribed risperidone long-acting injection: factors predicting favourable outcome. *Int J Neuropsychopharmacol*, **9**(6), 685–94.

Taylor M, Currie A, Lloyd K, Price M, Peperell K. (2008). Impact of risperidone long acting injection on resource utilization in psychiatric secondary care. *J Psychopharmacology*, **22**(2), 128–3.

Thyssen A, Rusch S, Herben V, Quiroz J, Mannaert E. (2010). Risperidone long-acting injection: Pharmacokinetics following administration in deltoid versus gluteal muscle in schizophrenic patients. *J Clin Pharmacol*, Jan 23. [Epub ahead of print].

Turner M, Eerdekens E, Jacko M, Eerdekens M. (2004). Long-acting injectable risperidone: safety and efficacy in stable patients switched from conventional depotFG-LAI antipsychotics. *Int Clin Psychopharmacol*, **19**(4), 241–9.

Uchida H, Mamo DC, Kapur S, Labelle A, Shammi C, Mannaert EJ, et al. (2008). Monthly administration of long-acting injectable risperidone and striatal dopamine D2 receptor occupancy for the management of schizophrenia. *J Clin Psychiatry*, **69**(8), 1281–6.

van Os J, Bossie C, Lasser R. (2004). Improvements in stable patients with psychotic disorders switched from oral conventionaloral FGA antipsychotics therapy to long-acting risperidone. *Int Clin Psychopharmacol*, **19**(4), 229–32.

van Os J, Burns T, Cavallaro R, Leucht S, Leucht S, Peuskens J, Helldin L, et al. (2006). Standardized remission criteria in schizophrenia. *Acta Psychiatr Scand*, **113**(2), 91–5.

Vehof J, Postma MJ, Bruggeman R, De Jong-Van Den Berg LT, Van Den Berg PB, Stolk RP, et al. (2008). Predictors for starting depot administration of risperidone in chronic users of antipsychotics. *J Clin Psychopharmacol*, **28**(6), 625–30.

Vieta E, Nieto E, Autet A, Rosa AR, Goikolea JM, Cruz N, et al. (2008). A long-term prospective study on the outcome of bipolar patients treated with long-acting injectable risperidone. *World J Biol Psychiatry*, **9**(3), 219–24.

Viner MW, Matuszak JM, Knight LJ. (2006). Initial dosing strategies for long-acting injectable risperidone. *J Clin Psychiatry*, **67**(8), 1310–1.

Weiden PJ, Schooler NR, Weedon JC, Elmouchtari A, Sunakawa A, Goldfinger SM. (2009). A randomized controlled trial of long-acting injectable risperidone vs continuation on oral atypical antipsychotics for first-episode schizophrenia patients: initial adherence outcome. *J Clin Psychiatry*, **70**(10), 1397–406.

Willis M, Svensson M, Löthgren M, Eriksson B, Berntsson A, Persson U. (2010). The impact on schizophrenia-related hospital utilization and costs of switching to long-acting risperidone injections in Sweden. *Eur J Health Econ*, Jan 19. [Epub ahead of print].

Yang YK, Tarn YH, Wang TY, Liu CY, Laoi YC, Chou YH, et al. (2005). Pharmacoeconomic evaluation of schizophrenia in Taiwan: model comparison of long-acting risperidone versus olanzapine versus depot haloperidol based on estimated costs. *Psychiatry Clin Neuroscience*, **59**(4), 385–94.

Yatham LN, Fallu A, Binder CE. (2007). A 6-month randomized open-label comparison of continuation of oral atypical antipsychotic therapy or switch to long acting injectable risperidone in patients with bipolar disorder. *Acta Psychiatr Scand*, **434**, 50–6.

Yatham LN, Kennedy SH, Schaffer A, et al. (2009). Canadian Network for Mood and Anxiety Treatments (CANMAT) and International Society for Bipolar Disorders (ISBD) collaborative update of CANMAT guidelines for the management of patients with bipolar disorder: update 2009. *Bipolar Disord*, **11**(3), 225–55.

Young CL, Taylor DM. (2006). (2006). Health resource utilization associated with switching to risperidone long-acting injection. *Acta Psychiatr Scan*, **114**(1), 14–20.

Chapter 6

Recently approved long-acting antipsychotic injections: paliperidone LAI and olanzapine LAI

John Lauriello and Niels Beck

Correspondence: laurielloj@health.missouri.edu

Introduction: the case for additional long-acting agents

Antipsychotic long-acting injections (LAIs) were introduced into clinical practice in the 1960s but until recently all those available were preparations of first-generation antipsychotic (FGA) drugs, also known as typical or conventional antipsychotics. A major problem with these drugs is their liability to cause extrapyramidal effects (EPS) and tardive dyskinesia (TD), problems that are particularly marked with the more potent D_2 blocking agents such as haloperidol; comparative studies with oral antipsychotics show that second-generation antipsychotics (SGAs), or atypical antipsychotics, offer reduced rates of extrapyramidal symptoms and tardive dyskinesia (Correll et al. 2004). A proviso is that these comparisons are largely based on trials where haloperidol was the FGA comparator and the EPS advantage of SGAs is less pronounced when they are compared to low potency FGAs such as chlorpromazine (Leucht et al. 2009). Preliminary evidence also suggests that SGAs may have an advantage in cognitive improvement and possibly brain plasticity (Lieberman et al. 2008).

In the United States first-generation antipsychotic long-acting injections (FGA-LAIs) are limited to fluphenazine decanoate and haloperidol decanoate (see Chapter 4). The introduction of risperidone LAI ushered in an era of second-generation antipsychotic long-acting injections (SGA-LAIs) (see Chapter 5) and has offered the reduced extrapyramidal advantages of an SGA in a long-acting form. In some countries, notably Spain and Australia, the introduction of risperidone LAI has increased the usage of LAIs, whereas in the United States the relative usage of LAIs has remained static somewhere between 3% and 5% (IMS-MIDAS) (see Chapter 10). Risperidone LAI has several disadvantages, including an initial minimal 3-week need for oral antipsychotic coverage, a fixed 2-week dosing interval, and a limited range of unit dosing options. In 2009 long-acting injectable paliperidone (the 9-OH metabolite of risperidone) was approved in the United States and other countries. Paliperidone LAI promises to remedy many of the drawbacks of risperidone LAI, allowing immediate loading, monthly injection frequency, and a greater dose range.

An obvious limitation of having risperidone and paliperidone as the only available SGA-LAIs is their shared pharmacology and likely overlapping efficacy and side-effect profiles. An example would be prolactin elevation, which although possibly less marked with these long-acting agents compared to their oral preparations, will still present in some patients. Switching between risperidone and paliperidone LAI would most likely offer little advantage in terms of efficacy or tolerability, although future comparative studies would be informative. In patients who show an inadequate response to risperidone and paliperidone or who do not tolerate these drugs, the availability of an unrelated SGA-LAI would be an advance. In this regard, the recent development of olanzapine LAI should represent a useful addition to a clinician's armamentarium (Lauriello et. al. 2008).

In this chapter we will describe the current body of knowledge on both paliperidone LAI and olanzapine LAI. At the time of writing these medications have only been available in specific countries for a short time. Complete information on these two medications is lacking, but there are several studies under way that should help clarify their efficacy and tolerability. As we have seen with other newly introduced medications, widespread clinical use of these agents will also provide important data on their effectiveness and safety in real world practice.

Paliperidone long-acting injection

Paliperidone palmitate (Invega® Sustenna® in the United States) is an LAI formulation of 9-hydroxyrisperidone, the active metabolite of risperidone. Paliperidone oral, marketed under the trade name Invega®, has been available since 2006. Invega® is a once-a-day extended-release OROS capsule that utilizes osmotic pressure to physically push paliperidone at a controlled rate through small openings in the capsule thereby achieving more stable plasma levels than would be achieved with an immediate release preparation. Because it does not undergo significant liver metabolism, paliperidone is not expected to be affected by inhibitors or inducers of P450 isoenzymes (Janssen, Division of Ortho-McNeil-Janssen Pharmaceuticals, Inc. 2010).

A recent study showed oral paliperidone and risperidone to have similar effects on prolactin elevation in a clinical dosing range (Berwaerts et. al. 2009). In many ways paliperidone LAI was developed to overcome the shortcomings seen with risperidone LAI. Table 6.1 compares these two LAIs.

Pharmacology

Release of 9-OH paliperidone from paliperidone LAI occurs by day 1, whereas significant release of risperidone from risperidone LAI does not occur for 3 to 4 weeks. The lag period with risperidone LAI is because the risperidone is embedded in biodegradable polymer microspheres that need to break down before risperidone is released. In contrast, paliperidone LAI is based on the palmitate ester of 9-OH paliperidone in a highly refined crystalline preparation that starts to break down and release 9-OH paliperidone as soon as it is administered (see Chapter 2). With paliperidone LAI maximum plasma concentration occurs in approximately 2 weeks and can last as long

Table 6.1 Comparison of paliperidone LAI and risperidone LAI

	Paliperidone LAI	Risperidone LAI
Formulation	Palmitate (crystal-base)	Microspheres
Initiation (Loading) Strategy	2 injections in first week	Not possible
Injection Interval	Every 4 weeks	Every 2 weeks
Injection Site	Deltoid or gluteal	Gluteal (later approved for deltoid)
Available Doses	39 mg, 78mg,117mg, 156mg, 234mg[b]	12.5mg[a], 25mg, 37.5 mg, 50mg
Reconstitution	No:pre-filled syringes	Yes:powder in vials
Refrigeration	No	Yes

[a] The 12.5mg dose of risperidone LAI is available in the United States but not in Europe
[b] See footnote 1 on page 133 regarding dosage of paliperidone LAI

as 18 weeks. In order to reach therapeutic levels in a short period, the first two doses of paliperidone LAI are given one week apart, 234 mg on day 1 and then 156 mg on day 8; both these initiation or loading doses are administered in the deltoid muscle. From then on the recommended maintenance dose is 117 mg starting on day 36 and every 4 weeks thereafter with dosage adjusted based on efficacy and tolerability. Maintenance doses can be administered at either the deltoid or gluteal site. Table 6.2 shows approximate equivalent doses of paliperidone LAI prescribed monthly and daily oral paliperidone (Janssen, Division of Ortho-McNeil-Janssen Pharmaceuticals, Inc 2010).

Efficacy Studies[1]

As Fleischhaker (2009) indicated, paliperidone LAI represents a relatively recent introduction to the marketplace, and hence much of the extant efficacy data are limited to conference presentations and a handful of very recently published articles (e.g. Kramer et al. 2009; Hough et al. 2010).

The Kramer et al. (2009) study was designed as a 9-week, randomized, double-blind investigation which included three groups of persons with diagnoses of schizophrenia, and Positive and Negative Symptom Scale (PANSS) scores in the 60 to 120 range at baseline. All subjects who were part of this study were hospitalized for the first 14 days. During this interval, which included a 7-day open-label period, subjects (n =266) received extended release OROS paliperidone (6 or 12 mg), or immediate release paliperidone (2 or 4 mg). Following this phase, subjects who met eligibility criteria

[1] Commercially in the United States, paliperidone LAI (Invega® Sustenna®) is available in milligrams of paliperidone palmitate. Dosages used in the clinical trials data are often reported as milligram equivalents (mg.eq.) to paliperidone. The equivalence between mg eq. of paliperidone and mg of paliperidone palmitate is as follows: 25, 50, 75, 100 and 150 mg. eq. paliperidone covert to 39, 78, 117, 156 and 234 mg. paliperidone LAI, respectively.

Table 6.2 Approximate equivalent doses of oral paliperidone and paliperidone LAI (Janssen, Division of Ortho-McNeil-Janssen Pharmaceuticals, Inc. 2010)

Oral paliperidone (mg/day)	Maintenance dose of paliperidone LAI (mg/4 weekly)[a]
12	234
6	117
3	39-78

[a] See footnote 1 on page 133 regarding dosage of paliperidone LAI.

($n = 247$) were then randomized to 50 mg eq. paliperidone LAI, 100 mg eq. paliperidone LAI, or placebo. Gluteal injections occurred on days 1, 8, and 36 and then at 64 days. At 9 weeks, the percentage of subjects who had completed the double-blind period differed, with both the 50 and 100 mg eq. paliperidone LAI groups completing more frequently than placebo controls (59%, 61%, and 32%). With regard to PANSS scores, the paliperidone LAI 50 mg eq. and 100 mg eq. groups were statistically significant and superior to placebo with regard to PANSS total scores as well as the PANSS subscales measuring Positive Symptoms, Negative Symptoms, Anxiety/Depression, Disorganized Thoughts, and Hostility/Excitement.

From a treatment-emergent side-effect point of view, the three groups did not differ significantly with regard to overall event rates, although Parkinsonian-related adverse events (extrapyramidal disorder, drooling, hypertonia) occurred more frequently in the paliperidone LAI groups (8%, 5%, and 1% in the 100 mg. eq., 50 mg eq., and placebo groups, respectively). However, no significant differences were observed between the three groups on Abnormal Involuntary Movement Scale (AIMS), Barnes Akathisia Scale (BAS), or Simpson Angus Scale (SAS) scores.

Hough et al. (2010) reported on the results of placebo-controlled recurrence prevention study. This design began with a 33-week transition and maintenance period, followed by a 9-week, open-label, flexible dose phase. The first two (gluteal) injections (50 mg eq.) were given 1 week apart. Patients were then given injections every 4 weeks, and dose could be adjusted between 25 mg eq., 50 mg eq., and 100 mg eq. Patients with total PANSS scores of less than 75 at week 9 continued into a 24-week maintenance phase. During the first 12 weeks of this period, flexible dosing continued, followed by the second 12 weeks, where a fixed dosing schedule was implemented.

Patients who were judged clinically stable at this point in the study were then randomly assigned to their current fixed dose of paliperidone LAI, or to placebo, and then monitored on an ongoing basis for symptom recurrence. Recurrence of symptoms was defined by such events as psychiatric hospitalization, deliberate self-injury or violent behaviour, suicidal or homicidal ideation, and/or predefined increases in PANSS total scores. An independent Data Monitoring Board conducted an interim analysis (n = 312 patients) of recurrence events (n = 68 events), which indicated a clear advantage of the drug condition over placebo, and therefore the study was terminated early,

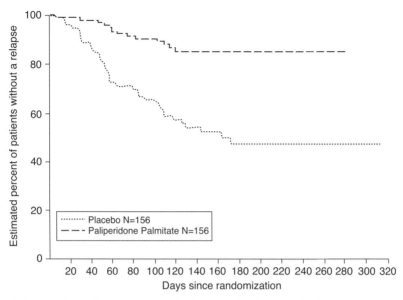

Fig. 6.1 Percentage of patients without relapse in placebo-controlled recurrence prevention study of paliperidone palmitate.
Reprinted from Hough et al (2010), Copyright (2010) with permission from Elsevier.

approximately 160 days into the study (10% vs. 34% recurrence events in the paliperidone LAI and placebo groups, respectively (Figure 6.1).

In terms of adverse events, significant weight increase occurred in 7% of paliperidone LAI in comparison to 1% of placebo subjects, although overall, weight gain in both groups was minimal, with mean weight increase in the paliperidone LAI group on the order of 1 kg.

Nasrallah et al. (2008) compared patients receiving one of three doses of paliperidone LAI (25, 50, 100 mg eq.) to placebo in a 13-week, randomized double-blind study. This study included patients with a diagnosis of schizophrenia, and baseline PANSS total scores in the 70 to 120 range. The first two injections (gluteal) were given a week apart, followed by 4-week injection intervals. A total of 518 patients were randomized, and 51% of these completed the full 13 weeks, with 38% of placebo, as contrasted with 53%, 54% and 57% completing in the 25, 50, and 100 mg eq. groups, respectively.

At end point (LOCF), data analysis indicated significant differences between all of the paliperidone LAI groups and controls with regard to PANSS total scores and CGI-S scores. In terms of adverse events, significant weight gain occurred in 4% of paliperidone LAI subjects, as opposed to 0% of placebo subjects. Somnolence also occurred somewhat more frequently in paliperidone LAI subjects (4% vs. 1% for placebo); Parkinsonian symptoms occurred at virtually identical rates (6% and 5% for paliperidone and placebo subjects, respectively).

Fleischhacker et al. (2008) reported on a randomized, 53-week, multicentre trial of patients with acute exacerbations of schizophrenia that compared flexibly dosed paliperidone LAI (25, 50, 75, 100 mg. eq.) supplemented with oral placebo to flexibly dosed risperidone LAI supplemented with oral risperidone. All injections given during this study were gluteal. Following a screening/washout/oral tolerability test period of 7 days, the initiation dose for the paliperidone group was two 50 mg eq. injections 1 week apart, and injections then followed at 4-week intervals. For LAI risperidone, the subjects received a placebo injection at day 1, 25 mg risperidone LAI on days 8 and 22, then injections every 2 weeks (25, 37.5, or 50 mg). Oral risperidone supplementation was given for 4 weeks initially, and for 3 weeks after each dose increase of risperidone LAI. Of 749 patients randomized, 45% completed the entire 53-week trial (41% paliperidone LAI, 50% risperidone LAI).

Results of this study indicated both groups manifested improved PANSS total scores over the course of the trial, but the non-inferiority analysis indicated somewhat lower levels of improvement manifested by paliperidone LAI subjects, as compared to risperidone LAI subjects. Overall adverse event rates were similar (76% paliperidone LAI, 79% risperidone LAI) as were rates of AEs leading to discontinuation (7% and 6% for paliperidone LAI and risperidone LAI, respectively) and weight gain (both groups in the ± 1 kg average weight change range). Relative to the finding regarding less improvement in the paliperidone LAI group, pharmacokinetic data collected during the study indicated that plasma concentrations of paliperidone in paliperidone LAI subjects lagged behind those of the risperidone LAI group, such that subjects on 50 mg eq. paliperidone LAI did not achieve comparable plasma levels until day 260. The authors speculated that this may have resulted from the study employing lower initiation (loading) doses of paliperidone LAI (i.e. 50 mg eq. at day 1 and 8) compared to the higher doses (150 and 100 mg eq.) subsequently approved by the FDA. Another possible explanation is that the gluteal injection site was used for all injections, including the two initiation injections, and this site provides slower release than the deltoid injection site.

In a companion study to test the hypothesis that an initial deltoid, rather than gluteal injection would result in more rapid achievement of therapeutic plasma levels of paliperidone, Pandina et al. (2009) conducted an investigation that entailed a 7-day screening/washout/oral tolerability period, followed by randomization to a placebo control group, or three groups that received day 1 deltoid injections of 150 mg eq. paliperidone LAI (1 or 1.5 inch needles were used depending on subject body weight). These groups then subsequently received injections (on days 8, 36, and 64) of 150, 100, or 25 mg eq. paliperidone LAI, in either deltoid or gluteal sites, at the discretion of the investigator. All patients in this study carried schizophrenia diagnoses and were experiencing a symptom exacerbation. The double-blind phase of the study was conducted over a 13-week interval. In all, 652 subjects were randomly assigned.

Results of this study indicated that within the first 8 days after having received the deltoid injection of 150 mg eq. of drug, mean PANSS total scores decreased sharply, and by end point all three paliperidone LAI groups differed significantly from placebo although the 100 mg eq. and 150 mg eq. groups improved more over the course of the study than the 25 mg eq. group. An examination of treatment emergent adverse effects (TEAEs) revealed similar rates across all groups (60% vs.63% vs. 65% for the paliperidone LAI and placebo groups, respectively). Serious TEAEs occurred more frequently in the placebo group than in the paliperidone LAI groups (14% vs. 8% to 13%, respectively).

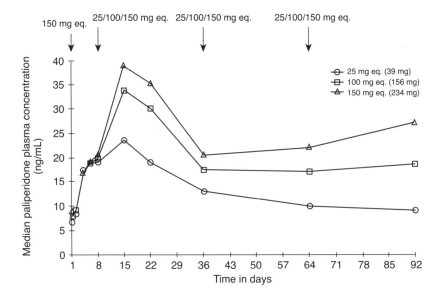

Fig. 6.2 Plasma concentrations following initiation (loading) dose of paliperidone palmitate (day 1) followed by successive injections (day 8, 36, and 64) with three doses of paliperidone palmitate.
Reproduced from Pandiana et al. (2009) with permission from the author.

Consistent with these findings, pharmacokinetic data revealed that following the initial 150 mg deltoid injection, subjects' paliperidone plasma levels reached what apparently was a therapeutic level by day 8, and remained relatively stable for each of the three groups that received paliperidone LAI for the duration of the study (Figure 6.2).

Approval status and formulation

Currently, paliperidone LAI is approved in the United States for the acute and maintenance treatment of schizophrenia. Pre-filled syringes are available in unit doses ranging from 39 mg to 234 mg.

Olanzapine long-acting injection

It would be fair to say that the SGA olanzapine, developed by Eli Lilly under the proprietary name Zyprexa®, has been an important, if not sometimes controversial, medication. Orally administered olanzapine became commercially available in 1996, and a series of clinical trials have established its effectiveness in the treatment of schizophrenia (Davis et al. 2003) and subsequently in the treatment of bipolar disorder (Tohen et al. 2003). However, early after olanzapine's introduction concern arose over excessive weight gain in patients and subsequently about glycemic and metabolic effects either primary or secondary to weight gain (Newcomer 2005). Indeed, the marketing of several other oral SGAs highlighted their reduced weight and metabolic liabilities compared to olanzapine.

In practice, matters are not quite as simple; although mean weight gain and mean elevation of glucose and lipids are greater with olanzapine than many antipsychotics, there is a marked individual variation in the extent of these adverse effects and not all patients experience significant weight gain or metabolic disturbance with olanzapine. Furthermore, other antipsychotics can cause weight gain and metabolic disturbance in vulnerable individuals. Most important, patients show different symptomatic responses to different antipsychotics, emphasizing the need for a range of available treatments. For these reasons the introduction of olanzapine in a long-acting form, despite its adverse effects, is a useful development as it increases the choices available to patients and clinicians.

Olanzapine LAI was recently approved in Europe and the United States as well as in several other countries. In the following sections we review the current data regarding its efficacy and side-effect profile, including the post-injection syndrome.

Pharmacokinetics

Olanzapine LAI or Olanzapine pamoate is a crystal salt made up of olanzapine and pamoic acid. Pamoic Acid salts are seen in other medical drugs, including hydroxyzine pamoate and imipramine pamoate. The crystals are suspended in water and the resulting compound has a distinct neon yellow colour. Each 15 mg of olanzapine LAI must be dissolved in 0.1 ml of water. Standard clinical practice limits any individual intramuscular injection dose to approximately 3.0 ml of solution or 450 mg per dose (Eli Lilly 2008). Patients can be switched abruptly from oral olanzapine to olanzapine LAI without the need for oral olanzapine supplementation at the start of treatment with the LAI. An initiation or loading strategy is recommended for the first two months before the dose of olanzapine LAI is reduced (Eli Lilly et al 2010). The recommended dosing scheme when switching between oral olanzapine and olanzapine LAI is given in table 6.3. Another way to estimate equivalency between maintenance doses of olanzapine LAI and oral olanzapine is to simply divide the injection dose by the interval in days (e.g. 210 mg/14 days = 15 mg/day, 300 mg/2 weeks =20 mg/day, and 405 mg/4 weeks = 15 mg/day.)

When injected into muscle, olanzapine LAI slowly breaks down into the original constituents, olanzapine and pamoic acid, and both are distributed into the circulation. This rate of dissolution is slow, allowing a dosing interval from 2 to 4 weeks.

Table 6.3 Dosing of olanzapine LAI based on correspondence to oral olanzapine dose (Eli Lilly and Company 2010)

Target oral olanzapine dose	Dosing of olanzapine LAI during the first 8 weeks	Maintenance dose after 2 months of treatment with olanzapine LAI
10 mg/day	210 mg/2 weeks or 405 mg/4 weeks	150 mg/2 weeks or 300 mg/4 weeks
15 mg/day	300 mg/2 weeks	210 mg/2 weeks or 405 mg/4 weeks
20 mg/day	300 mg/2 weeks	300mg/2 weeks

Randomized clinical trials

To date two randomized clinical trials of the efficacy of olanzapine LAI have been published (Kane et. al., 2009; Lauriello et al. 2008). Lauriello et al. (2008) randomly assigned patients with schizophrenia diagnoses, male or female, 18 to 75 years old, to receive 210 mg/2 weeks, 300 mg/2 weeks, or 405 mg/4 weeks olanzapine LAI, or a placebo for 8 weeks. Patients received either active or placebo injections every 2 weeks, those randomized to 405 mg/4 weeks received placebo injections at every other 2-week intervals.

The study included 404 subjects conducted from June 2004 to April 2005 in the United States ($N = 315$), Russia ($N = 61$), and Croatia ($N = 28$). All subjects were obligated to remain hospitalized for the first 2 weeks and then discharged if appropriate. Most patients (83%) stayed in the hospital for the entire 8-week period. Patients were pre-selected for moderate-to-high levels of symptom severity as measured by the BPRS, but individuals with significant risk of harm to self or others, or substance dependence within 30 days of study entry were excluded. In contrast to the risperidone LAI pivotal trials, patients were not allowed antipsychotic supplementation or cross titration and were placed directly on their assigned treatment. Concomitant psychotropic medications were restricted to benzodiazepines/sedative hypnotics and anticholinergic rescue medications as warranted.

The primary efficacy measurement was mean baseline to end of the 8 weeks PANSS scores, utilizing an LOCF analysis. Secondary efficacy measures included the PANSS positive, negative, and general subscales as well as PANSS-derived BPRS scores and CGI-Severity of Illness scale. Clinical improvement was defined as a CGI score of less than or equal to 3 ('minimal improvement'). An a priori 40% or greater reduction in the total PANSS score was set as a response cut-off.

Mean baseline-to-end point decreases in PANSS total scores were significantly greater for all of the olanzapine LAI regimens when compared to placebo. Reductions in PANSS scores were 22.5 in the 210 mg/2 weeks group, 26.3 in the 300 mg/2 weeks group, 22.6 in the 405 mg/4 weeks group, and 8.5 points in the placebo group. There was no significant statistical difference in active dose groups. Response to olanzapine LAI was relatively rapid, with separation from the placebo group as measured by the PANSS occurring within 3 to 7 days.

Measures of sedation and increased appetite were numerically greater in all the active treatment arms but met statistical significance only when the placebo and 300 mg/2 weeks groups were compared. Of the 25 sedation reports in the active arms, 11 occurred a day after the first injection, and none was rated as severe. Injection-site reactions were mild and at a low rate (3.6%), and did not lead to any patient discontinuations. Fasting glucose measures did not change over the 8-week trial. Hyperglycemia is generally understood to be a relatively late clinical event when it occurs. There was a statistical elevation in aspartate aminotransferase in the 300 mg/2 week arm compared to placebo. This is not surprising because many SGAs show an initial rise in liver enzymes that resolves over the first few months. Mean baseline-to-end point weight gain across all the olanzapine LAI groups differed significantly from placebo; 4.8 kg in the 210 mg/2 weeks group, 3.8 kg in the 300 mg/2 weeks group, 3.9 kg in the 405 mg/4 weeks group, and 0.3 kg in the placebo group. No significant group differences were noted in electrocardiogram data. Extrapyramidal symptoms were low at the start of the study and there were minimal elevations during the study as measured by the AIMS, SAS, and BAS.

The second study has been published recently by Kane et al. (2009). The design entailed random assignments to five treatment groups, including doses of olanzapine LAI of 405 mg/4 weeks ('high' dose), 300 mg/2 weeks ('medium dose'), 150 mg/ 2 weeks ('low'dose), 45 mg/4 weeks ('very low dose'), or a final group that received an oral olanzapine dose of 10 to 20 mg per day. The 45 mg/4-week treatment regimen was a sub-therapeutic dose of drug that was used for comparison purposes and substituted for a placebo control group. Subjects comprised patients with schizophrenia diagnoses who at the time of randomization were on oral olanzapine and clinically stable.

Comparisons between groups over a 24-week period focused on several measures of time to exacerbation of symptoms, including comparisons of BPRS scores recorded periodically during the course of the study to BPRS scores at baseline and the incidence of hospitalization. Over the course of the evaluation period, the number of patients free of exacerbation was 93% for patients receiving oral olanzapine, 95% for the high-dose group, 90% for the medium-dose group, and 84% for the low-dose group, as contrasted with a rate of 69% for the very low-dose group. Time to exacerbation was longer for all three standard LAI groups (high, medium, and low) relative to the very low-reference group. Furthermore, all three standard dose long-acting groups showed superiority to the very low-dose group in terms of PANSS total score baseline-to-end point changes. From the standpoint of PANSS total score ranges, all three standard dose long-acting groups, together with the oral treatment group, maintained mean PANSS total scores in the mid-50s, indicating sufficient symptom control, whereas the very low-dose group evinced significant worsening over time, with PANSS total scores increasing into the mid-60s.

Partial data are also available on a third study that appears to have recruited patients from the two randomized clinical trials reported above into a long-term safety and efficacy study with a planned follow-up period of 4 years (Eli Lilly; FDA Briefing Document 2008). This design involved starting all study participants on 210 mg of olanzapine LAI for the first injection period, which was of 2 weeks duration. Following that, a flexible dosing schedule is being used, confined within the range of 45 to 405 mg in terms of dose, with time intervals ranging from 2 to 4 weeks.

The first interim report on this study, which included 880 patients, indicated a small but statistically significant decrease in PANSS total scores, demonstrating that patients remained stable and minimally symptomatic; analysis of CGI scores indicated persistence of effect, with low levels of rated symptom severity. All-cause discontinuation data based on Kaplan–Meier estimates projecting over an 18-month period produced estimates of 27.8% and 34% at 12 and 18 months, respectively. These rates compare favourably with the CATIE study, in which the rate of discontinuation at 18 months for oral olanzapine, which had the lowest rate of discontinuation of all the antipsychotics evaluated, was 64% (Lieberman et al. 2005).

Post-injection syndrome

In the pre-marketing phase of development for olanzapine LAI a unique post-injection phenomenon occurred that has been termed Post-Injection Syndrome (PIS) or

Post-Injection Delirium Sedation Syndrome (PDSS)—also described in Chapter 3 of this book. The first reported case illustrates many of the hallmark signs and symptoms as reported in the FDA Briefing Document (Eli Lilly 2008). Below is an abridged description:

> Patient was a 31-year-old male who began to experience severe sedation 45 minutes after his second injection of 300 mg/4 weeks. The patient experienced weakness, sleepiness, and tension in his legs; he was slightly disoriented, spoke briefly, and immediately fell asleep. Six hours after the injection he was still experiencing sleepiness. Olanzapine plasma concentration measured at 6 hours post-injection were unexpectedly elevated. The next day the sedation had decreased in severity to mild. Sedation was fully resolved after 48 hours after the injection. The patient completed the 6-month study at a lower dose of 200 mg/4 weeks.

Similar presentations were seen in subsequent patients, some with agitation significant enough to merit sedation in several cases. Nearly 80% of the cases were hospitalized for observation and supportive care. Two cases required proactive intubation to allow adequate control of the agitation; there were no cases of respiratory depression. All patients' PDSS resolved within 72 hours. Seventy per cent of the patients remained on olanzapine LAI post-event.

An analysis of trial data available as of May 2008 showed that 29 PDSS events had occurred in 28 patients (one patient had two events). The rate per injection was approximately 29 out of 40 000 injections equivalent to a rate of 0.07% (Citrome 2009). This translated to a 1% rate in patients enrolled in all studies to date.

As described in the case vignette above, the symptoms of PDSS appear to mimic those of an olanzapine overdose. Symptoms include sedation, dizziness, slurred speech, agitation, confusion, ataxia, weakness, and unconsciousness. The vast majority of cases occurred within the first hour post-injection with some progressing from mild to more severe presentations. There does not appear to be a period of unique liability to PDSS, with episodes occurring from the first to as late as the sixty-sixth injection. With the possible exception of one case, symptom onset was within the first 3 hours post-injection.

Measurement of vital signs did not show any significant perturbations of heart rate, blood pressure, or respiration. There does not appear to be any relationship between occurrence and specific gender, race, or concomitant medication; in short, it appears that that predicting new cases is very challenging.

The presumed mechanism for PDSS lies in the difference in solubility of olanzapine LAI in blood compared to its solubility in muscle. When exposed to blood, olanzapine LAI is highly soluble, and it is theorized that this leads to the elevation in olanzapine blood level (Psychopharmacologic Drugs Advisory Committee, Eli Lilly, 2008). Figure 6.3 shows the olanzapine blood levels in one of the patients who had a PDSS, in which blood levels were sampled before and after the event.

Of special note is the high peak of olanzapine after the injection that immediately preceded the PDSS event. Although not completely proven, it is hypothesized that the event is caused either by a direct or by a partial injection into the vasculature or bleeding around the injection site leading to direct contact between olanzapine LAI and blood.

Because each injection has the potential for inadvertent vascular injection, continued good clinical practice for injection technique (i.e. syringe aspiration to check for blood) must always be maintained. In addition, there are specific requirements in the product

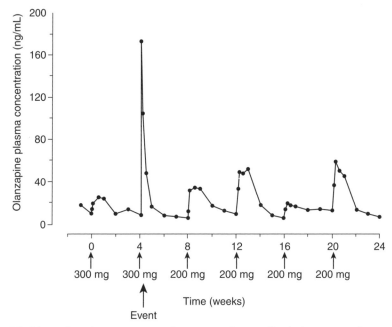

Fig. 6.3 Olanzapine plasma-concentrations versus time profile during a case of
post-injection delirium sedation syndrome
Figure reproduced from FDA website (http://www.fda.gov) accessed May 2010.

license to help manage the risk of PDSS. These are discussed in the next section and include
an observation period of at least 3 hours in a healthcare facility after each injection.

Approval status

Olanzapine LAI is approved in the European Union under the brand name Zypadhera
for maintenance treatment of adults with schizophrenia who have been sufficiently
stabilized during acute treatment with oral olanzapine. Currently olanzapine LAI is
marketed in Ireland, Finland, Germany, Norway, and Denmark with other European
countries to follow. As a condition for European Union approval, Eli Lilly has developed
a risk minimization plan for identifying and managing PDSS (European Medicines
Agency 2008). The plan includes health care provider training and education and
specific requirements for the administration of olanzapine LAI. The latter include
the patient being observed in a healthcare facility, by an appropriately qualified
person, for at least 3 hours after each injection for signs and symptoms consistent with
PDSS. If PDSS is suspected, medical supervision and monitoring should continue until
all symptoms have resolved. Patients should not travel home alone after the injection.
For the reminder of the day after injection they should not drive or operate machinery,
and should be informed to be observant for symptoms of PDSS and be able to
obtain assistance if required (Eli Lilly and Company 2010; European Medicines
Agency 2008).

Olanzapine LAI has also been approved in the United States, Australia, and
New Zealand under the name Zyprexa Relprevv. As in Europe, there are specific

requirements to reduce the risk of harm associated with PDSS, including that patients are observed for at least 3 hours post-injection and are accompanied home. In addition, Eli Lilly agreed with the US FDA to develop a Risk Evaluation and Mitigation Strategy (REMS). This includes a patient medication guide and a mandatory patient registry, which restricts prescribing to enrolled clinicians and pharmacies.

Conclusions

The introduction of paliperidone LAI and olanzapine LAI are significant pharmaco-therapeutic developments. Each antipsychotic offers the advantages of up to once a month injection intervals—an improvement over twice monthly risperidone LAI. Paliperidone LAI was developed in part to overcome some of the problems seen with risperidone LAI, especially the need to supplement risperidone LAI for at least 3 weeks with oral medication. Olanzapine LAI offers an alternative for those patients who have had a good response to oral olanzapine but have a history of poor adherence. In addition, there are clearly a number of patients who do not tolerate or respond to the risperidone family of medications and may respond to olanzapine and vice versa. Olanzapine LAI poses a unique challenge in its association with PDSS, but risk mitigation programmes should allow its use. Although the addition of these two medications is long overdue, the psychiatric field is in need of more long-acting antipsychotics and several others are in development, including an LAI of aripiprazole. These are welcome events as they increase the choice of medications available to patients and clinicians.

References

Berwaerts J, Cleton A, Rossenu S, Talluri K, Remmerie B, Janssens L, et al. (2009). A comparison of serum prolactin concentrations after administration of paliperidone extended-release and risperidone tablets in patients with schizophrenia. *J Psychopharmacol,* 2009 Oct 13 [Epub ahead of print].

Citrome L. (2008). Olanzapine pamoate: a stick in time? A review of the efficacy and safety profile of a new depot formulation of a second-generation antipsychotic. *Int J Clin Prac,* **63**, 140–50.

Correll CU, Leucht S, Kane JM. (2004). Lower risk for tardive dyskinesia associated with second-generation antipsychotics: A systematic review of 1-year studies. *Am J Psychiatry,* **161**, 414–25.

Davis JM, Chen N, Glick ID. (2003). A meta-analysis of the efficacy of second-generation antipsychotics. *Arch Gen Psychiatry,* **60**, 553–64.

Eli Lilly and Company (3 January 2008). *Zyprexa Olanzapine Pamoate (OP) Depot, Psychopharmacological Drugs Advisory Committee Briefing Document.* http://www.fda.gov/ ohrms/dockets/ac/08/briefing/2008-4338b1-03-Lilly.pdf (accessed 20 May 2010).

Eli Lilly and Company (2010). Zypadhera (olanzapine pamoate) Summary of Product Characteristics. Electronic Medicines Compendium. Electronic Medicines Compendium.http://www.medicines.org.uk/emc/medicine/21361/SPC/ZYPADHERA

European Medicines Agency. (2008). Pre-authorisation evaluation of medicines for human use. Assessment report for Zypadhera. International Nonproprietary Name: olanzapine. London: EMEA.

Fleischhacker WW, Gopal S, Samtani MN, Quiroz JA, Pandina G, Vermeulen A, et al. (2008). Optimization of the dosing strategy for the long-acting injectable antipsychotic paliperidone palmitate: Results of two randomized double-blind studies and population pharmacokinetic simulations. Poster presented at the American College of Neuropsychopharmacology, Dec.6–11, 2008.

Fleischhacker WW. (2009). Second-generation antipsychotic long-acting injections: Systematic review. *Br J Psychiatry* **195** (suppl 52) S20–28.

Hough D, Gopal S, Vijapukar U, Lim P, Morozova M, Eerdekens M. (2010). Paliperidone palmitate maintenance treatment in delaying the time-to-relapse in patients with schizophrenia: a randomized, double-blind, placebo-controlled study. *Schizophr Res,* **116**, 107–17.

IMS MIDAS. [Internet]. IMS Health, Inc. Available from http://www.ims-international.com (accessed 20 May 2010).

Janssen, Division of Ortho-McNeil-Janssen Pharmaceuticals, Inc (2010), Invega® Sustenna® (paliperidone palmitate) Extended-Release Injectable Suspension. United States Prescribing information. Available from: http://www.invegasustenna.com/invegasustenna/shared/pi/invegasustenna.pdf (accessed August 2010).

Kane JM, Detke HC, Naber D, Sethuraman G, Lin DY, Bergstrom RF, et al. (2009). Olanzapine long-acting injection: a 24-week, randomized, double-blind trial of maintenance treatment in patients with schizophrenia. *Am J Psychiatry,* **167**(2), 181–9.

Kramer M, Litman R, Hough D, Lane R, Lim P, Liu Y, Eerdekens M. (2009). Paliperidone palmitate, a potential long-acting treatment for patients with schizophrenia. Results of a randomized, double-blind, placebo-controlled efficacy and safety study. *Int J Neuropsychopharmacol,* **13**, 635–47.

Lauriello J, Lambert T, Andersen S, Lin D, Taylor CC, Mcdonnell D. (2008). An 8-week, double-blind, randomized, placebo-controlled study of olanzapine long-acting injection in acutely ill patients with schizophrenia. *J Clin Psychiatry,* **69**, 790–9.

Leucht S, Corves C, Arbter D, Engel RR, Li C, Davis JM. (2009). Second generation versus first-generation antipsychotic drugs for schizophrenia: a meta-analysis. *Lancet,* **373**(9657), 31–41.

Lieberman JA, Bymaster FP, Meltzer HY, Deutch AY, Duncan GE, Marx CE, et al. (2008). Antipsychotic drugs: comparison in animal models of efficacy, neurotransmitter regulation, and neuroprotection. *Pharmacoly Rev,* **60**(3), 358–403.

Lieberman JA, Stroup TS, McEvoy JP, Swartz MS, Rosenheck RA, Perkins DO, et al. for Clinical Antipsychotic Trials of Intervention Effectiveness (CATIE) Investigators. (2005). Effectiveness of antipsychotic drugs in patients with chronic schizophrenia. *N Engl J Med,* **353**, 1209–23.

Nasrallah HA, Gopal S, Quiroz JA, Gassmann-Mayer C, Lim P, Eerdekens M, et al. (2008). Efficacy and safety of three doses of paliperidone palmitate, an investigational long acting injectable antipsychotic, in schizophrenia [poster]. Presented at American Psychiatric Association 161st Annual Meeting; Washington, DC; May 3–8.

Newcomer JW. (2005). Second-generation (atypical) antipsychotics and metabolic effects: A comprehensive literature review. *CNS Drugs,* **19**, 1–93.

Pandina GJ. Lindenmayer J-P, Lull J, Lim P, Gopal S, et al. (2009). A randomized, placebo-controlled study to assess the efficacy and safety of three doses of paliperidone palmitate in adults with an acute exacerbation of schizophrenia. Presented at the International Congress on Schizophrenia Research. San Diego, CA: 28 March –1 April 2009.

Tohen M, Ketter TA, Zarate CA, Suppes T, Frye M, Altshuler L, et al. (2003). Olanzapine versus divalproex sodium for the treatment of acute mania and maintenance of remission: A 47-week study. *Am J Psychiatry,* **160**(7), 1263–71.

Chapter 7

Long-acting injectable antipsychotics in early psychosis

Robin Emsley, Bonga Chiliza, Laila Asmal, and Mathias de Fleuriot

Correspondence: rae@sun.ac.za

Introduction

Traditionally antipsychotic long-acting injections (LAIs) or depots have primarily been used as maintenance agents in patients with schizophrenia who have repeatedly relapsed owing to poor adherence with oral antipsychotic medication. Usually these patients have suffered from schizophrenia for many years, and many have accrued marked social disabilities owing to their illness. Recently there has been increased interest in using LAIs early in the course of schizophrenia. In this chapter we explore the rationale for this and then review the key studies of LAIs that have been conducted in this group.

Schizophrenia imposes a disproportionate burden on patients, their families, health care systems, and society because of its early onset, devastating effects, and usually life-long course (Mueser & McGurk 2004). Referred to as 'youth's greatest disabler', its onset is typically in adolescence or early adulthood (WHO,2008.http://www.searo.who.int/en/section1174/section1199/section1567_6744.htm.internet.RefType:ElectronicCitation). An encouraging development has been the increased research attention that is focusing on aspects such as identifying high-risk individuals prior to the onset of frank psychosis, treatment strategies for preventing such individuals from undergoing transition to psychosis, shortening the period between the onset of psychotic illness and initiation of effective treatment, and providing comprehensive management for individuals with a first episode of psychosis. There is a growing body of evidence to indicate that prompt diagnosis and effective management are of critical importance in achieving optimal long-term outcomes, at least in the short term (McGorry et al. 2005).

It is during the early stages of illness that patients are particularly responsive to treatment (Lieberman et al. 1993). For example, Robinson et al. (1999b) reported that 87% of their first-episode cohort had achieved a clinical response (much or very much improved) in the first year of treatment, with a median time of 8 weeks to response. In addition to their more favourable response to antipsychotic treatment, young individuals in the early stages of the illness are likely to be more integrated into aspects of society such as families, relationships, schools, and employment. However, despite the favourable initial response to treatment, the longer-term outcome remains poor.

In the same cohort mentioned above, after 5 years of treatment only 47% had achieved symptom remission, 26% had adequate social functioning, and 13.7% met full recovery criteria (symptomatic and functional) for 2 years or longer (Robinson et al. 2004). The problem therefore is not so much in achieving a response but in maintaining it. This same point was demonstrated in a secondary analysis that was conducted on a large sample of early psychosis patients ($N = 462$) who had participated in a multinational, randomized controlled trial comparing oral risperidone and haloperidol. At some time point in the study 323 (70%) of the 462 subjects had a reduction to mild levels on the key symptoms as measured by the Positive and Negative Syndrome Scale (PANSS), indicating a robust initial response to treatment. However, only 109 (23.6%) were able to maintain this level of improvement for at least 6 months to meet operationally defined criteria for remission (Emsley et al. 2007). Results of these research studies mirror the high rates of relapse and partial response that are observed in clinical practice.

Relapse and medication adherence

Relapse rates are very high in the early stages of schizophrenia. In the Robinson et al. (1999a) cohort the cumulative first-relapse rate was 82% after 5 years, with the vast majority of these patients going on to experience multiple relapses. These high-relapse rates are likely to be closely associated with non-adherence and partial adherence to medication. Discontinuation of antipsychotic medication was found to be the strongest predictor of relapse by far in this study, increasing the risk nearly fivefold (Robinson et al. 1999a). In another study of first-episode patients in a clinical setting, it was found that in the first year of treatment 39% were non-adherent and a further 20% were judged to be inadequately adherent (assessed as taking <70% of their prescribed medication). Non-adherent patients were more symptomatic and experienced more relapses. They also had poorer insight, more substance abuse, and poorer quality of life (Coldham et al. 2002). However, the true extent of poor medication adherence is likely to be even greater than is reported in the literature, as all of the current methods of assessing adherence are likely to underestimate its prevalence (Velligan et al. 2006).

Poor medication adherence is one of the most important potentially modifiable barriers to a favourable outcome in schizophrenia. Therefore it would seem prudent for clinicians to focus attention on all possible methods of improving adherence. There are multiple factors that determine medication adherence, some of which may be unique to early psychosis patients. In a secondary analysis of data from first-episode patients who participated in a 52-week randomized, controlled trial comparing the oral second-generation antipsychotics (SGAs) olanzapine, quetiapine, and risperidone, 115 of 400 (29%) patients discontinued treatment against medical advice (Perkins et al. 2008). Factors associated with poor adherence were substance abuse, persistent depression, poor treatment response, higher cognitive performance, ethnicity (black), and achieving remission status. Experiencing side-effects was not associated with poor adherence (Perkins et al. 2008). These risk factors differ somewhat from those reported for poor adherence in multi-episode samples (Perkins 2002). In particular, the associations with higher cognitive function and achieving remission status have not been described in other samples. It may be that after a single psychotic episode patients who respond well and have good cognitive function may believe that they have recovered and are not in need of ongoing treatment.

It was hoped that the introduction of the SGAs, with their relatively low risk of extrapyramidal symptoms, would improve adherence. However, although they have been reported to be moderately more effective than the first-generation antipsychotics (FGAs) in reducing relapse rates in schizophrenia, they have not been shown to significantly improve patient adherence (Diaz et al. 2004).

Partial adherence and partial response

Apart from the risk of relapse, inadequate or partial medication adherence is likely to lead to incomplete or partial response to treatment. Patients who experience persistent symptoms and fail to achieve sustained remission have been referred to as partial responders and may represent the majority of patients with schizophrenia seen in an outpatient setting (Breier et al. 1994).

Consequences of relapse and partial response

There is now considerable evidence indicating that schizophrenia is a progressive brain disease. First, neuroimaging studies indicate that, contrary to an earlier belief that structural brain changes in schizophrenia are static, progressive loss of brain matter occurs, with accelerated loss of particularly frontal and temporal brain matter over time (Hulshoff Pol & Kahn 2008). The loss appears most pronounced in patients with a poorer outcome (Cahn et al. 2009). Second, studies of the relationship between duration of untreated psychosis (DUP) and outcome in schizophrenia indicate a significant association between longer DUP and poorer outcome. This association has been shown to be independent of other possible confounders such as pre-morbid adjustment (Marshall et al. 2005). Third, there is also some evidence to suggest that relapses may result in progressive deterioration in the level of functioning. The first few years of the illness have been proposed as a 'critical period' during which an aggressive relapsing course may lead to accruing morbidity and persistent deficits (Birchwood et al. 1998). Each relapse from a remitted state may be associated with a substantial risk of incomplete remission and persisting disability (Wiersma et al. 1998).

Regardless of the putative neurodegenerative consequences of relapse, the psychosocial consequences are extremely important, particularly in the early stages of the illness. Young individuals recovering from a first psychotic illness often have 'more to lose' than multi-episode patients as they are more frequently still living with their families, have friendships and relationships, are at school or college, or are employed. Whether through neurodegenerative effects or psychosocial consequences, relapse or a partial response to treatment may have devastating effects including evolving treatment refractoriness and poor overall outcome, psychiatric and general medical complications, and death from co-morbid medical conditions or suicide. For these reasons vigorous efforts to achieve and maintain remission should begin immediately after the first episode (Kane 2006).

Antipsychotic LAIs

The LAIs of antipsychotics, or depots, were developed in the 1960s, specifically to address the problem of poor adherence in the maintenance treatment of psychosis. The single most important advantage of LAIs over their oral counterparts is that they provide assured medication delivery, thereby effectively addressing the problem of covert non-adherence or partial adherence. First-generation antipsychotic long-acting injections (FGA-LAIs) have been demonstrated to be superior to oral FGAs, although the evidence was not always clear-cut (Kane et al. 2003). These agents were used extensively in many countries. However, they were traditionally reserved for patients who were known to be, or suspected to be poorly adherent, uncooperative, or refractory to treatment and in the chronic phase of the illness (Emsley et al. 2008c). Furthermore, the considerable safety and tolerability concerns with the FGA-LAIs, particularly with regard to extrapyramidal symptoms (EPS) and tardive dyskinesia (TD) limited their use once the oral SGAs became available. These agents offered clinicians another treatment option, and FGA-LAIs, despite their adherence advantages, never came to be considered as a first-line or even early treatment option. The availability of second-generation antipsychotics long-acting injections (SGA-LAIs) (currently risperidone, olanzapine, and paliperidone with aripiprazole in development) offers further options, combining the low EPS risk of SGAs with adherence benefits of an LAI preparation.

Rationale for using antipsychotic LAIs in the early stages of schizophrenia

Patients who are in the early stages of their illness may be ideal candidates for treatment with an antipsychotic LAI, as poor adherence is a major problem in the early stages of the illness (Coldham et al. 2002) and relapse rates are very high (Robinson et al. 1999a). Modern public health principles dictate early intervention and prevention of accruing morbidity. It makes good sense therefore to intervene with an agent designed to improve adherence and reduce the risk of relapse *before* such relapses occur. Why wait for patients to 'prove' that they are poorly adherent and suffer the consequences of relapse? Another possible advantage of antipsychotic LAIs is that they may be associated with fewer side-effects than their oral counterparts owing to their different pharmacokinetic profile. Antipsychotic LAIs achieve steady state at lower doses, and without the large fluctuations observed with oral medication, thus avoiding the peaks and troughs associated with oral antipsychotics—the high peak values have been associated with an increased risk of some side-effects (e.g. EPs and prolactin elevation; Ereshefsky & Mannaert 2005). Improved tolerability would be particularly useful for patients in the early stages of the illness as these young and antipsychotic medication naïve patients are very sensitive to the effects of antipsychotics (Chatterjee et al. 1995). In the following two sections we review key studies that have investigated FGA-LAIs and risperidone long-acting injections (SGA-LAIs) in early psychosis.

Studies of FGA-LAIs in early psychosis

Given the fact that depot antipsychotics or LAIs have not traditionally been regarded as first-line treatment for schizophrenia it is not surprising that there are only a few studies investigating the use of these agents in the early stages of the illness.

In an early study evaluating an FGA-oral and an FGA-LAI, 28 patients who had recovered from an acute first-episode of schizophrenia were randomized to either fluphenazine hydrochloride, fluphenazine decanoate, or placebo for a 12-month period in a double-blinded study. Seven of the 17 patients (41%) who received placebo experienced a relapse, whereas none of the 11 fluphenazine-treated patients relapsed. Eighteen (69%) of 26 patients who were available for follow-up (mean interval, 3.5 years) experienced a second relapse, and 14 (50%) of the original sample experienced a third relapse. Six patients receiving fluphenazine discontinued (3 owing to adverse events and 3 owing to withdrawal of consent) compared with seven in the placebo group (all owing to withdrawal of consent; Kane et al. 1982). The small sample size and the combined reporting of oral and depot fluphenazine results in the study make it difficult to draw any firm conclusions.

In a prospective cohort study using national central registers in Finland, the association between prescribed antipsychotic drugs and outcome was investigated. The sample comprised 2230 consecutive first hospitalizations owing to schizophrenia and schizoaffective disorder. Initial use of clozapine (adjusted relative risk 0.17, 95% CI 0.10–0.29), perphenazine depot (0.24, 95% CI 0.13–0.47), and olanzapine (0.35, 95% CI 0.18–0.71) were associated with the lowest rates of discontinuation for any reason and current use of perphenazine depot (0.32, 95% CI 0.22–0.49), olanzapine (0.54, 95% CI 0.41–0.71), and clozapine (0.64, 95% CI 0.48–0.85) were associated with the lowest risk of rehospitalization (Tiihonen et al. 2006).

We are currently conducting an open-label, non-comparative, prospective study of patients with first-episode psychosis treated with flupentixol decanoate, a long-acting FGA, according to a fixed protocol over 12 to 24 months. Inclusion criteria are DSM IV diagnosis of schizophrenia, schizophreniform disorder, or schizoaffective disorder for no more than 12 months, age 16 to 45 years, and with less than 12 weeks of cumulative lifelong exposure to antipsychotics. Exclusion criteria were another Axis I diagnosis including substance dependence or abuse; the need for mood stabilizers or antidepressants at enrolment; serious or unstable medical illness; or previous depot antipsychotic treatment. Subjects initially received oral flupentixol 1 to 3 mg/day for 7 days. On day 7 the first injection of 10 mg of flupentixol decanoate was given and subsequently every 2 weeks. The dose could be increased to 40 mg 2-weekly if required. Interim results from the first 20 participants over the first 3 months have been reported. Mean±SD PANSS total scores reduced by 41% from 104±20 at baseline to 60 at 3 months. The mean CGI-S scores improved from 5±4 at baseline to 3±1 at 3 months. The Calgary Depression Scale for Schizophrenia (CDSS) scores reduced from 4.4± 4.0 at baseline to 0.9±2.0 at 3 months. The mean Extrapyramidal Symptom Rating Scale (ESRS) scores were 9.9±6.5 at baseline and 8.1±8.1 at 3 months. The highest mean ESRS score was 14.0±8.7 at 4 weeks. Mean weight and BMI at baseline were

59.8±11.5 kg and 22.4±4.7 kg/m² respectively, and mean weight and BMI at 3 months were 63.8 ±11.5 kg and 23.9±4.5 kg/m². Although these results are preliminary, overall the treatment of first-episode psychosis patients with flupentixol decanoate appears to be effective and fairly well tolerated (Chiliza et al. 2008).

Studies of RLAI in early psychosis

The only SGA-LAI to have been studied in early psychosis is risperidone long-acting injection (RLAI), which has been investigated in several studies. In a secondary analysis of a larger study (Moller et al. 2005) conducted in Europe, the efficacy and safety of RLAI were investigated in a subset of patients in the early phases of schizophrenia and schizoaffective disorders (Parellada et al. 2005). Early phase was defined as 3 years or less and maximum allowed age was 45 years. Patients were included in the study if they had been symptomatically stable, treated with the same dose of an antipsychotic therapy for at least 1 month before study entry, and if the investigator felt that a treatment change was indicated. The main reasons for treatment change were non-compliance (42%) and insufficient efficacy (31%) of previous medication. Previous medications were mainly atypical antipsychotics (70%) and depot neuroleptics (24%). A total of 382 participants received 2-weekly gluteal injections of RLAI 25, 37.5, or 50 mg (without an oral risperidone run-in phase) over 6 months in an open-label design.

As many as 73% of patients completed the study. The reported reasons for discontinuation were as follows: withdrawal of consent (10%), adverse events (6%), insufficient response (4%), poor adherence (3%), lost to follow-up (3%), ineligibility to continue (<1%), and other reasons (2%). The total PANSS and all its subscale scores improved significantly ($p < .0001$) with 40% of patients showing more than 20% improvement on total PANSS. Global Assessment of Functioning, quality of life, and patient satisfaction also improved significantly. Tolerability of RLAI was generally good, and no unexpected adverse events were reported.

Most of the patients (88%) received a starting dose of 25 mg of RLAI. At the end of the 6-month study period, 45% were still on 25 mg, and 27% and 28% received 37.5 and 50 mg, respectively. Oral risperidone was prescribed as supplemental medication at some point for 73 (19%) patients. Of the 156 (41%) patients who were hospitalized at baseline, most (81%) had been discharged at end point. Eighteen patients (5%) were newly hospitalized during the study. Significant improvements in quality of life were recorded at each assessment point. Patient satisfaction with treatment improved significantly from baseline to end point.

The most frequently reported treatment emergent adverse events (AEs) were insomnia (7%) and exacerbation of psychosis (6%). Injection-site pain was reported by 6 patients (2%) and one (0.3%) had new-onset diabetes mellitus. There were six reports of sexual dysfunction; gynaecomastia, hyperprolactinaemia, and galactorrhoea were each reported by one patient. None of these AEs led to discontinuation from the study. ESRS total and subscale scores improved significantly from baseline to end point. Mean body weight and mean BMI increased by 1.8 kg and 0.6 kg/m², respectively, from baseline to end point ($p < .001$). The authors concluded that RLAI treatment was effective and well tolerated by these patients in the early stage of their illness. They suggested that RLAI might represent a novel option for patients in the early phases of schizophrenia and schizoaffective disorder but cautioned that further studies need to be conducted in this patient population to draw firm conclusions.

In another secondary analysis of a larger 12-month, open-label study with RLAI (Fleischhacker et al. 2003) a subset of 100 young adults (men ≤ 25 years and women ≤ 30 years) was studied (Lasser et al. 2004). The completion rate was 58%. Reasons for discontinuation were insufficient response (9%), withdrawal of consent (15%), AEs (7%), poor adherence (3%), and other reasons (9%). PANSS total scores decreased from baseline to end point by −9.8±1.7 (p < .001) and clinical improvement (>20% reduction in PANSS total score) was seen in 62% of patients. The most commonly reported AEs were insomnia (27%), psychosis (22%), anxiety (21%), depression (17%), and rhinitis (15%). Patient ratings of injection-site pain were made using a 100-mm visual analogue scale (0 = no pain; 100 = unbearably painful) and decreased from 23.3±21.7 to 14.4 ≤ 18.3 from baseline to end point. Significant reductions in ESRS scores were observed.

Preliminary results of an ongoing randomized controlled trial to compare RLAI with oral SGAs were presented in two posters at the 46th annual meeting of the ACNP (Schooler et al. 2007; Weiden et al. 2007). The study investigated patient acceptance and adherence behaviour during the first 12 weeks following randomization. Thirty-seven patients with first-episode schizophrenia, schizophreniform, or schizoaffective disorder were randomized in a 2:1 ratio to the recommendation of either RLAI (n = 26) or oral SGAs (n = 11). Eight patients refused maintenance medication (6 refused any medication and 2 refused injectable medication specifically). Adherence behaviour was measured using All Source Verification (ASV), which integrates information from pharmacy records, injection administration, oral medication administration (date of prescription), clinician, and family and patient report. Non-adherence was defined as a medication gap of 14 days or more. The sample comprised 76% males, with a median age of 23 years at first hospitalization. The likelihood of any medication gap during the first 12 weeks was 27%, emphasizing the fact that poor adherence is a problem from the outset. There were no significant differences between groups either in the intention to treat or in the treatment acceptor populations, although there was a difference based on verification of whether they actually accepted and received RLAI even during this initial 12-week interval. Most of the subjects (19 of 26, 73%) randomized to the RLAI recommendation accepted this recommendation. Of note was that almost all of these subjects were initially reluctant to accept an LAI but were willing to try upon completion of a tailored psycho-education programme. Although the results of this study are preliminary, they suggest that the majority of first-episode patients are willing to accept injectable formulations of medication if properly informed.

A prospective, naturalistic, controlled open-label study was conducted in 50 patients who were treated over 2 years either with RLAI (n = 22) or with oral risperidone (n = 28; Kim et al. 2008). Medication adherence and relapse rates were compared. There were no demographic or clinical differences between the treatment groups at baseline. There was a significantly lower relapse rate and higher adherence rate for the patients treated with RLAI compared with those treated with oral risperidone. Kaplan–Meier survival analysis indicated that time to non-adherence was greater with RLAI.

Cox proportional survival analysis revealed that the time from baseline to relapse was associated with time to non-adherence. The authors felt that the results of this study suggest that RLAI could be effective in maintaining medication adherence and preventing relapse.

Emsley et al. (2008c) conducted a study to assess whether RLAI could be used safely and effectively as a first-line treatment in first-episode psychosis This was a 24-month, single-site, open-label study. After pre-screening, 51 participants aged 15 to 43 years were entered into the study. One patient was excluded prior to receiving study treatment as he no longer met the inclusion criteria. Inclusion criteria were schizophrenia, schizophreniform disorder, or schizoaffective disorder for no more than 12 months, and with less than 12 weeks of cumulative exposure to antipsychotics. Patients were excluded if they had another Axis I diagnosis including substance dependence or abuse; required mood stabilizers or antidepressants at enrolment; had a serious or unstable medical illness; or had received previous depot antipsychotic treatment. All participants and in the case of minors their parents provided informed written consent before entering the study.

Participants initially underwent a 4- to 7-day drug washout period before receiving rapidly dissolving oro-dispersible risperidone 1 to 3 mg/day for 7 days. On day 7 the first injection of 25 mg of RLAI was given and subsequently every 2 weeks. Oro-dispersible risperidone was continued for a further 21 days after the first RLAI. RLAI dose could be increased to 37.5 mg and 50 mg if patients did not respond according to specific criteria. For acute exacerbations between the scheduled visits, oro-dispersible risperidone could be given at the investigator's discretion. Concomitant psychotropic medications allowed were orphenadrine or biperiden for EPS, propranolol for akathisia, and antidepressants for co-morbid depressive or anxiety disorders.

The study sample comprised 32 men and 18 women aged 25.3±7.3 years with schizophreniform disorder ($n = 23$) or schizophrenia ($n = 27$) and a mean duration of illness of 129±199 days. Most subjects ($n = 39$) were racially mixed and were antipsychotic naïve ($n = 27$). The completion rate for the 2-year study was 72%. Reasons for discontinuation were withdrawal of consent ($n = 5$), insufficient response ($n = 3$), subject relocated ($n = 3$), lost to follow-up ($n = 2$), and relapse ($n = 1$). Whereas 38 patients were hospitalized at baseline, only 6 were hospitalized at some later stage. The RLAI dose at the end of the study was 25 mg for 54% of patients, 37.5 mg for 30, and 50 mg for 16%.

PANSS total, positive, negative, and general psychopathology subscales as well as the Clinical Global Impressions Severity (CGI-S) and Change (CGI-C) scores, Social and Functional Assessment Scale (SOFAS), and Short Form-12 (SF-12) Mental Component all showed robust improvements. Clinical response defined as at least 20% or at least 50% reduction of baseline PANSS total scores was obtained by 84% and 78% of patients, respectively. The relapse rate in patients who had responded was 8% (Figure 7.1). Of note, no patient relapsed in the second year of the study. Low levels of EPS were observed. Mean maximum changes on the ESRS were as follows: ESRS total score 1.4 (SD 2.60; CI 0.61–2.10, $n = 50$), Parkinsonism subscale score 1.36 (SD 2.60; CI 0.62–2.10, $n = 50$), dystonia subscale score 0, dyskinesia subscale score 0.18 (SD 0.94; CI –0.09 to 0.45, $n = 50$), and akathisia score 10 (SD 0.54; CI –0.05 to 0.25, $n = 50$).

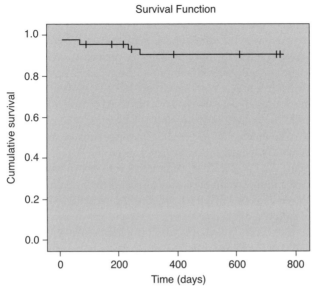

Fig. 7.1 Kaplan–Meier survival analysis of time to relapse in patients treated with risperidone long acting injection.
Reproduced with permission from Emsley et al. (2008) *J Clin Psychopharmacology* **28**, 210–13.

Anticholinergic medication was prescribed in 10 patients. One patient developed emergent, persistent dyskinesia. Considerable weight gain was observed, particularly in the first 12 months of treatment. This is consistent with the fact that first-episode patients appear to be particularly vulnerable to weight gain effects of antipsychotics (Strassnig et al. 2007). Blood glucose increases were reported in 2 patients, and cholesterol increases were reported in 5 patients. Eighteen patients had elevated prolactin levels, with four reporting prolactin-related AEs (amenorrhea, $n = 1$; galactorrhea, $n = 1$; both amenorrhea and galactorrhea, $n = 1$; and both amenorrhoea and delayed menses, $n = 1$). No injection site AEs were reported. Other observed AEs in at least 10% of patients at some stage in the study were headache ($n = 13$), sedation ($n = 9$), influenza ($n = 9$), aggression ($n = 6$), insomnia ($n = 5$), depression ($n = 5$), and psychotic disorder ($n = 5$). One patient suffered a cerebrovascular accident.

   This study has several limitations, particularly its open-label nature, the absence of a comparator, and the small sample. However, its strengths include the selection of a first-episode sample with limited antipsychotic exposure, use of operationalized and validated assessment instruments, the relatively long duration of the study, and the fact that antipsychotic medication was assured throughout. Although the results of this study need to be interpreted with caution, they do suggest that RLAI can be used safely and effectively as a first-line treatment in first-episode schizophrenia. Patients responded very well in terms of symptom reductions and functional outcome measures. The drug was generally well tolerated, although considerable weight gain and hyperprolactinaemia were observed. The high study retention rate suggests that RLAI is an effective method of keeping early psychosis patients in treatment.

In a secondary analysis in the same cohort, remission as an outcome measure was investigated (Emsley et al. 2008b). Specifically, rates, predictors, and clinical correlates of remission were examined. A definition for remission in schizophrenia proposed by the 'Remission in Schizophrenia Working Group' (RSWG; Andreasen et al. 2005) was used, where remission is defined according to a threshold of symptom severity (absent, borderline, or mild) for a minimum duration of 6 months. Whereas the definition is based purely on symptomatic improvement, achieving remission has been associated with other favourable outcomes including better social and occupational functioning (Helldin et al. 2007; van Os et al. 2006; Wunderink et al. 2007), fewer relapses, better quality of life, and a more favourable attitude towards their treatment (Emsley et al. 2007). Previously reported rates of remission according to the RSWG criteria in samples treated with oral antipsychotics range between 22% and 55% in multi-episode samples and between 23.6% and 48% in first-episode schizophrenia (Emsley et al. 2008b).

Thirty-two (64%) of the RLAI-treated patients achieved remission at some stage in the study. Of these, 31 (97%) maintained this status for the duration of the study. An additional three patients met symptom criteria for remission but not duration criteria. The median time until remission was 301 (standard error 0.77) days. Compared to the non-remission group, patients who achieved remission improved significantly more on CGI-S and PANSS total, factor, and insight item scores. They also showed improvement in ESRS scores, whereas the non-remitted subjects showed worsening, required lower doses of RLAI, showed more improvement on the SOFAS, and remained longer in the study.

Likelihood of achieving remission was increased ($p < .10$) by being a woman, having higher BMI, higher CGI-S rating, lower negative and disorganized symptoms, and higher anxiety and depression symptoms at baseline. At the multivariate level after including the variables significant at the bivariate level only sex revealed significance. Early symptom improvement (as assessed by change on PANSS total scores) was also examined as a potential predictor of remission. A large and significant between-group difference was observed starting at week 2, with a –12-point advantage for the remission group that was maintained at weeks 4 and 6. Change to week 2 was significantly associated with remission, with less reduction on PANSS being associated with reduced likelihood of remission (hazard ratio = 0.95; $p = .002$), although adding in change at weeks 4 and 6 was not significant.

These results suggest that a majority of patients with first-episode schizophrenia are able to achieve RSWG-defined remission when antipsychotic treatment is assured by means of an LAI. The remission rate of 62% compares favourably with that reported in studies with oral medication. The results also provide further evidence that patients achieving symptomatic remission do better in other outcome domains. This study identified female sex and early treatment response as significant predictors of remission. The results suggest that using a depot antipsychotic earlier rather than later in the course of the illness may have significant benefits over oral antipsychotics and may contribute to achieving sustained remission in the majority of these patients.

Finally, the same cohort of patients was used in a cross-study comparison of RLAI versus oral antipsychotic medication in first-episode schizophrenia (Emsley et al. 2008a). We had an opportunity to indirectly compare the effects of oral versus depot antipsychotics by comparing patients who had participated in two similar studies conducted at the Early Psychosis Unit, University of Stellenbosch, Cape Town, South Africa. In the first study, patients were treated with oral antipsychotics (risperidone and haloperidol; Schooler et al. 2005), and in the other, reported above, they received RLAI (Emsley et al. 2008c). The two studies were similar in terms of inclusion and exclusion criteria, assessment instruments used, assessment time intervals, dosing strategy (flexible, low dose), and concomitant medications allowed. In addition, patients were recruited from the same catchment area, so that socioeconomic conditions were similar, and the principal investigator was the same for both studies. No patient participated in both studies. This meant that some of the potential confounding variables associated with cross-study comparisons were removed.

The RLAI study, conducted between February 2004 and December 2006, was an open-label, non-comparative study. The oral antipsychotic study was a multinational, randomized, double-blind controlled trial that compared oral risperidone and haloperidol (Schooler et al. 2005). Only participants from our site in Cape Town ($n = 47$) were included in the analysis. Patients underwent a 0- to 7-day drug washout period and were randomly allocated to receive flexible doses of either oral risperidone or haloperidol. For both oral risperidone and haloperidol, the starting dose was 1 mg/day, increased if necessary to a maximum daily dose of 4 mg/day (and 8 mg/day in exceptional cases). Concomitant medications similar to those in the RLAI study were allowed. To increase the sample size for the oral antipsychotic group in the efficacy analysis, the risperidone- and haloperidol-treated patients were combined because no efficacy differences were found between them. For the tolerability analyses, RLAI was compared with oral risperidone and oral haloperidol separately because of the known differences in AE profiles.

Demographic and baseline clinical characteristics for the two groups were similar regarding sex, age, DSM-IV diagnosis, proportion that was previously antipsychotic naïve, and baseline PANSS total scores, ESRS total scores, and BMI. However the RLAI group had a significantly higher score on the PANSS positive subscale. The end-point doses for RLAI were 25 mg (54%), 37.5 mg (30%), and 50 mg (16%) 2-weekly. For the oral antipsychotic group, the mean modal total daily dose was 3.99 mg for risperidone and 3.58 mg for haloperidol. Response rates (defined as >20% decrease in PANSS total score) were similar for the two groups. However, the RLAI group showed significantly fewer all-cause discontinuations at 12 and 24 months (20%, 26% vs. 49%, 70%, $p < .005$), greater reduction of PANSS total-score from baseline to end point (−39.7 SD 21.1 vs. −25.7 SD 30.2, $p = .009$), higher remission rates (64% vs. 40%, $p = .028$), and lower relapse rates (9.5% vs. 42%, $p = .001$) (Table 7.1).

There were significant group differences for the tolerability assessments (Table 7.2). The RLAI group had significantly lower values for maximum change in ESRS total scores, Parkinsonism subscale, and akathisia scores compared with both the oral risperidone and oral haloperidol groups, and lower dyskinesia and dystonia subscale scores compared with oral haloperidol but not oral risperidone. Prolactin-related AEs

Table 7.1 Effectiveness and efficacy comparisons for the patients treated with risperidone long-acting injection versus those treated with oral risperidone and haloperidol

Outcome	RLAI (*n* = 50)	Oral Risperidone and Haloperidol (*n* = 47)	*p*[a]
All-cause discontinuation, 12 months	10 (20.0%)	23 (48.9%)[b]	<0.005
All-cause discontinuation, 24 months	13 (26.0%)	33 (70.2%)[c]	<0.005
PANSS total-score change at end point, mean (SD)	−39.7 (21.1) (*n* = 50)	−25.7 (30.2) (*n* = 46)[d]	0.009 (*t* = 2.65, *df* = 94)
Remission[e]	32 (64.0%)	19 (40.4%)[f]	0.028
Clinical response at any point (20% decrease in PANSS)	42 (84.0%)	38 (80.9%)[g]	0.790
Relapse (among responders, *n* = 43)[h]	4/43 (9.3%)	16/38 (42.1%)[i]	0.001

PANSS = Positive and Negative Syndrome Scale.
[a] The Fisher exact test was used for categorical variables; *t* test for continuous variables.
[b] Risperidone 13/23 (56.5%) versus haloperidol 9/24 (37.5%); *P* = 0.21.
[c] Risperidone 17/23 (73.9%) versus haloperidol 16/24 (66.7%); *P* = 0.59.
[d] Risperidone −23.3 (SD, 25.8; *n* = 23) versus haloperidol −28.0 (SD, 34.4; *n* = 23); *P* = 0.61.
[e] Remission at any time point according to operationally defined criteria.[6]
[f] Risperidone 9/23 (39.1%) versus haloperidol 10/24 (41.7%); *P* = 0.99.
[g] Risperidone 18/23 (78.3%) versus haloperidol 20/24 (83.3%); *P* = 0.66.
[h] Relapse according to operationally defined criteria.[21]
[i] Risperidone 5/18 (27.8%) versus haloperidol 11/20 (55.0%); *P* = 0.11.
Reproduced with permission from *Clinical Therapeutics* 2008, **30**, 2378–86.

were similar for the three groups when related to duration of antipsychotic exposure. After 6 months of treatment, BMI had increased in the RLAI group by 3.9 (1.9) kg/m², in the risperidone group by 3.4 (2.0) kg/m², and in the haloperidol group by 2.2 (1.3) kg/m².

These results suggest advantages in terms of efficacy and overall outcome for RLAI compared to oral risperidone or haloperidol in treating patients with early-stage psychosis. A more favourable outcome for RLAI treated patients was indicated by the higher-study retention rate, greater degree of symptom reduction, lower-relapse rate, and greater remission rate. These results may be a consequence of a greater degree of adherence in the RLAI patients compared with those treated with oral medication. The findings regarding tolerability were not as clear-cut. Although the lower levels on the ESRS that were observed in the RLAI group support the claim that long-acting injectable antipsychotics are better tolerated than their oral counterparts, no advantages were observed regarding weight gain and prolactin-related adverse events. There are important limitations to this study. Although the patients were from the same site, the two studies were conducted over different periods. Also, more patients may discontinue treatment in a double-blind study, where they are not sure what medication they are taking, than in an open-label study. Furthermore, although the times of assessment visits were similar, the RLAI group had more frequent contact because they received 2-weekly injections throughout the trial. In additon, the sample sizes were small, increasing the chances of a type II error.

Table 7.2 Maximum changes from baseline in total and subscale scores on the Extrapyramidal Symptom Rating Scale for the patients treated with risperidone long-acting injection versus oral risperidone and haloperidol

ESRS Score	RLAI (n = 50)	Oral Risperidone (n = 23)	Oral Haloperidol (n = 23)	P (t Test) RLAI vs Risperidone	RLAI vs Haloperidol	Risperidone vs Haloperidol
Total maximum change	1.40 (2.60)	5.61 (5.22)	9.04 (6.21)	0.001	<0.001	0.04
Dyskinesia	0.18 (0.94)	0.04 (0.21)	1.26 (1.86)	0.32	0.002	0.003
Parkinsonism	1.36 (2.60)	5.43 (5.24)	8.70 (6.33)	<0.001	<0.001	0.06
Dystonia	0	0.26 (0.62)	0.70 (1.33)	<0.06	<0.001	0.16
Akathisia	0.10 (0.54)	0.87 (1.18)	1.09 (1.00)	<0.006	<0.001	0.50

Reproduced with permission from *Clinical Therapeutics* 2008; **30**, 2378–86.

In a sub-analysis of pooled data eight countries from an observational study investigating outcomes before and after RLAI treatment (the electronic Schizophrenia Treatment Adherence Registry, or e-STAR), patients with recent-onset schizophrenia (duration 2 years or less) compared with those with longer-term illness (duration >2 years). The recent onset group showed significantly greater global symptom severity improvement (CGI-S) and a greater decline in the proportion of patients hospitalized, number of hospital stays, and length of hospital stay compared with the group with longer-term illness (Olivares et al. 2009).

Conclusions

Accumulating evidence suggests that early, effective intervention in schizophrenia is critical to achieving optimal long-term outcomes. However, although the initial response to treatment is often favourable, the long-term outcome is poor. Most patients experience frequent relapses or achieve only a partial response to treatment. Poor adherence to medication is a major factor here. Using an antipsychotic LAI to address poor adherence is an option that should be considered early in the illness, in keeping with modern public health principles of prevention of accruing morbidity. Several studies have evaluated LAIs in the early stages of illness. Results suggest good efficacy and tolerability. Clearly, long-term, prospective, blinded, randomized, controlled trials with larger samples comparing oral and LAI antipsychotic treatments in early psychosis patients are indicated. Such studies would more clearly determine the relative benefits and risks of antipsychotic LAIs in the early stages of the illness. Nevertheless, preliminary evidence suggests that, by assuring delivery of antipsychotic medication, the use of antipsychotic LAIs in the early phases of the illness could result in the majority of patients achieving sustained remission. If we were to achieve this, we would be providing these individuals with their best chance of an optimal outcome in terms of symptom remission, improved functionality and quality of life, and individual autonomy.

Given the need for early, effective intervention in schizophrenia (McGorry et al. 2005) together with the fact that that poor adherence is a major problem from the outset (Coldham et al. 2002), all possible methods of ensuring sustained adherence should be considered, including psychosocial interventions, optimizing treatment tolerability and efficacy, and considering the option of depot antipsychotics. The latter option requires a shift in our thinking, away from reserving antipsychotic LAIs for the chronic stages of the illness. This would also necessitate revision of current treatment guidelines.

References

Andreasen NC, Carpenter WT Jr, Kane JM, Lasser RA, Marder SR, Weinberger DR. (2005). Remission in schizophrenia: proposed criteria and rationale for consensus. *Am J Psychiatry*, **162**(3), 441–9.

Birchwood M, Todd P, Jackson C. (1998). Early intervention in psychosis. The critical period hypothesis. *Br J Psychiatry Suppl*, **172**(33), 53–9.

Breier A, Buchanan RW, Kirkpatrick B, Davis OR, Irish D, Summerfelt A, et al. (1994). Effects of clozapine on positive and negative symptoms in outpatients with schizophrenia. *Am J Psychiatry*, **51**(1), 20–6.

Cahn W, Rais M, Stigter FP, van Haren NE, Caspers E, Hulshoff Pol HE, et al. (2009). Psychosis and brain volume changes during the first five years of schizophrenia. *Eur Neuropsychopharmacol*, **19**(2), 147–51.

Chatterjee A, Chakos M, Koreen A, Geisler S, Sheitman B, Woerner M, et al. (1995). Prevalence and clinical correlates of extrapyramidal signs and spontaneous dyskinesia in never-medicated schizophrenic patients. *Am J Psychiatry*, **152** (12), 1724–9.

Chiliza B, Schoeman R, Emsley R, Oosthuizen PP, Koen L, Niehaus, DJ, et al. (2008). Treatment of first-episode psychosis: efficacy and tolerability of a long-acting typical antipsychotic. *Early Intervention in Psychiatry*, **2**, A81.

Coldham EL, Addington J, Addington D. (2002). Medication adherence of individuals with a first episode of psychosis. *Acta Psychiatr Scand*, **106**(4), 286–90.

Diaz E, Neuse E, Sullivan MC, Pearsal, HR, Woods SW. (2004). Adherence to conventional and atypical antipsychotics after hospital discharge. *J Clin Psychiatry*, **65**(3), 354–60.

Emsley R, Oosthuizen P, Koen L, Niehaus DJ, Medori R, Rabinowitz J (2008a). Oral versus injectable antipsychotic treatment in early psychosis: post hoc comparison of two studies. *Clin Ther*, **30**(12), 2378–86.

Emsley, R, Oosthuizen, P, Koen, L, Niehaus, DJ, Medori, R, Rabinowitz, J. (2008b). Remission in patients with first-episode schizophrenia receiving assured antipsychotic medication: a study with risperidone long-acting injection. *Int Clin Psychopharmacol*, **23**(6), 325–31.

Emsley R, Medori R, Koen L, Oosthuizen PP, Niehaus DJ, Rabinowitz J. (2008c). Long-acting injectable risperidone in the treatment of subjects with recent-onset psychosis: a preliminary study. *J Clin Psychopharmacol*, **28**(2), 210–13.

Emsley R, Rabinowitz J, Medori R. (2007). Remission in early psychosis: rates, predictors, and clinical and functional outcome correlates. *Schizophr Res*, **89**(1–3), 129–39.

Ereshefsky L Mannaert E. (2005). Pharmacokinetic profile and clinical efficacy of long-acting risperidone: potential benefits of combining an atypical antipsychotic and a new delivery system. *Drugs RD*, **6**(3) 129–37.

Fleischhacker WW, Eerdekens M, Karcher K, Remington G, Llorca PM, Chrzanowski W, et al. (2003). Treatment of schizophrenia with long-acting injectable risperidone: a 12-month open-label trial of the first long-acting second-generation antipsychotic. *J Clin Psychiatry*, **64**(10), 1250–7.

Helldin L, Kane JM, Karilampi U, Norlander T, Archer T (2007). Remission in prognosis of functional outcome: a new dimension in the treatment of patients with psychotic disorders. *Schizophr Res*, **93**(1–3), 160–8.

Hulshoff Pol HE, Kahn RS. (2008). What happens after the first episode? A review of progressive brain changes in chronically ill patients with schizophrenia. *Schizophr Bull*, **34**(2), 354–66.

Kane, JM. (2006). Utilization of long-acting antipsychotic medication in patient care. *CNS Spectr*, **11**(Suppl 14), 1–7.

Kane JM, Eerdekens M, Lindenmayer JP, Keith SJ, Lesem M, Karcher K. (2003). Long-acting injectable risperidone: efficacy and safety of the first long-acting atypical antipsychotic. *Am J Psychiatry*, **160**(6), 1125–32.

Kane JM, Rifkin A, Quitkin F, Nayak D, Ramos-Lorenzi J. (1982). Fluphenazine vs placebo in patients with remitted, acute first-episode schizophrenia. *Arch Gen Psychiatry*, **39**(1), 70–3.

Kim B, Lee SH, Choi TK, Suh S, Kim YW, Lee E, et al. (2008). Effectiveness of risperidone long-acting injection in first-episode schizophrenia: in naturalistic setting. *Prog Neuropsychopharmacol Biol Psychiatry*, **32**(5), 1231–5.

Lasser R, Bossie CA, Zhu Y, et al. 21 AD. (2004). Long acting risperidone in young adults with schizophrenia and schizo-affective disorder. Presented at the 157th American Psychiatric Association Annual Meeting. 1–6 May 2004, New York, USA.

Lieberman J, Jody D, Geisler S, Alvir J, Loebel A, Szymanski S, et al. (1993). Time course and biologic correlates of treatment response in first-episode schizophrenia. *Arch Gen Psychiatry*, **50**(5), 369–76.

Marshall M, Lewis S, Lockwood A, Drake R, Jones P, Croudace T. (2005). Association between duration of untreated psychosis and outcome in cohorts of first-episode patients: a systematic review. *Arch Gen Psychiatry*, **62**(9), 975–83.

McGorry P, Nordentoft M, Simonsen E. (2005). Introduction to 'Early psychosis: a bridge to the future'. *Br J Psychiatry Suppl*, **48**, S1–S3.

Möller HJ, Llorca PM, Sacchetti E, Martin SD, Medori R, Parellada E. (2005). Efficacy and safety of direct transition to risperidone long-acting injectable in patients treated with various antipsychotic therapies. *Int Clin Psychopharmacol*, **20**(3), 121–30.

Mueser KT, McGurk SR. (2004). Schizophrenia. *Lancet*, **363**(9426), 2063–72.

Olivares JM, Peuskens J, Pecenak J, Resseler S, Jacobs A, Akhras KS; e-STAR Study Group. (2009). Clinical and resource-use outcomes of risperidone long-acting injection in recent and long-term diagnosed schizophrenia patients: results from a multinational electronic registry. *Curr Med Res Opin*, **25**(9), 2197–206.

Parellada E, Andrezina R, Milanova V, Glue P, Masiak M, Turner MS, et al. (2005). Patients in the early phases of schizophrenia and schizoaffective disorders effectively treated with risperidone long-acting injectable. *J Psychopharmacol*, **19** (Suppl 5), 5–14.

Perkins, DO. (2002). Predictors of noncompliance in patients with schizophrenia. *J Clin Psychiatry*, **63**(12) 1121–8.

Perkins DO, Gu H, Weiden PJ, McEvoy JP, Hamer RM, Lieberman, JA. (2008). Predictors of treatment discontinuation and medication nonadherence in patients recovering from a first episode of schizophrenia, schizophreniform disorder, or schizoaffective disorder: a randomized, double-blind, flexible-dose, multicenter study. *J Clin Psychiatry*, **69**(1), 106–13.

Robinson D, Woerner MG, Alvir JM, Bilder R, Goldman R, Geisler S, et al. (1999a). Predictors of relapse following response from a first episode of schizophrenia or schizoaffective disorder. *Arch Gen Psychiatry*, **56**(3) 241–7.

Robinson DG, Woerner MG, Alvir JM, Geisler S, Koreen A, Sheitman B, et al. (1999b). Predictors of treatment response from a first episode of schizophrenia or schizoaffective disorder. *Am J Psychiatry*, **156**(4) 544–9.

Robinson DG, Woerner MG, McMeniman M, Mendelowitz A, Bilder RM. (2004). Symptomatic and functional recovery from a first episode of schizophrenia or schizoaffective disorder. *Am J Psychiatry*, **161**(3) 473–9.

Schooler NR, Weiden PJ, Sunakawa A, Weedon JC. (2007). An RCT of long-acting vs oral antipsychotics in 'first-episode' schizophrenia: preliminary results for adherence behaviour. Program and abstracts of the 46th Annual Meeting of the American College of Neuropsychopharmacology; 9–13 December 2007, Boca Raton, Florida.

Strassnig M, Miewald J, Keshavan M, Ganguli R. (2007). Weight gain in newly diagnosed first-episode psychosis patients and healthy comparisons: one-year analysis. *Schizophr Res*, **93**(1–3), 90–8.

Tiihonen J, Wahlbeck K, Lonnqvist J, Klaukka T, Ioannidis JP, Volavka J, et al. (2006). Effectiveness of antipsychotic treatments in a nationwide cohort of patients in community care after first hospitalisation due to schizophrenia and schizoaffective disorder: observational follow-up study. *BMJ*, **333**(7561), 224.

van Os J, Drukker M, à Campo J, Meijer J, Bak M, Delespaul P. (2006). Validation of remission criteria for schizophrenia. *Am J Psychiatry*, **163**(11), 2000–2.

Velligan DI, Lam YW, Glahn DC, Barrett JA, Maples NJ, Ereshefsky L, et al. (2006). Defining and assessing adherence to oral antipsychotics: a review of the literature. *Schizophr Bull*, **32**(4), 724–42.

Weiden PJ, Schooler NR, Weedon JG, Goldfinger SM, Elmouchtari A, Sunakawa A. 9 AD. (2007). An RCT of long-acting vs oral antipsychotic route in 'first-episode' schizophrenia: effects on acceptance and attitudes, Program and abstracts of the 46th Annual Meeting of the American College of Neuropsychopharmacology; 9–13 December 2007; Boca Raton, Florida. Abstract 23.

Wiersma D, Nienhuis FJ, Slooff CJ, Giel R. (1998). Natural course of schizophrenic disorders: a 15-year followup of a Dutch incidence cohort. *Schizophr Bull*, **24**(1),75–85.

Wunderink L, Nienhuis FJ, Sytema S, Wiersma D. (2007). Predictive validity of proposed remission criteria in first-episode schizophrenic patients responding to antipsychotics. *Schizophr Bull*, **33**(3), 792–6.

Chapter 8

Health professionals' and patients' attitudes to LAIs

Maxine X. Patel

Correspondence: Maxine.Patel@kcl.ac.uk

Introduction

In this chapter, the attitudes of psychiatrists, psychiatric nurses, and patients regarding antipsychotic long-acting injections (LAIs) are examined. Psychiatrists' and nurses' attitudes are important as they prescribe and administer LAIs, respectively. Patients' attitudes are explored in detail in terms of preferences, attitudes, and perspectives on medication adherence. Consideration is given to the potential roles of side-effects, insight, and beliefs about medication as well as coercion. The implications of the findings are discussed in the context of the concepts of medication choice and the therapeutic alliance. Attitudinal differences towards LAI use may partly explain the disparate patterns of oral and LAI use seen in different countries (Patel & David 2005) (see Chapter 10). Glazer (2007) stated that 'clinicians' decision-making can be, to put it mildly, bizarre'.

For the purpose of this review, 'attitude' is taken to mean a hypothetical construct of summary evaluation of an object or thought. Attitudes are usually based on direct experience or observational learning. Attitudes can change with experience or by persuasion (where a person is guided to adoption of an idea or attitude by rational or symbolic means). 'Belief' is a psychological state in which a person holds a proposition statement to be true. Beliefs of others around us are often internalized for the self. 'Knowledge' is the expertise or skills acquired by experience or education with theoretical or practical understanding of a subject matter. Acquisition involves complex cognitive processes including perception, learning, communication, and reasoning. With knowledge a statement is justified, true and believed.

Psychiatrists' attitudes

There are very few published data on psychiatrist's attitudes to LAIs (Nasrallah 2007). An early study investigated the attitudes of 170 mental health professionals, including a small sample of 42 psychiatrists in Australia (Lambert et al. 2003). They developed a questionnaire with 12 statement items assessed with Likert scales, based on pilot interviews with clinicians. Reliability and validity testing were not conducted, and no correction was made for multiple statistical comparisons. Interprofessional differences were considered, and this is a key point of interest for LAIs as psychiatrists usually prescribe, whereas nurses usually administer LAIs. Psychiatrists were more likely to consider the use of LAIs as 'about right' or 'too high', unlike the majority of the 88 nurses respondents who said 'about right' or 'too little'. Most psychiatrists (94%) reported that they were confident in prescribing SGA orals but only 65% were confident in prescribing first-generation antipsychotic long-acting injections (FGA-LAIs). Concerns reported regarding side-effects of FGA-LAIs included extrapyramidal symptoms (EPS), sedation, and tiredness. Only 29% of the psychiatrists reported patient preference as an important indication for LAI use (vs. 54% of nurses), and 69% of psychiatrists stated patient dislike of LAIs as an important problem with using LAIs. The authors suggest that this may reflect a paternalistic stance and that psychiatrists 'who are entrenched in the medical model may be less consumer-focussed than other mental health workers' (Lambert et al. 2003). Glazer and Kane (1992) suggested that clinicians may want to save the patient from the fear and pain of injections or that they may feel that giving an injection, if the patient must disrobe, is a psychological intrusion.

Heres et al. (2006) reported on a survey of 246 mostly German psychiatrists. This study used an opportunistic sampling method for delegates self-selecting to attend a conference on biological psychiatry and so the authors acknowledge that their sample may not be representative of all psychiatrists. A novel 16-item scale was used regarding factors that influenced them against the prescription of an LAI (FGA or SGA) but details of the development and psychometric testing of the scale were not provided. Indeed as hypotheses were not stated, it is difficult to identify the rationale behind the questions considered. Nonetheless, Heres et al. (2006) reported that for 80% of the psychiatrists, 'presumed sufficient adherence' with oral antipsychotics was an important factor opposing an FGA-LAI prescription. Heres et al. further reported that 83% of psychiatrists said their recommendation of an FGA-LAI had frequently been rejected by patients. A recent study in Japan reported that 86% of psychiatrists who prescribed FGA-LAI did so for patients with a tendency to refuse drugs and that their main reason for choosing LAI was 'to improve adherence' (56.1%) (Kanazawa et al. 2008). However, research shows that psychiatrists in general are not good at identifying patients who have poor adherence with medication and those who do not (Byerly et al. 2005; Gilmer et al. 2004). Indeed, less than 36% of the participant psychiatrists' patients in the study by Heres et al. (2006) had ever been offered antipsychotic LAI treatment, and this may be because psychiatrists are concerned that the LAI formulation does not overcome overt non-adherence. Alternatively, they may not even bother to prescribe for the presence of covert oral non-adherence, simply because they falsely believe that the non-adherence rate for oral medication in one's own patient group is less than that reported by others.

Patel et al. (2003b) reported on a cross-sectional study to investigate attitudes and knowledge regarding antipsychotic LAIs for 143 systematically sampled psychiatrists in 2001 from South-East England. The questionnaire comprised item statements with Likert scales grouped into four subscales. It was designed for purpose based on a brainstorming exercise and the existing literature; psychometric testing was conducted for test–retest reliability. The cut-off between knowledge and attitudes subscales was, to a certain extent, arbitrary but this is reflective of the lack of a definitive evidence base regarding LAIs. It is noted that some effects of presumed social desirability may have influenced responding. A substantial minority of psychiatrists believed that FGA-LAIs were old-fashioned (40%), stigmatizing (48%), and associated with more side-effects than FGA orals (38%). Many believed that FGA-LAIs were as efficacious as oral medication (91%) but were less acceptable than oral antipsychotics for patients (69%) and relatives (66%). This sample stated that they said they would be persuaded to prescribe LAIs in patients where adherence is an issue. This provides supporting ongoing evidence that clinicians consider non-adherence as a key selection criterion for LAI formulations and is contrary to claims by Glazer (2007). Furthermore, psychiatrists believed that LAIs have more side-effects than is commonly reported including direct weight gain, local inflammation, and pain on administration. Lambert et al. (2003) reported that one of the key barriers to prescribing LAIs was the perception of long-term side-effects. Patel et al. (2003b) were the first to report that psychiatrists' knowledge about LAIs was positively associated with attitudes (see Figure 8.1).

In considering a change in antipsychotic medication for a hypothetical patient with sub-optimal functioning described in a case vignette, older and more experienced psychiatrists were more conservative as few suggested changing the treatment, whereas younger psychiatrists recommended change if the patient was on an FGA-oral or FGA-LAI (approximately equal numbers changed from an SGA to an FGA; Patel et al. 2003a). Similar results were reported by Heres et al. (2006). This may not necessarily

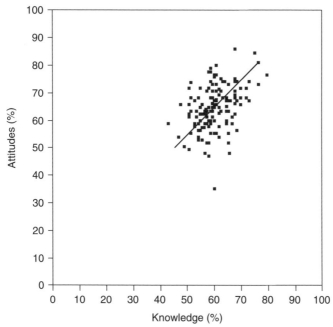

Fig. 8.1 Psychiatrists' total attitudes (%) against total knowledge (%)[1].
Reproduced with permission from Patel, M.X., Nikolaou, V. & David, A.S. (2003b) Psychiatrists attitudes to maintenance medication for patients with schizophrenia. *Psychological Medicine*, **33**, 83–89 Cambridge University Press.

[1]Total attitudes percentage score is summation of all the attitudinal items divided by number of attitude items and this was plotted against the total knowledge percentage score.

reflect ideal clinical decision-making. The younger group was nevertheless experienced but a greater proportion of their working lives would have taken place in the era of the SGA drugs so they are presumably more comfortable with their use. Thus if younger psychiatrists prescribe LAIs only as the 'last resort', it would not be surprising if psychiatrists did not always feel confident and competent to use LAIs. The case vignette method also elicited the underlying assumption that FGAs (oral or LAI) are bound to cause side-effects, whereas SGAs virtually never do.

In a more recent study, using an updated version of the same questionnaire, attitudes of 102 psychiatrists in North-West England were explored (Patel et al. 2009c). As many as 50% reported a decrease in their use of LAIs over the preceding 5 years, approximately the same period that an SGA-LAI has been available. The most common reason for prescribing an LAI was a history of poor adherence with oral medication leading to relapse (82%), followed by patient request for an LAI (14%). LAI prescribing was evenly split between FGA-LAIs and SGA-LAIs although it was also evident that psychiatrists want a range of SGA-LAIs to choose from. 'Having more SGAs available in LAI form' (43%) was the factor most likely to persuade them to use LAIs more (see Figure 8.2; Patel et al. 2009c). It may be that psychiatrists want a similar level of choice for antipsychotic LAIs as they currently have for oral formulations. Patel et al. (2009c) also noted that half of the psychiatrist participants believed that LAIs were less acceptable to patients than oral medication and 33% believed that patients *always* prefer to have oral medication instead of an LAI. It appears that it is the inappropriate overemphasis of patients' presumed dislike of LAIs that was the key factor.

Compared to a sample investigated 5 years previously (Patel et al. 2003b), the more recent sample (Patel et al. 2009c) scored more favourably on the subscale regarding attitudes about the patient for whom LAI is considered (60.4% vs. 63.5%, $t = 2.13, p = .034$). There were no significant differences in the other three subscales highlighting that psychiatrists' knowledge and attitudes regarding LAIs are relatively stable and consistent in the United Kingdom. In other words, the introduction of an SGA-LAI has not yet led to a major shift in attitudes and knowledge (see Figure 8.3; Patel et al. 2009c). Item-by-item analysis revealed significantly fewer participants regarding LAIs as being stigmatizing (mean 1.88 vs. 2.42, $p = .002$) and old-fashioned (1.49 vs. 2.04, $p = .002$). However, concerns regarding patient fear of injections being a common reason for LAI rejection increased (3.44 vs. 3.01, $p = .005$), and there was no difference in perceived patient acceptance of LAIs (3.24 vs. 3.03, $p = .170$) or in prescribing LAIs as being

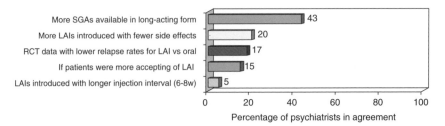

Fig. 8.2 Persuading factors for more LAI use.
Reproduced with permission from Patel et al. (2009a).

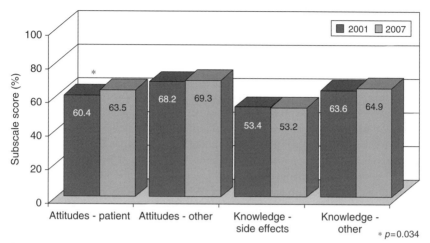

Fig. 8.3 Subscales scores (%)—SE England 2001 versus NW England 2007. Reproduced with permission from Patel et al. (2009a).

coercive (1.29 vs. 1.58, p = .064). The comparisons between the two samples should be interpreted with caution as it was not one sample tested twice but two different samples from two different geographical locations within the United Kingdom.

Nurses' attitudes

In most countries, psychiatric nurses, including community psychiatric nurses (CPNs), usually administer LAIs and so their attitudes regarding LAIs are also important. In a systematic review by Walburn et al. (2001), six studies were identified, for the period 1966 to May 1999, which specifically investigated nurses' opinions of antipsychotic LAIs. A variety of methods including simple questionnaires, qualitative interviews, or focus groups were used. None of the studies considered nurse attitudes to LAIs as their primary research question; most were concerned about training courses for primary care nurses (Burns et al. 1998; Cantle 1997; Kendrick et al. 1998). Two studies explored mental health service provision and staff competency with regard to LAI administration (Brooker et al. 1996; Warren et al. 1998). Only the study by Bennett et al. (1995) provided description of attitudes held by psychiatric nurses although primarily examining monitoring of side-effects. This study was conducted in the United Kingdom, had no stated hypotheses, and an opportunistic method of sampling of 50 direct clinical team CPN colleagues. All the same, the sample size was larger than most and details of the development of the 20-item questionnaire were provided. The authors reported that attitudes of psychiatric nurses were mostly positive about LAI administration but rated it as a task of low importance. Some felt that LAI administration did not utilize their skills and could be done by other nurses. Not all CPNs routinely assessed side-effects; those who did, only monitored an average of three to four side-effects (Bennett et al. 1995). As nurses regularly administer LAIs to the same group of patients, they are ideally placed to do more than just give an injection, and this could and perhaps should include systematic monitoring of side effects.

The subsequent follow-on systematic review by Waddell and Taylor (2009), for the period June 1999 to February 2008, reported on four studies for nurses (Harris et al. 2007; Lambert et al. 2003; Patel et al. 2005, 2008b). Lambert et al. (2003) reported on interprofessional group differences between nurses, psychiatrists, and allied health professionals regarding their attitudes to LAIs as outlined above. This included a reasonably sized sample of psychiatric nurses but with a low response rate (52%). Nurses were more inclined than psychiatrists to say that (i) patient preference was an indication for LAI use (54% vs. 29%) and limitation of rights is a problem in using LAIs (73% vs. 44%; Lambert et al. 2003). In the study by Harris et al. (2007) attitudes to antipsychotics for people with schizophrenia were explored for a sample of a group of students who were also mental health professionals ($N = 50$) including nurses, occupational therapists, and social workers. The response rate and hypotheses were not stated and only two item statements on attitudes to LAIs were considered. They found that 70% felt that patients 'should be given the choice between LAI and oral medication', although 58% agreed with the statement that 'if a person agrees to take oral medication, this is the preferred treatment method'.

The two studies conducted by Patel et al. aimed specifically to investigate psychiatric nurses' attitudes, beliefs, and knowledge regarding LAIs and used adapted and updated versions of a questionnaire for psychiatrists (Patel et al. 2003b). The first study was for CPNs attending either of two academic meetings in London and also included statistical comparisons with data previously obtained from psychiatrists (Patel et al. 2005). The second study was for psychiatric nurses based in Hong Kong attending an academic meeting and included international comparisons (Hong Kong nurses vs. London CPNs) (Patel et al. 2008b). As these studies are for nurses who self-selected to attend the academic meetings, they are likely to be over-inclusive of those who actively seek to update their knowledge and consequently, the samples may not be truly representative of all psychiatric nurses. Thus, these studies will need replicating for an epidemiologically defined systematically sampled group of psychiatric nurses. London nurses were more specialized as CPNs than were Hong Kong nurses.

These studies reported nurses have several strongly endorsed attitudes towards LAI medication (Patel et al. 2005, 2008b). Most nurses had positive views regarding their role in LAI administration and reported that they had sufficient training but international differences existed in that significantly fewer Hong Kong psychiatric nurses than London CPNs felt involved in treatment decision-making. This may reflect differences between the United Kingdom and Hong Kong in the nursing role. It is interesting to note that most Hong Kong nurses reported that patients' friends and family were more accepting of LAI (vs. oral) (69%). As many as 80% of Hong Kong nurses believed most patients always prefer to have oral rather than LAI medication and 40% agreed that force is sometimes required when administering an LAI. This is a matter of concern as it is generally considered unsafe to give LAIs while the patient is being physically restrained owing to the risk of accidentally administering the LAI intravenously rather than intramuscularly. It was also noted that some London CPNs seldom asked their patients about side-effects and did not feel that they had sufficient time for consultations. It is of interest that for both cohorts, their knowledge of side-effects was positively associated with favourable attitudes. The studies were conducted some

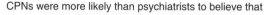

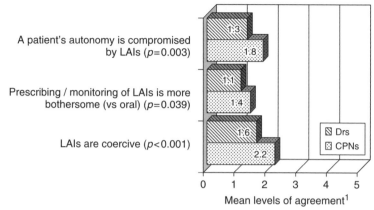

Fig. 8.4 Some key significant differences between London CPNs and psychiatrists.
[1]Mean score on question answered using Likert scale for level of agreement.

years apart (London 2003 vs. Hong Kong 2006) but this is not necessarily a cause for concern as both were sampled at approximately the same time that risperidone LAI was licensed in each place and the issue of LAIs and staff attitudes to LAIs became more topical.

Interprofessional comparison between nurses and psychiatrists (London CPNs 2003 vs. SE England psychiatrists 2001) was also conducted (Patel et al. 2003b, 2005). However, it should be noted that the differing sampling methods (with psychiatrists being sampled from a larger geographical region) means that the interpretation of these findings is limited as the potential remains for confounding by differences in local policies and so on. Compared to psychiatrists in 2001, London CPNs in 2003 did not statistically significantly differ in subscales scores for attitudes or knowledge about side-effects. However, for individual items, London CPNs believed more than psychiatrists that LAIs compromised patient autonomy (28%, $p = .003$) and were coercive (42%, $p < .001$; see Figure 8.4; Patel et al. 2005). These differences may be reflective of the fact that CPNs actually administer LAIs, whereas psychiatrists are more likely to prescribe them rather than routinely administer them. Interprofessional differences in attitudes could result in conflicting messages for patients and thereby undermine the treatment process. That said, nurses also share some attitudes to LAIs with psychiatrists e.g. LAIs are old-fashioned and stigmatizing. It therefore seems that LAIs have an 'image' problem among CPNs as well as psychiatrists, and this is perhaps reflective of the adverse attitudes of some service-users towards an injectable formulation. Thus multi-disciplinary cohesive teamwork is critical.

Patients' attitudes

Systematic reviews: attitudes to LAIs

As with clinicians, patient preferences for LAIs versus oral antipsychotics also vary. In a systematic review of attitudes to antipsychotic LAIs by Walburn et al. (2001),

12 main studies were identified, for the period 1966 to May 1999, which detailed specific data on patient attitudes or preferences. Six studies compared LAIs with oral antipsychotics and in five of these patients showed a preference for LAIs. Quality analysis, based on 13 criteria, revealed that four of the six studies were very poorly reported. Of the remaining two, Hoencamp et al. (1995) reported on outpatients in the Netherlands receiving LAI or oral antipsychotics who were compared using the specially designed 'Neuroleptic Evaluation and Attitude Scale'. Both groups were found to have similar attitudes towards their disease and medication use. However, patients were clearly biased towards the medication that they were receiving at that time. Desai et al. (1999) sampled patients who were recently switched from an FGA-LAI to oral risperidone owing to side-effects with their former LAIs and then reported that most patients preferred oral medication. Walburn et al. (2001) concluded that patient-reported satisfaction with LAIs is high but studies invariably target LAI clinic attendees. They suggested that asking about LAI formulation preference in both oral and LAI groups could be a method for overcoming this selection bias with over-representation of LAI compliers. The real issue therefore is to ensure that a representative view of patients is obtained.

The subsequent follow-on systematic review by Waddell and Taylor (2009), for the period June 1999 to February 2008, reported on five more studies (Bradstreet & Norris 2004; Castle et al. 2002; Heres et al. 2007; Patel et al. 2008a, 2009b). Castle et al. (2002) conducted a large study on attitudes to psychotropic medication for 1126 people sampled in 1997. Of all the psychotropics, antipsychotic LAIs were least likely to be rated as being helpful and more so by those lacking insight. Bradstreet and Norris (2004) surveyed patients in Scotland who had changed psychotropic medication in the previous 3 years; of those who had used LAIs, 43% found them unhelpful. The most recent study on patients' attitudes to LAIs, worthy of more considered comment, is that by Heres et al. (2007). They sampled inpatients (response rate 62%) shortly before discharge from hospital but the sampling method is unknown. The questionnaire was described as entailing 'items on demographics, anamnestic data, experience with antipsychotic treatment, and various rating scales' but the development of the questionnaire and its psychometric testing was not reported. Indeed, with this evident lack of detail, one is left wondering what the exact aims of the study were. That said, Heres et al. (2007) did perform interesting comparisons between three groups of patients, LAI naïve ($n = 145$), currently on LAI ($n = 60$), and currently on oral but with former LAI experience ($n = 95$) and reported that patients prefer their current formulation (see Figure 8.5; Heres et al. 2007). Thus, this study re-confirmed that most patients already taking an LAI do accept it and many prefer this formulation to tablets. It is also interesting to note that approximately a quarter of LAI naïve patients think an LAI is acceptable.

Attitudes to oral antipsychotics

Five other studies, not summarized in systematic reviews, have considered patients' attitudes to oral (but not LAI) antipsychotics and used the Drug Attitude Inventory (Hogan et al. 1983) and explored associated factors. More negative attitudes were associated with presence of symptoms, poor insight, and being employed but not with

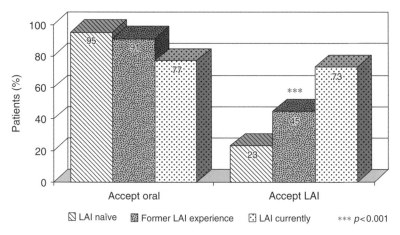

Fig. 8.5 Inpatient attitudes—acceptance of formulations (data from Heres et al. 2007).

class of antipsychotic (FGA vs. SGA; Adewuya et al. 2006; Freudenreich et al. 2004; Hofer et al. 2002; Sajatovic et al. 2002). Day et al. (2005) reported that attitudes were positively associated with levels of insight and degree of good therapeutic alliance (with the psychiatrist); in turn, both of these were inversely associated with coercion regarding the admission experience. Evidence regarding the association between patients' attitudes to antipsychotics and side-effects is mixed with findings suggesting attitudes are (i) inversely related to dyskinesia and sedation; (ii) unrelated to EPS in another; and (iii) unrelated to a global rating of side-effects (Adewuya et al. 2006; Day et al. 2005; Freudenreich et al. 2004; Hofer et al. 2002).

Attitudes and adherence: LAIs versus oral

In a two-part cross-sectional study, patients' perspectives regarding antipsychotics were explored, including factors influencing medication adherence (Patel et al. 2008a, 2009b). This study was novel in using a catchment-area-based sample with schizophrenia/schizoaffective disorder on oral or LAI medication, who are more symptomatically stable and voluntarily treated patients in the community. As stated previously, this issue was highlighted by Walburn et al. (2001) as being a primary concern and as a method for overcoming the selection bias with over-representation of LAI compliers that was evident in previous studies. It is acknowledged that this was not a randomized controlled trial (i.e. formulation was not randomized) and so comparison of attitudes and beliefs between groups of patients is liable to various biases.

In stage 1 ($n = 222$), it was found that LAIs were preferred by 43% (33/76) on LAI versus 6% (8/146) on orals ($p < .001$) (see Figure 8.6), thus preference for LAI medication was very strongly related to current formulation as seen in former studies (Patel et al. 2009b). In the first systematic review (Walburn et al. 2001), endorsement of LAIs in those currently taking LAIs had a range of 23% to 93% (median 61%), and the reported finding of 43% preferring LAI (Patel et al. 2009b) falls within the lower end of this range. Concerns regarding perceived force on LAI commencement were noted

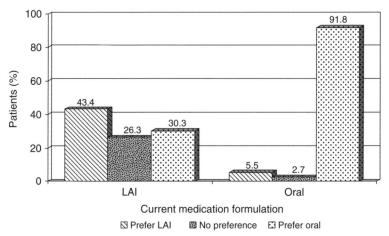

Fig. 8.6 Formulation preference according to current medication formulation.

as were feelings that there was more reason to feel ashamed or embarrassed if someone has an LAI rather than tablets.

The questionnaire for stage 1 included reliable and validated self-report tools with minimal and systematic adaptation. These included the Drug Attitude Inventory (DAI; Hogan et al. 1983), Insight Scale (Birchwood et al. 1994), and Liverpool University Neuroleptic Side-Effect Rating Scale (LUNSERS; Day et al. 1995) that included seven items regarding extrapyramidal symptoms. Attitudes (DAI scores) regarding current formulation were inversely associated with extrapyramidal symptoms; positively associated with the insight subscales of symptom attribution and need for treatment as well as illness duration. Other side-effects, the insight subscale of illness awareness, and current medication formulation (LAI vs. oral) were not predictive of DAI scores. Thus, when voluntary patients on maintenance antipsychotics are asked about their attitudes to their current medication, those on LAI respond similarly to those on oral. However, when asked to state a preference for formulation (LAI vs. oral), patients tend to favour their current formulation. Specific insight regarding the need for treatment was found to be a separable and more clinically relevant dimension than illness awareness.

Stage 1 also included within-participant comparisons for a subsample of 136 patients with experience of both formulations, to explore whether patients always prefer their current formulation (current LAI n =70, current oral n = 66), thereby controlling for individual differences. It also meant that participants were reporting on DAI scales for medication that had not suited them as well as their current medication. Participants currently on orals scored LAIs less favourably than oral ($p < .001$); those on LAI did not differentiate ($p = .101$) (see Figure 8.7; Patel et al. 2009b). Thus, adverse reporting was found in that patients currently on oral medication have negative attitudes to their former LAI. Whatever leads some to switch from LAI to oral leaves a lasting negative impression of the LAI, and this may limit uptake of newer LAIs. This subsample analysis also endorses the previous finding (Walburn et al. 2001), among patients prescribed an LAI, that they generally preferred their current formulation (but avoids

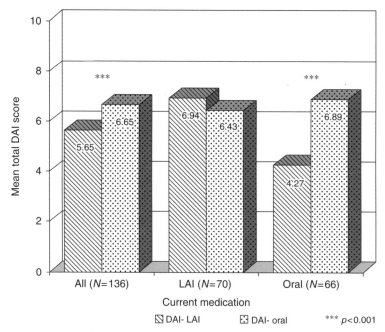

Fig. 8.7 Comparison of DAI scores for LAI and oral, according to current formulation.

the reliance solely on LAI compliers that undermined older studies), although the differentiation was not statistically significant.

Stage 2 of the study, entailed in-depth interviews in a random subsample of 73 patients from stage 1 and investigated attitudes to antipsychotic adherence and influencing factors (Patel et al. 2008a). Although there are numerous studies on medication adherence for oral antipsychotics and potentially associated factors such as insight and side-effects, as summarized in systematic reviews (Fenton et al. 1997; Lacro et al. 2002), these have not been considered for LAI adherence. Self-report tools were used including the 20-item Rating of Medication Influences scale (ROMI; Weiden et al. 1994) with two subscales: compliance and non-compliance. The lack of use of an objective measurement for adherence may attract criticism but objective measures are fraught with problems and there is no true 'gold standard' measure of adherence, objective or subjective. The Beliefs about Medicines Questionnaire (BMQ; Horne et al. 1999) was also included as it facilitates differentiation of beliefs regarding specific medication from beliefs about medication in general (e.g. doctors use too many medications). Other measures used considered psychopathology, side-effects, quality of life, and functional ability. Limitations of this study include lack of measurement of substance and alcohol misuse that are predictive factors of non-adherence, and so ideally they should also have been formally assessed. Furthermore, FGA and SGA oral and clozapine were considered together as a single group in the analyses and were compared to those on FGA-LAIs.

Participants on LAI (vs. oral) had higher ROMI non-compliance subscale scores ($t = 2.41$, $p = .019$) but there were no differences between the two formulation groups

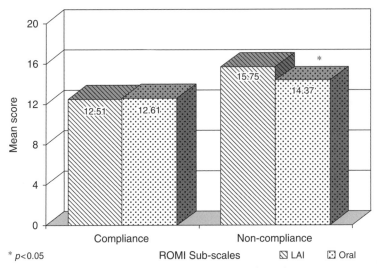

Fig. 8.8 ROMI subscale mean scores according to current formulation.

on the ROMI compliance subscale (see Figure 8.8; Patel et al. 2008a). Common reasons for compliance included fear of rehospitalization (oral: 47%; LAI: 67%) and relapse prevention (oral: 78%; LAI: 71%). Common reasons for non-compliance included denial of illness (oral: 33%; LAI: 14%) and deeming the medication unnecessary (oral: 24%; LAI: 42%). The two formulation groups did not differ in baseline measures of sociodemographic characteristics and clinical factors of diagnosis and duration of illness and evidence of recent admission. These findings endorse the study reported by Weiden et al. (1995) who found an initial benefit in adherence attitudes and behaviour for those discharged from hospital on LAI (vs. oral) but was not maintained at 12 months. Participants who were more likely to be non-adherent may have subsequently been prescribed LAIs but their reasons for non-adherence would not have changed.

In an exploratory multivariate linear regression, predictive factors for influences on non-compliance included poor insight, concern regarding their specific medication, and more beliefs regarding overuse of medication in general (BMQ subscales) but not extrapyramidal symptoms. Being on oral medication (vs. LAI) remained inversely associated with ROMI non-compliance ($\beta = -1.05$, $p = .043$) when these other factors were taken into consideration; in other words participants on LAI scored more on ROMI non-compliance than did participants on oral medication. This model predicted 51.5% of the variance in non-compliance (ROMI) scores. Symptom severity, function, and quality of life were predictive of neither ROMI compliance nor non-compliance, which endorses findings by others (Hofer et al. 2004; Lacro et al. 2002). ROMI compliance scores were positively associated with presence of extrapyramidal symptoms and greater beliefs regarding the need the medication (necessity BMQ subscale).

Previously, side-effects were considered to be a reason for non-adherence to LAIs more than for orals, but the current findings do not support this. Insight was predictive of ROMI non-compliance scores but not of compliance scores. In current clinical practice, many consider insight primarily to mean that a patient is able to verbalize their awareness of their current illness process (Olfson et al. 2006) but illness awareness and the need for treatment are not the same (David 1990). Thus, helping patients to accept a mental illness label is not essential for adherence (Freudenreich et al. 2004; Hughes et al. 1997). Beliefs and attitudes appear more important than side-effects in predicting self-reported adherence and the need to be considered for patients on LAI as well as those on oral.

Coercion

As coercion regarding medication has not been investigated by previous studies, this was also explored (Patel et al. 2009a) as concern had been identified in a significant minority of clinicians. The *Concise Oxford English Dictionary* defines coercion as 'persuasion of an unwilling person to do something by using force or threats' (Persall 2001). In this study, the term coercion was used to refer not to a legal detention but to a sense of external force as perceived by the patient that impedes otherwise true free will, choice, desire, or action. This is in keeping with concept of coercion regarding hospital admission as considered by Hoge et al. (1997) who found that coercion was reported by some voluntarily admitted patients but not by all of those involuntarily admitted (10% vs. 65%). The MacArthur Admission Experience Survey Short Form 1 (Gardner et al. 1993; Lidz et al. 1995), comprising self-report items in three subscales on perceived coercion, negative pressure, and voice, was adapted for purpose to specifically address coercion regarding medication rather than hospital admission. Only 9 (12.5%) participants gave a score of zero, indicating no concerns about coercion. LAIs were reported to be more coercive than oral antipsychotics (LAI: total score mean 4.39; oral: 2.80, $t = 2.26$, $p = .027$), as were subscales for perceived coercion ($p = .041$) and negative pressures respectively ($p = 0.009$) (see Figure 8.9; Patel et al. 2009a).

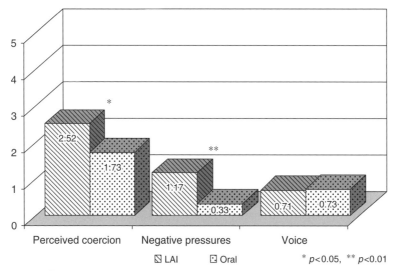

Fig. 8.9 Medication Experience Scale—subscale mean scores according to formulation.

No significant differences were found for the 'voice' subscale and affective reactions. The apparent association between increased coercion and ROMI non-adherence scores did not hold when other factors were considered. Here, formulation (i.e. LAI) is the likely explanatory factor with significant associations with both coercion and ROMI non-adherence scores. An inverse relationship between coercion in general and adherence has been previously identified (Day et al. 2005; McPhillips & Sensky 1998). Although forced medication may sometimes be required, the experience of coercion should be minimized by giving patients a fair say in treatment decisions, regardless of formulation. As LAIs are 'given' rather than 'taken' this sense of power may be seen as more potent.

Implications

Attitudes and preferences

One of the main causes for variation in LAI utilization seems to be that psychiatrists assume that patients simply do not like or want an LAI injection, or psychiatrists believe that patients cannot possibly prefer to have LAI medication. In light of this assumption, some clinicians believe that the LAI formulation is not a good treatment option even though prescribers have their own biases, resistances, and negative thoughts about the LAI route (Glazer & Kane 1992). Glazer and Kane postulated that these attitudes are often conveyed to the patient, resulting in poor patient acceptance. Thus it is likely that many psychiatrists do not even think to discuss antipsychotic LAIs for patients to then consider in the context of an informed choice. This goes against the spirit of the patient choice agenda which is evident in the United Kingdom and elsewhere. It also further reinforces the belief that patients always prefer oral medica-tion, precisely because they are not given the option to prefer anything else. Furthermore, if psychiatrists only prescribe LAIs as the 'last resort' their initiation will often be for legally detained inpatients. Consequently it would not be surprising if psychiatrists did not always feel confident and competent to include an LAI in the choice of medications that are offered to less ill patients who are able to make an informed choice about their treatment. However, some patients really do prefer LAI injections, and this is at serious risk of being overlooked by clinicians. Reasons for LAI preference might include (i) LAIs being a 'safety-net' providing protection against relapse and rehospitalization; (ii) injections being easier to remember than daily tablets; and (iii) feeling more comfortable with less frequent medication administra-tion as this minimizes the need for regular conflict with poor insight into illness (Svedberg et al. 2003; Wistedt 1995). Also, the concept that 'LAIs are less acceptable to patients' should not be over-emphasized as the overall difference in patients' attitudes to the two formulations is relatively modest (Patel et al. 2009b). Furthermore, where there are interprofessional differences in attitudes between psychiatrists and psychiatric nurses, these could result in conflicting messages for patients and thereby undermine the treatment process. Thus patient involvement in the decision-making process should take place with a background of cohesive multidisciplinary teamwork, with due attention paid to differences in clinician opinion.

Knowledge

Patients who were switched from LAI to oral seem to retain their negative views about LAI in spite, or perhaps because, of their more favourable experience of oral medication (Patel et al. 2009b). This may be because the clinicians involved in the switch believed at the time that the newer SGA oral medication was somehow superior in efficacy and side-effect profile; this is no longer as strongly believed. However, it is interesting to speculate that where the clinician believes and emotionally invests in a form of medication, the patient might be more likely to willingly follow. This relates back to the notion that clinicians need an enhanced evidence base regarding antipsychotic LAIs as well as the skills to openly discuss the option of LAIs with patients. Admittedly, the evidence for superior relapse prevention with LAIs (vs. oral formulations) is not definitive (Adams et al. 2001; see also Chapters 4 and 5). Even worse, the evidence for the comparative efficacy and side-effect profiles of LAIs (LAI 1 vs. LAI 2; LAI vs. oral), is virtually non-existent. Studies that do exist are, in general, variously old, of poor methodological quality, short in follow-up duration, and/or underpowered. The studies on staff's attitudes also reveal that not all clinicians have good knowledge about antipsychotic LAIs. For example, Heres et al. (2006) reported that 70% of psychiatrists expected a 'poorer control of the antipsychotic effect' with FGA-LAIs compared to oral formulation of the same drug. Poor knowledge is a barrier to LAI prescribing but blaming this on the poor quality evidence base alone seems insufficient. When contemplating prescribing LAI medication, suboptimal knowledge coupled with a poor evidence base may cause the clinician to not adequately consider the comparative risk and benefits for LAI (vs. oral) for an individual patient. Also as FGA-LAIs are used less frequently than previously, the knowledge base and skills associated with prescribing these drugs is questionable, especially among the younger generation of psychiatrists. If clinicians are unsure of their knowledge, or choose to ignore what evidence there is, then it is perhaps unsurprising that LAIs are not as regularly considered as a prescribing option as might otherwise be the case. In turn this may drive less than ideal attitudes and further deterioration in knowledge and so a vicious circle continues. By updating clinicians' knowledge about LAIs, in turn some of their more adverse attitudes may become more positive and clinical practices may subsequently change. In the longer term, how prescribers will choose between future LAIs also remains unknown. Factors used by prescribers to differentiate between oral drugs may not necessarily translate to the equivalent LAI formulations. Even if equivalent efficacy is assumed, LAIs may differ in other ways e.g. need for initial oral supplementation and injection interval. These issues also need to be confirmed by data-driven research.

Predictors of preference

In recent years, the clinician's perspective on antipsychotic formulation preference has focussed on side-effects, stigma, and fear of injection. The findings reviewed here do not support this. Current medication formulation (LAI vs. oral) was the strongest predictor of formulation preference (Patel et al. 2009b). It is possible that preferences are more indicative of medication-taking behaviour than attitudes alone. Thus evidence to be presented to clinicians should not only focus on side-effects or even attitudes of patients but also the stated preferences of patients. This is important as it also means that psychiatrists should ask the patient what they want or prefer rather than surmise this from statements regarding attitudes alone. Further emphasis should be directed towards the patient's beliefs about medication (specific medication concern and general medication overuse) and lack of insight as these were factors associated with non-adherence (Patel et al. 2008a). It is also particularly noteworthy that the two formulation groups did not differ in baseline measures, and this would suggest that those prescribed LAIs are not always selected differentially by clinicians, on the basis of certain sociodemographic or clinical factors, and this contradicts findings of others. Shi et al. (2007) reported on data from the United States (1997–2003) and found that a stereotypic pattern of prescribing an FGA-LAI for patients who were young unmarried African-American men with a history of drug/alcohol use and were more likely to have been previously arrested. They also had more psychopathology with psychotic symptoms and disorganized thinking, lower functional ability scores and more hospitalizations in the year prior to study enrolment. Prescribing for patient stereotypes is not ideal as LAI prescribing decision-making should be based on the indications of non-adherence and the predictors thereof. That said, at least some of the characteristics highlighted by Shi et al. (2007) are also predictors of non-adherence. Heres et al. (2008) similarly identified that prior history of patient non-adherence and relapses were not only likely to cause psychiatrists to consider an LAI, but they also identified an illuminating second cluster of attributes which included the patient's high level of insight, openness to drug treatment, and profound knowledge about the disease.

Therapeutic alliance

It is possible that at the root of all of this is the perspective of the clinician that they know better than the patient; this is in keeping with a paternalistic stance and the notion of compliance (patient does as they are told) rather than adherence (partnership agreement in context of a therapeutic alliance between psychiatrist and patient). Here a therapeutic alliance is a relationship between the clinician–with expertise in medication and illness, and patient–with expertise in their illness, personal preferences and perspectives, and how they feel when they take medication. A related concept to this is when the clinician thinks they have a poor therapeutic alliance they may feel they have little option but to tell the patient what to do. This may more commonly occur where communication is compromised by a lack of shared understanding owing to cultural and/or language differences. This may also explain why studies have reported on LAI use being higher for patients from migrant or ethnic subpopulations (Shi et al. 2007).

In a critique of the CATIE study (Liebermann et al. 2005), Weiden (2007) noted that when a clinician disagrees with the patient, the reason for medication discontinuation is *not* recorded as being on account of poor efficacy or the presence of a side-effect. Thus the clinician is deemed to be more 'correct' than the patient. The same could be said for everyday clinician–patient interactions regarding medication and non-adherence whereby clinicians may listen more to themselves than their patients.

Patient beliefs need to be considered seriously by doctors and not dismissed lightly. This also includes concerns about medication in general such as the belief that doctors use too many medications. Thus the discussion between clinician and patients regarding the benefits of adherence should also include other aspects such as achievement of personal future goals to consider and balance the individual costs against the potential benefits. It is not sufficient to consider only the case where the patient is perceived to accept what the clinician says rather it is critical that the patient has a shared responsibility within the decision-making process for true medication adherence to ensue. Psychological interventions for adherence should also be considered for LAIs (rather than only for orals). Ultimately, it is imperative that clinicians continue to strive to understand their patients' individual perspectives, including the opportunity to express concerns regarding the use of force during voluntary treatment and beliefs about medication. LAIs are perceived by some to be a coercive measure and thus would be seen to compromise any therapeutic alliance that did exist. This may be because LAIs are clinician administered and LAIs are prescribed for those less able to adhere to oral treatment (i.e. confounding or reverse causality). However, this does not mean they should not be used if the overall harm–benefit analysis is favourable. This seems particularly true for when LAIs are used in conjunction with supervised community treatment (Lambert et al. 2009). The experience of coercion should be minimized by giving patients a fair say in treatment decisions, regardless of formulation.

Choice

If clinicians are equipped with the ability to discuss true medication choice with patients for both antipsychotic orals and LAIs, not only will the therapeutic alliance potentially improve but also the perspective of the clinician regarding the false belief that patients will never freely accept an LAI. It may also shift the clinician's perspective from the stance of 'I personally would never accept an LAI and I can't imagine that any of my patients would either, so there is no point in even discussing it' to 'I wonder whether Mr Smith will choose an LAI or an oral antipsychotic, once I have facilitated and enabled him to express an informed choice.' It is interesting to speculate as to whether in the future, psychiatrists will eventually be assessed on their 'compliance' with patient choice regarding antipsychotic medication.

Limitations

It is acknowledged that the studies considered here failed to consider the attitudes of carers and family members of people with schizophrenia regarding LAIs. A literature search found only one study from Korea (Han et al. 2005). As coercion regarding medication is perceived as originating from family as well as clinicians this should be considered further. Furthermore, these studies reviewed here did not examine the potential relationship between a psychiatrist's attitudes of LAIs and those of a patient with whom an LAI has been discussed. The key concept here continues to be that of the treatment alliance. Indeed, Day et al. (2005) noted an association between therapeutic alliance and attitudes to medication. Even without directly connecting patient and psychiatrist participants, the individual perspective on therapeutic alliance regarding medication choice needs to be explored further.

Conclusions

This chapter has considered the preferences, attitudes, and perspectives of clinicians and patients regarding antipsychotic LAIs. Various factors have been considered including medication coercion in addition to those previously reported in the literature. Clinical guidelines suggest that LAIs are indicated where there are concerns regarding medication adherence. In essence, staff and patient acceptance of LAI medication is variable, and the mode of delivery seems to be a major stumbling block. It is true that the evidence base for comparative effectiveness of antipsychotic LAIs (vs. oral) is not definitive (Adams et al. 2001). However, the LAI formulation also seems to have an 'image' problem, even though many patients already receiving LAI medication like it. This is especially true for FGA-LAIs. However, SGA-LAIs attempted to avoid this by rejecting the name of 'depot', which was perceived to be stigmatizing. The collective term LAIs, for both FGAs and SGAs in this formulation, is partly an attempt to move away from stigmatizing stereotypes (Patel et al. 2009d).

If LAIs are underutilized and variation in rate of use suggests this to be the case at least in some areas, then reasons for this might include patients' concerns about coercion and erroneous assumptions by clinicians that they 'know' that patients will not accept an LAI. Psychiatrists are also likely to underestimate the numbers of patients who are non-adherent with oral medication. In turn, this adversely affects on offering patient choice especially if LAIs, that may offer enhanced relapse prevention, are not even discussed. Also as FGA-LAIs are used less frequently than previously, the working knowledge base is at risk of becoming diminished. The new clinical guidelines for schizophrenia in the United Kingdom (NICE 2009) states that clinicians should 'consider offering depot/long-acting injectable antipsychotic medication to people with schizophrenia who would prefer such treatment after an acute episode'. Thus, clinicians need to have competence and confidence with providing patient choice for antipsychotic medication and this also includes LAIs.

In relation to prescribing, it is not the presence or absence of a needle that should determine the quality of the clinician-patient therapeutic alliance or the degree of patient autonomy. Rather it is how the clinician approaches patients and involves them in decision making, including antipsychotic LAI medication where appropriate.

References

Adams CE, Fenton MKP, Quraishi S, David AS. (2001). Systemic meta-review of depot antipsychotic drugs for people with schizophrenia. *Br J Psychiatry*, **179**, 290–9.

Adewuya AO, Ola BA, Mosaku SK, Fatoye FO, Eegunranti AB. (2006). Attitudes towards antipsychotics among out-patients with schizophrenia in Nigeria. *Acta Psychiatr Scand*, **113**, 207–11.

Bennett J, Done J, Hunt B. (1995). Assessing the side-effects of antipsychotic drugs: a survey of CPN practice. *J Psychiatr Ment Health Nurs*, **2**, 177–82.

Birchwood M, Smith J, Drury V, Healy J, MacMillan F, Slade M. (1994). A self-report Insight Scale for psychosis: reliability, validity and sensitivity to change. *Acta Psychiatr Scand*, **89**, 62–7.

Bradstreet S, Norris R. (2004). *All you need to know? Scottish survey of people's experience of psychiatric drugs.* www.samh.org.uk (accessed 21 May 2010).

Brooker C, Faugier J, Gray C. (1996). *An Audit of Depot Clinics in the North West Region*. Sheffield: University of Sheffield/NHS Executive N.W. Regional office.

Burns T, Millar E, Garland C, Kendrick T, Chisholm B, Ross F. (1998). Randomised controlled trial of teaching practice nurse to carry out structured assessments of patients receiving depot antipsychotic injections. *Br J Gen Pract*, **48**, 1845–8.

Byerly M, Fisher R, Whatley K, Holland R, Varghese F, Carmody T, et al. (2005). A comparison of electronic monitoring vs clinician rating of antipsychotic adherence in outpatients with schizophrenia. *Psychiatry Res*, **133**, 129–33.

Cantle F. (1997). Management of depot neuroleptics. *Practice Nursing*, **8**, 118–47.

Castle D, Morgan V, Jablensky A. (2002) Antipsychotic use in Australia: the patients' perspective. *Aust N Z J Psychiatry*, **36**, 633–41.

David AS. (1990). Insight and psychosis. *Br J Psychiatry*, **156**, 798–808.

Day JC, Bentall RP, Roberts C, Randall F, Rogers A, Cattell D, et al. (2005). A comparison of patients' and prescribers' beliefs about neuroleptic side-effects: prevalence, distress and causation. *Arch Gen Psychiatry*, **62**, 717–24.

Day JC, Wood G, Dewey M, Bentall RP. (1995). A self-rating scale for measuring neuroleptic side-effects: validation in a group of schizophrenic patients. *Br J Psychiatry*, **166**, 650–3.

Desai N, Huq Z, Martin SD, McDonald G. (1999). Switching from depot antipsychotics to risperidone: results of a study of chronic schizophrenia. *Adv Ther*, **16**, 78–88.

Fenton WS, Blyler CR, Heinssen RK. (1997). Determinants of medication compliance in schizophrenia: empirical and clinical findings. *Schizophr Bull*, **23**, 637–51.

Freudenreich O, Cather C, Evins AE, Henderson DC, Goff DC. (2004). Attitudes of schizophrenia outpatients toward psychiatric medications: relationship to clinical variables and insight. *J Clin Psychiatry*, **65**, 1372–6.

Gardner W, Hoge SK, Bennett N, Roth LH, Lidz CW, Monahan J, et al. (1993). Two scales for measuring patients' perceptions for coercion during mental hospital admission. *Behav Sci Law*, **11**, 307–21.

Gilmer TP, Dolder CR, Lacro JP, Folsom DP, Lindamer L, Garcia P, et al. (2004). Adherence to treatment with antipsychotic medication and health care costs among Medicaid beneficiaries with schizophrenia. *Am J Psychiatry*, **161**, 692–9.

Glazer WM. (2007). The depot paradox. *Behav Healthcare*, **27**, 44–6.

Glazer WM, Kane JM. (1992). Depot neuroleptic therapy: An underutilized treatment option. *J Clin Psychiatry*, **53**, 426–33.

Han C, Lee B-H, Kim Y-K, Lee H-J, Kim S-H, Kim L, et al. (2005). Satisfaction of patients and caregivers with long-acting injectable risperidone and oral atypical antipsychotics. *Prim Care and Com Psychiatry*, **10**, 119–24.

Harris N, Lovell K, Day JC. (2007). Mental health practitioner's attitude towards maintenance neuroleptic treatment for people with schizophrenia. *J Psychiatr Mental Health Nurs*, **14**, 113–9.

Heres S, Hamann J, Kissling W, Leucht S. (2006). Attitudes of psychiatrists toward antipsychotic depot medication. *J Clin Psychiatry*, **67**, 1948–53.

Heres S, Hamann J, Mendel R, Wickelmaier F, Pajonk F-G, Leucht S, et al. (2008). Identifying the profile of optimal candidates for antipsychotic depot therapy: A cluster analysis. *Prog Neuropsychopharmacol Biol Psych*, **32**, 1987–93.

Heres S, Schmitz FS, Leucht S, Pajonk F-G. (2007). The attitude of patients towards antipsychotic depot treatment. *Int Clin Psychopharmacol*, **22**, 275–82.

Hoencamp E, Knegtering H, Kooy JJ, Van der Molen AE. (1995). Patient requests and attitude towards neuroleptics. *Nord J Psychiat*, **49**(Suppl 35), 47–55.

Hofer A, Kremmler G, Eder U, Edlinger M, Hummer M, Fleischhacker WW. (2004). Quality of life in schizophrenia: The impact of psychopathology, attitude toward medication and side effects. *J Clin Psychiatry*, **65**, 932–9.

Hofer A, Kremmler G, Eder U, Honeder M, Hummer M, Fleischhacker WW. (2002). Attitudes toward antipsychotics among outpatient clinic attendees with schizophrenia. *J Clin Psychiatry*, **63**, 49–53.

Hogan TP, Awad AG, Eastwood R. (1983). A self-report scale predictive of drug compliance in schizophrenics: Reliability and discriminative validity. *Psychol Med*, **13**, 177–83.

Hoge SK, Lidz CW, Eisenberg M, Gardner W, Monahan J, Mulvey EP, et al. (1997). Perceptions of coercion in the admission of voluntary and involuntary psychiatric patients. *Int J Law Psychiatry*, **20**, 167–81.

Horne R, Weinman J, Hankins M. (1999). The beliefs about medicines questionnaire: the development and evaluation of a new method for assessing the cognitive representation of medication. *Psychol Health*, **14**, 1–24.

Hughes I, Hill B, Budd R. (1997). Compliance with antipsychotic medication: from theory to practice. *J Ment Health*, **6**, 473–89.

Kanazawa T, Tsutsumi A, Nishimoto Y, Yoneda H. (2008). The questionnaire of the usage of depot injection in Japan. *Eur Neuropsychopharmacol*, **18** (Suppl 4), S418.

Kendrick T, Millar E, Burns T, Ross F. (1998). Practice nurse involvement in giving depot neuroleptic injections: Development of a patient assessment and monitoring checklist. *Prim Care Psychiatry*, **4**, 149–54.

Lacro JP, Dunn LB, Dolder CR, Leckband SG, Jeste DV. (2002). Prevalence of and risk factors for medication nonadherence in patients with schizophrenia: A comprehensive review of recent literature. *J Clin Psychiatry*, **63**, 892–907.

Lambert T, Brennan A, Castle D, Kelly DL, Conley RR. (2003). Perception of depot antipsychotics by mental health professionals. *J Psychiatr Practice*, **9**, 252–60.

Lambert TJ, Singh B, Patel MX. (2009). Community treatment orders and antipsychotic long-acting injections. *Br J Psychiatry*, **195** (Suppl 52), S57–62.

Lidz CW, Hoge SK, Gardner W, Bennett NS, Monahan J, Mulvey EP, et al. (1995). Perceived coercion in mental hospital admission. Pressures and process. *Arch Gen Psychiatry,***52**, 1034–9.

Lieberman JA, Stroup TS, McEvoy JP, Swartz MS, Rosenheck RA, Perkins DO, et al; for the Clinical Antipsychotic Trials of Intervention (CATIE) Investigators. (2005). Effectiveness of antipsychotic drugs in patients with chronic schizophrenia. *N Engl J Med*, **353**, 1209–23.

McPhillps M, Sensky T. (1998). Coercion, adherence or collaboration? Influences on compliance with medication. In T Wykes, N Tarrier, S Lewis (eds), *Outcome and Innovation in Psychological Treatment of Schizophrenia*. Chichester, England: John Wiley, pp. 161–77.

Nasrallah HA. (2007). The case for long-acting antipsychotic agents in the post-CATIE era. *Acta Psychiatr Scand*, **115**, 260–7.

National Institute for Clinical Excellence (NICE). (2009). *Schizophrenia: core interventions in the treatment and management of schizophrenia in adults in primary and secondary care. CG82*. http://www.nccmh.org.uk/downloads/Schizophrenia_update/CG82NICEGuideline.pdf (accessed 20 May 2010).

Olfson M, Marcus SC, Wilk J, West JC. (2006). Awareness of illness and nonadherence to antipsychotic medications among persons with schizophrenia. *Psychiatr Serv*, **57**, 205–211.

Patel MX, David AS. (2005). Why aren't depots prescribed more often, and what can be done about it? *Adv Psychiat Treatment*, **11**, 203–13.

Patel MX, deZoysa N, Baker D, David, AS. (2005). Antipsychotic depot medication and attitudes of community psychiatric nurses. *J Psychiatr Ment Health Nurs*, **12**, 237–44.

Patel MX, deZoysa N, Bernadt M, Bindman J, David AS. (2009a). Are depot antipsychotics more coercive than tablets? The patient's perspective. *J Psychopharmacol*, (published online ahead of print 20 March 2009, doi: 10.1177/0269881109103133).

Patel MX, deZoysa N, Bernadt M, David AS. (2008a). A cross-sectional study of patients' perspectives on adherence to antipsychotic medication: depots versus oral. *J Clin Psychiatry*, **69**(10), 1548–56.

Patel MX, deZoysa N, Bernadt M, David AS. (2009b). Depot and oral antipsychotics: Patient preferences and attitudes are not the same thing. *J Psychopharmacol*, **23**, 789–96.

Patel MX, Haddad PM, Chaudhry IB, McLoughlin S, Husain N, David AS. (2009c). Psychiatrists' use, knowledge and attitudes to first and second generation antipsychotic long-acting injections: comparisons over five years. *J Psychopharmacol*, (published online ahead of print 28 May 2009, doi: 10.1177/0269881109104882).

Patel MX, Nikolaou V, David AS. (2003a). Eliciting psychiatrists' beliefs about side effects of typical and atypical antipsychotic drugs. *Int J Psychiatry Clin Pract*, **7**, 117–20.

Patel MX, Nikolaou V, David AS. (2003b). Psychiatrists attitudes to maintenance medication for patients with schizophrenia. *Psychol Med*, **33**, 83–9.

Patel MX, Taylor M, David AS. (2009d). Antipsychotic long-acting injections— Mind the gap. [editorial] *Br J Psychiatry*, **195** (Suppl 52), s1–4.

Patel MX, Yeung FKK, Haddad P, David AS. (2008b). Psychiatric nurses' attitudes to antipsychotic depots in Hong Kong and comparison with London. *J Psychiatr Ment Health Nurs*, **15**, 758–66.

Persall J. (2001). *Concise Oxford English Dictionary* (10th Edition revised) Oxford: Oxford University Press.

Sajatovic M, Rosch DS, Sivec HJ, Sutana D, Smith DA, Alamir S, et al. (2002). Insight into illness and attitudes towards medications among inpatients with schizophrenia. *Psychiatr Serv*, **53**, 1319–21.

Sanz M, Constable G, Lopez-Ibor I, Kemp R, David A. (1998). A comparative study of insight scales and their relationship to psychopathological and clinical variables. *Psychol Med*, **28**, 437–46.

Shi L, Ascher-Svanum H, Zhu B, Faries D, Montgomery W, Marder SR. (2007). Characteristics and use patterns of patients taking first-generation depot antipsychotics or oral antipsychotics for schizophrenia. *Psychiatric Services*, **58**, 482–8.

Svedberg B, Backenroth-Ohsako G, Lutzen K. (2003). On the path to recovery: Patients' experiences of treatment with long-acting injections of antipsychotic medication. *Int J Ment Health Nurs*, **12**, 110–18.

Waddell L, Taylor M. (2009). Attitudes of patients and mental health staff to long acting injections of antipsychotic medication—a systematic review. *Br J Psychiatry*, **95** (Suppl 52), S43–S50.

Walburn J, Gray R, Gournay K, Quraishi S, David AS. (2001). A systematic review of patient and nurse attitudes to depot antipsychotic medication. *Br J Psychiatry*, **179**, 300–7.

Warren B. (1998). Developing practice through clinical audit. *J Clinl Effectiveness*, **3**, 151–5.

Weiden PJ. (2007). Discontinuing and switching antipsychotic medications: Understanding the CATIE schizophrenia trial. *J Clin Psychiatry*, **68** (Suppl 1), 12–19.

Weiden PJ, Olfson M. (1995). Cost of relapse in schizophrenia. *Schizophr Bull*, **21**, 419–29.

Weiden PJ, Rapkin B, Mott T, Zygmunt A, Goldman D, Horvitz-Lennon M, et al. (1994). Rating of medication influences (ROMI) scale in schizophrenia. *Schizophr Bull*, **20**, 297–310.

Wistedt B. (1995). How does the psychiatric patient feel about depot treatment, compulsion or help? *Nord J Psychiat*, **49** (Suppl 35), 41–6.

Chapter 9

Patient choice and improving the uptake of long-acting injectable medication

Mary Jane Tacchi, Jennifer Nendick, and Jan Scott

Correspondence: Mary-Jane.Tacchi@ntw.nhs.uk

Introduction

This chapter considers the importance of patient choice, examines the practicalities of implementing patient choice in clinical practice, and outlines a health belief model that may aid clinicians in enhancing clinician–patient collaboration and shared understanding of the patients' problems. We relate these aspects to the prescription of antipsychotic long-acting injections (LAIs) for an individual seen in outpatient settings. Next, we review the evidence supporting the use of a variety of interventions to improve medication adherence whether this be oral medication or an LAI. Finally, we highlight some practical approaches that have been applied successfully in clinical settings

Patient choice

According to Rankin (2005) 'Making choices is a manifestation of the rights and responsibilities of adulthood' and choice is a basic human right. This is particularly important to remember in mental health, where the illnesses, symptoms, medication, and associated stigma can have a great impact on many areas of an individual's life.

Many international initiatives over the last decade have highlighted the need for patient choice in mental health service users. For example, the UK government has attempted to establish the rights of the patient, in particular, introducing 'expert patient' panels to advise on acceptable treatments for a range of persistent physical disorders such as diabetes and now establishing similar panels for mental disorders. Although the conceptualization of patient choice described in the first National Health Service (NHS) constitution (Department of Health 2009) also describes possible situations where exclusion of patients with mental disorders may rarely be deemed appropriate, the document emphasizes the rights of all mental health service users to be involved in discussions and decisions about health care and to be given information to enable this. The UK Royal College of Psychiatrists' Good Psychiatric Practise Guidelines (2009) suggest a framework through which this can occur and stipulate the importance of the therapeutic alliance with patient and carers, the need to maximize patient participation in assessment, and treatment planning and effective communication. Furthermore, the Schizophrenia Guideline from the National Institute for Clinical Excellence (NICE 2009) specifically recommends collaborative informed decision-making in antipsychotic prescribing.

In mental health complex issues such as compulsory treatment, capacity, capability, and safety arise for the patient and the general public. However, it is vital that clinicians do not jump too quickly to the conclusion that an individual is unable make choices about lifestyle and illness management (Samele et al. 2007), and the provision of choice should be an essential part of everyday consultation and prescribing practice. It is likely that only a relatively small subgroup of patients are truly unable to participate in some choices about their care and treatment, and choice even when restricted to a 'limited menu of options' is still preferable if the clinician is trying to maintain a collaborative working relationship with a patient (Scott 2001). Even patients who are detained in forensic settings or who are subject to long-term community treatment orders may be able to exercise choice about some aspects of their care and treatment even if no choice is permitted in other areas.

What happens when no choice is permitted?

The original definition of compliance was 'a patient doing what their doctor tells them'. Thankfully, such ideas have largely been eradicated but that does not mean we have yet reached the era where all prescribers genuinely promote patient choice. The difficulty is that many clinicians are unaware that their didactic style may stifle a patient's ability to ask questions as they fear being labelled as challenging the authority and 'being difficult'. Patients may be reluctant to seek information to clarify clinical decisions for a number of other reasons. If patients feel they have not been listened to or given some choice in the management of 'their' problem, they may be less likely to report barriers to medication adherence and highly likely to default on appointments and ultimately disengage from the services. In the past, if the reasons for non-adherence or disengagement were not explored and understood, there was a high probability that these patients would be seen as the group who require LAI medication (Velligan et al. 2009). This further alienated the patient as they were left with even less sense of personal control. This approach to prescribing LAIs has largely disappeared but surveys of psychiatrists suggest that negative attitudes to the use of LAIs remain a significant psychological barrier for a new generation of psychiatrists who perceive LAIs as coercive (Patel et al. 2003, 2009). The attitudes of health professionals to LAIs are discussed in detail in Chapter 8.

Empowering individuals receiving mental health services has moved psychiatry firmly away from the coercive nature of its past and may also facilitate social change, destigmatizing people with mental health problems (Rankin 2005; Warner 2010). Clinicians and patients usually have similar goals in wanting to minimize the effects of illness. Time spent creating a truly collaborative therapeutic encounter with mutual understanding between clinician and patient is more likely to engender engagement.

In such a setting positive choices can be made by the patient, and the clinician is more confident that the patient will adhere to the treatment package offered.

Understanding how patient choice influences adherence and outcomes in mental health or other areas of health care is a relatively new focus for research, but so far the majority of publications indicate that enhancing patient choice does improve adherence to appointments and medication (Mendonca & Brehm 1983; Rennie et al. 2007; Scott 2004). Research indicates that patients identify in particular that the opportunity to choose a medication is highly important to them (Hill & Laugharne 2006). If the specific drug prescribed is not chosen by the patient, then having a choice in the frequency or timing of dosing (e.g. twice versus once per day; morning versus evening) and mode of delivery (liquid, tablet, oro-dispersible, injection) have been demonstrated to improve adherence (Horne & Weinman 1995).

Good outcomes are important to patients, carers, and clinicians alike but the terms 'effective' and 'acceptable' are value judgements, at least partially determined by the patient's own subjective opinions, background, and experiences (Hope 2002). Although clinicians may focus on symptoms, good outcomes for a patient or carer may be dictated by the level of social adjustment or functioning achieved. Even in patients who prioritize reduction in symptoms, the weighting of distress from symptoms will vary between individuals with similar presentations. As such even the most extensively validated treatments are not equally effective for a defined sub-population of patients. In recent years this idea has been encapsulated in the recovery model. This model recognizes the different meanings of wellness endorsed by patients or clinicians and emphasizes the need to achieve the personal treatment goals of the individual rather than generic illness outcomes (Gray et al. 2009; Warner 2010). The presentation to the patient of a wide range of treatments options is, therefore, essential if clinicians are to promote recovery (Lehman et al. 2004).

Making choice work

This section describes how clinicians may help promote 'effective choice' for an individual patient. The key elements of this approach involve establishing a positive therapeutic relationship and engaging the patient in the use of a health belief model that helps the development of a shared understanding of the patients' needs and the goals of treatment. We use the example of the prescription of antipsychotic medication to demonstrate how this approach might work in clinical settings.

For an individual to make an informed choice, he or she requires accessible, understandable, accurate, and relevant information. In the case of the prescription of antipsychotic medication the vehicle by which the patient is helped to make such a choice is the therapeutic alliance between prescriber and patient. Much has been written about the therapeutic relationship, but in this context two of the most important aspects of the interaction are the affective quality and communication style. The affective components of the relationship identified as particularly important include the qualities of warmth, positive regard, lack of tension, and non-verbal expressiveness (DiMatteo 1979). Communication is essential in the encounter; various styles can have a detrimental effect upon the relationship especially those that are one-sided or where the patient does not feel that they have been listened to. Psychotherapeutic principles

Box 9.1 Techniques to develop a positive therapeutic alliance (adapted with permission from Tacchi & Scott 2005)

1. Affective Qualities: warmth, positive regard, lack of tension, non-verbal expressiveness
2. Communication Style: ask not tell, listen
3. Patient Participation: answer patient concerns, allow discussion
4. Collaboration: mutual understanding and goal setting
5. Psychotherapeutic Qualities: empathy and respect
6. Time: don't rush

of ensuring that there is mutual respect in the relationship and showing empathy will strengthen the alliance and make it more effective. An important aspect of the interview that clinicians can plan is to create an atmosphere where the patient feels that open and honest communication can take place, which enables both the clinician and patient to explore any difficulties that the patient reveals so that appropriate problem solving and true choice can be implemented (box 9.1).

As important as finding out about the patient's beliefs and attitudes about the disorder and its treatment is the clinician being aware of his or her own beliefs and of not making assumptions for the patient. According to Patel et al. (2009) clinicians generally view LAIs as being less acceptable to patients than oral medication and, in one study, one-third of psychiatrists indicated that they believed that patients always prefer oral medication to LAIs (Patel et al. 2009). Such findings conflict with studies suggesting that patients' attitudes are frequently positive towards LAI medication and of those who remain on LAIs, the majority do so because they prefer that formulation over oral medications (Walburn et al. 2001). Such research highlights the importance of ensuring that individuals are not excluded from being offered all available formulations simply because their clinician believes that LAIs are less popular. When patients are given informed choices and active involvement in their treatment, LAIs may be the formulation that is most acceptable and, therefore effective, for that individual. The same is true with regard to side-effects where clinicians may believe that side-effects have a great influence on patients' acceptance or otherwise of treatment. It has been shown that patient attitudes and beliefs about medication appear to be better predictors of adherence than side-effects per se (Patel et al. 2008). Furthermore, their ability to manage side-effects, if they occur, is more important than the actual experience of the side-effect per se (Kikkert et al. 2006).

Establishing the patient's model

The recovery model is increasingly viewed as the accepted clinical approach in mental health. A health belief model that integrates well with this philosophy is the cognitive representation of illness model (Leventhal et al. 1992). This model describes how an individual constructs an internal representation of what is happening to him or her when he or she experiences physical or psychological symptoms and how he or she 'copes' or reacts to this. This health belief model draws on self-regulation theory, which is important when promoting patient choice as self-regulation theory assumes that an individual tries to be an active problem solver and that the behaviours represents his or her personal efforts to resolve the problem caused by the health threat. Horne and Weinman (1995) suggested that the individual's coping strategies represent an attempt to close the gap between his or her current health status and the desired future state and introduce the idea of 'intelligent non-adherence'. It describes someone whose concerns about taking a medication exceed his or her beliefs about the necessity of the medication for his or her recovery (Clatworthy et al. 2009).

The cognitive representation of illness model has three core elements: (i) a cognitive representation that reflects the meaning of the health threat to the individual, (ii) an action plan or coping strategy developed and instigated by the individual to deal with the threat, and (iii) the individual's appraisal of the outcome of the coping strategy. It is suggested that no matter what the nature of the symptoms, most individuals organize their thinking about any health threat around five key themes (Scott & Tacchi 2002). These themes are consistent across cultures, although the actual content of the thinking around the themes will vary e.g. beliefs that symptoms are caused by 'my inadequate personality', or externally controlled by 'my neighbour', by witchcraft, and so on. The five core themes that an individual uses to organize his or her thinking about a problem can be labelled as identity (what is it?), cause (what caused it?), timeline (how long will it last, will it recur?), consequences, and cure/control (can I solve the problem or can someone else cure it?).

The second component of the model suggests that if symptoms occur, individuals will make some attempt to cope with them. However, their individual coping strategy will clearly be influenced by what seems to be logical to them given their personal beliefs about the five areas such as the nature or cause of the problem. Finally, having instituted their preferred solution, the individuals appraise their coping strategy and decide how effective it has been. This will then be continued or modified depending on results, or the appraisal system will begin again and new solutions generated. This model also helps explain why some individual seek help at the first sign of any problems, whereas others may try many different approaches before viewing their difficulties as something that might be resolved by seeing a psychiatrist.

The model is not universally accepted and there are some criticisms about the notion that emotional and cognitive processes occur in parallel. However, classic cognitive models would postulate a direct link between emotions and cognitions and regard health beliefs as a reflection of other underlying beliefs and assumptions related to views of the self, world, and future (Scott 1999). The strength of the model is that it identifies the individual's pattern of behaviour as being logical to them and allows the clinician to understand the patient's behaviours in context. As part of developing the therapeutic alliance and working towards patient choice, we advocate the use of this model to establish the patient's view. In turn, this will help the clinician avoid from being judgemental about patients' behaviours that may appear to reduce rather than enhance their chances of recovery.

The next step is to integrate the patient's and clinician's goals. In reality clinicians cannot always endorse all the 'cure or control' choices expressed by patients. However, when the therapeutic alliance is positive and communication is open and honest, both parties are aware of each other's point of view, and this allows them to develop a shared understanding of the problem and negotiate the way forward. The task for the clinician is to use the patient's model as a starting point for reinforcing accurate information and perceptions and adaptive coping strategies using questions as a guide to the discovery of other important facts and providing information as necessary. Having incorporated both the patient's and clinician's models into the formulation of the patient's problems, it is then possible to put forward a logical set of treatment goals that make sense to the patient and from which informed choices can be made (Tacchi & Scott 2005). By doing this, the clinician can also ensure that the role of medication and its benefits are clearly defined and that 'tablets' or an LAI is understood to be one element of the overall approach and not the 'only' curative factor.

The choice of long-acting injectable medication

With regard to the choice of oral or long-acting injectable antipsychotic medication the patient needs to establish the pros and cons of each alternative. Such information should be given in an open and honest fashion and a collaborative decision can be made as to what will be best in terms of what is most acceptable, understandable, and manageable to this individual. It should be established what the patient needs to know to make the choice, how this information should be imparted, and by regular checking whether the patient has understood by asking questions. Information available to patients outside of the clinical setting, and particularly online resources, varies greatly in quality, and so the clinician has a responsibility to help the patient understand both the content and quality of the information (Hope 2002). Box 9.2 gives examples of the questions that could be asked with regard to the choice of medication.

A realistic appraisal of the pros and cons of each type of medication for the individual will help to inform choice. This can be made specific for the individuals taking into account their own model, their knowledge and what is important to them. Box 9.3 shows an example of a completed grid for an individual. The idea is that the blank grid is filled by the patient with the help of the clinician to make it personal to that patient.

Box 9.2 Questions regarding choice of medication (adapted with permission from Tacchi & Scott 2005)

1. How often does medication have to be taken?
2. How can I remember to take medication?
3. How do I obtain medication or who will give medication and from where?
4. What should I do if forget to take medication?
5. What are common side effects of the medication and how can I manage these?

Box 9.3 Patient's appraisal of pros and cons of medication (adapted with permission from Tacchi & Scott 2005)

Oral medication	Long-acting injectable medication
Positive	**Positive**
1. Flexibility and control	1. Control
2. Easy to take	2. Easy to remember
3. Convenient	3. Someone to prompt
4. Discrete	4. No prescription to organise
5. Rapid effects following change of dose is usual	5. No daily reminder of illness
6. No problems if going away from home on holiday for extended period	6. Regular contact with professionals
Negative	**Negative**
1. Daily reminder of condition	1. Lack of flexibility
2. Hassle to remember	2. Stigma of attending clinic or someone attending house
3. Need to organize prescription	3. Hassle
4. More difficult to remember/up to the individual	4. Pain at injection site
	5. Slow to change effects with dose change
	6. Needle phobia
	7. Have to travel to get injection
	8. May be difficult to arrange injection if on holiday away from home

The example shows some positives that may be viewed as negatives (and vice versa) by others showing the need to personalize this for a particular patient. It may be that the clinician and patient have different views about what are positive and negative, and such a grid allows a discussion to take place and for the likelihood of success of different medications to be established.

Adherence with antipsychotic LAIs

There are some myths about antipsychotic LAIs stemming perhaps from their prescription in the past when oral medication had failed. In particular there is an erroneous belief that the prescription of LAI medication will improve medication adherence (Tacchi & Scott 2005). Although it is true that once a patient has accepted the injection it is possible to know exactly how much medication they are receiving, the same issues need to be addressed with regard to whether the medication is acceptable to the patient in injectable form as would be the case with oral medication. Clinicians may feel that the observation in a large Scandinavian study (Tiihonen et al. 2006)—that inpatients who agreed to remain on injectable medication post-discharge had lower relapse rates than most of those receiving oral medications—would mean such an approach was logical for a patient with frequent admissions who forgets or actively omits medication. However, this assumes that the patient fully understands the 'timeline' of their disorder and is truly aware that it is a relapsing illness and that the patient also believes that an LAI can directly 'cure or control' symptoms without having negative consequences. It is very important that injectable medication is seen as a positive individual choice and not as a coercive measure for those who find taking oral medication difficult. Although at first glance the prescription of injectable medication may appear to solve some of the difficulties of adherence, patients still have to agree to have the injection and attend regularly; otherwise non-adherence may occur with appointments being missed and/or increasing intervals between injections. Long-acting injectables are no substitute for establishing a shared understanding, agreeing the treatment goals, and jointly agreeing which medication is likely to be most acceptable to the patient i.e. the same principles should be employed when establishing and improving adherence regardless of the type of medication that is prescribed.

Interventions to enhance medication adherence

Once the choice of medication has been made it is incumbent upon mental health professionals to enhance adherence to the chosen regimen for maximum effectiveness. Until recently this was an area that was neglected by clinicians. There is clear evidence that non-adherence to prescribed medication is a significant public health issue. At least 30% to 50% individuals with a persistent physical or mental disorder will be partially or fully non-adherent with medication prescribed for the long term (Velligan et al. 2009). In this section we give an overview of interventions that are specifically designed to improve adherence as well as those where adherence represents one of several key targets. As well as discussing interventions for schizophrenia we also review briefly the less well-developed field of adherence in bipolar disorders. We have not included every study but have noted some that are relevant as this is likely to become increasingly important and as there is widespread use of atypical antipsychotics in both the acute and continuation phases of bipolar disorders. Furthermore, there are published pilot studies and clinical case series on the use of LAIs as alternative mood stabilizers to the classic mainstays of lithium or anticonvulsant medications.

Psycho-education

The term psycho-education is now so common in clinical parlance as to be rendered almost meaningless. However, it can be defined as an intervention that increases a patient's knowledge and understanding of a disorder (Pekkala & Merinder 2002). The assumption is that this enables someone with schizophrenia to cope more effectively with their illness and as such it remains the most often recommended intervention in clinical practice (Velligan et al. 2009). Studies of psycho-education in schizophrenia use a range of interventions but most focus on the dissemination of knowledge about schizophrenia and treatment to achieve medication adherence without focusing on attitudinal and behavioural change. Psycho-education has been given to individuals, groups, and relatives of patients, and the programmes tend to use a multi-dimensional viewpoint including familial, social, biological, and pharmacological perspectives (Tacchi & Scott 2005).

Pekkala and Merinder (2002) examined 10 randomized control trials of psycho-education in schizophrenia. Only one intervention—that of Bauml et al. (1996)—led to improvements in adherence. In this study subjects were randomly allocated to a control group or to a group intervention providing verbal and written information delivered over eight sessions. At one year there was a significant advantage for the intervention group as demonstrated on a continuous measure of medication adherence. Within this review interventions that were not successful included an individual educational session (MacPherson et al. 1996), individual counselling sessions by hospital pharmacists in the presence of a key relative (Razali et al. 1995), group medication management (Goulet et al. 1993), an education group providing information and problem-solving skills (Atkinson et al, 1996), an eight-session education and intervention (Merinder 1999), and extended courses of group psycho-education (Streiker et al. 1986).

A further review by Dolder et al. (2003) shows only one of four educational interventions improved medication adherence. This was the study by Seltzer et al. (1980) where 67 inpatients with schizophrenia, bipolar disorder, and unipolar depression were allocated to a psycho-education programme comprising nine lectures about their disorder and its pharmacological treatment, combined with behavioural reinforcement for desirable medication routines, compared with a control group. It has been suggested that this intervention contained elements of behaviour modification and therefore was not purely psycho-educational. At 5 months it was found that the intervention group showed non-adherence rates of 6% to 9% (according to urine or pill counts) compared with 25% to 66% in the control group. However, this very successful study had substantial dropout rates in both groups, which raise concerns about biases if only completed analyses were undertaken. A study by Brown et al. (1987) that assigned patients to one of four different psycho-educational interventions showed that although patients' knowledge about medication improved with the interventions, it failed to translate into any change in adherence.

There have been a number of studies using family psycho-education interventions; again these have shown little benefits apart from one (Xiang et al. 1994), which was a teaching programme designed to provide family members with a basic knowledge of mental disorders and their treatment to allow them to understand the patient and help look after them. This was compared with treatment as usual. At 4 months the rates of full and partial adherence were significantly improved in the intervention group. However, other studies of family interventions have failed to demonstrate such improvement. Falloon et al. (1985) described a family-based approach aimed at enhancing the problem-solving capacity of the patient and family compared with an individual patient orientated approach of a similar intensity over 2 years. Medication adherence was one of the outcomes measured and was improved in the family intervention group; however, there was no evidence that the effects of family therapy were mediated only by increased adherence. Smith et al. (1992) evaluated a group educational intervention based on material developed for family psycho-education. The intervention was provided to patients divided into two groups according to the presence or absence of positive symptoms. Again it was found that there were significant improvements and knowledge in both groups but no change in adherence levels.

More encouragingly, Hogarty et al. (1991) studied patients from high-expressed emotional environments who had been assigned to one of four treatments: (i) family psycho-education, (ii) social skills training, (iii) both, or (iv) a control intervention comprising supportive therapy plus medication. The family treatment involved an education and management strategy intended to lower the emotional climate of the home through formal education about the disorder and strategies to encourage family members to become allies in the treatment process. The social skills training employed behavioural techniques of modelling instruction, role-play, and feedback and assigned homework assignments. Medication non-adherence was reduced significantly in the experimental conditions compared with the control group.

In bipolar disorders, Harvey and Peet (1991) examined the effect of a brief educational programme compared with treatment as usual on lithium adherence. The intervention was a simple 12-minute videotaped lecture with graphic illustrations of how lithium is used to treat affective disorder complemented with an illustrated transcript. Patients then received a visit 2 weeks later to discuss any difficulties they were having with lithium. No significant between-group difference was found.

Early group approaches are not clearly psycho-education but are most closely aligned to this type of intervention e.g. Shakir et al. (1979) undertook groups for long periods (>1 year) but hinted at marked improvements in medication adherence as measured by lithium levels and the course of the disorder. Van Gent and Zwart (1991) utilized five theme-orientated groups for the partners of patients with bipolar disorder and compared this with the usual input for partners but it failed to show any improvement in adherence in the patients as assessed by serum lithium levels. Clarkin et al. (1998) described a randomized control trial of marital intervention with the spouses of patients with bipolar disorder or severe unipolar disorders who were admitted to hospital. Patients were randomly assigned to receive medication plus 25 sessions of a manualized psycho-educational and marital therapy or medication alone. Adherence levels were significantly higher in the intervention group.

The above studies were of small sample size, non-randomized, or employed less sophisticated methodologies than would now be accepted. However, recent research in Barcelona has demonstrated that medication adherence is one of the benefits of 22 sessions of structured group psycho-education and was statistically significantly better than adherence rates in an unstructured support group led by the same clinicians meeting for the same duration (Colom et al. 2003). The psycho-education approach was broader than that described in studies of schizophrenia and included behavioural interventions and 'homework' that enabled patients to transfer skills they had learnt to the community. At 2 years the psycho-educational intervention was associated with a significant reduction in relapse and higher serum lithium levels than in the control group (Colom et al. 2005; Scott & Colom 2005).

Behavioural intervention

Behavioural interventions assume that behaviours are acquired through learning and conditioning and can be modified by targeting, shaping, rewarding, or reinforcing specific behavioural patterns. The types of intervention include skill building, practising activities, behavioural modelling, and reinforcing strategies. Several studies have shown behavioural interventions to be successful in improving medication adherence. Boczkowski et al. (1985) randomly assigned males with schizophrenia to behavioural training, didactic psycho-education, or standard treatment. The behavioural intervention included patients being told the importance of medication adherence and an individual regime adapted to their own habits and routines e.g. identifying a highly visible location for the replacement of medication and pairing daily medication intake with specific routine behaviour. The intervention was self-monitored using a specific calendar. At 3-month follow-up there was a significant improvement in the behavioural intervention group as measured by pill count compared with the other two groups. It has been noted that patient–observer reported adherence in this study did not improve suggesting that self-report was inaccurate or that patients had falsified the pill counting to demonstrate improved adherence.

A study comparing treatment as usual to the MUSE (Medication Usage Skills for Effectiveness) programme by Cramer and Rosenheck (1999) showed significant improvement in the intervention group. The MUSE programme teaches simple techniques of how to remember daily medication doses to patients with severe mental disorders. The intervention consisted of an initial session of 15 minutes where the patient was taught to develop cues to remember dose times. Electronic pill bottles with special caps displaying date and time of each bottle opening were used in the study, and patients were taught to check the dose cap to see when their next dose of medication was due. Five-minute meetings were held each month where the patient was provided with a calendar showing the number of times the bottle had been opened and when. The control group received several minutes of general instructions about the importance of medication.

Eckman et al. (1990) studied a behavioural programme in outpatients with schizophrenia. Groups of patients followed a structured module for about three hours per week over four months. The module used videotapes, demonstrations, focused instruction, specialized role-play, video feedback, and practice in the real world to focus on four skill areas i.e. information regarding the benefits of antipsychotic medication, correct self-administration, evaluation of medication effects and identifying side-effects, and negotiating medication issues with health care professionals. Adherence significantly improved from 60% pre-intervention to 80% post-intervention. However, it has been argued by Scott and Tacchi (2002) that this group had a high baseline adherence before intervention and was therefore likely to participate in research and may not represent a typical sample of those at high risk of non-adherence.

Razali et al. (2000) looked at a culturally modified behavioural family therapy compared with a standard version of behavioural family therapy. The culturally modified intervention provided an explanation of schizophrenia taking into account prevailing cultural beliefs concerning mental disorder, and it gave a rationale for various treatments; allowed the counsellor to provide a positive attitude to modern treatment; and provided clear instructions about dose, frequency, and side-effects of medication, and reminders of follow-up appointments. There was increased adherence in the culturally modified group compared with the control group that continued at one-year follow-up. Another study by Telles et al. (1995) failed to show an improvement in medication adherence at 12 months for behavioural family intervention compared with case management to a sample of 40 immigrant families suggesting that the cultural context may be important for success.

Tarrier et al. (1988) showed medication adherence as a secondary outcome in a study of two different types of behavioural intervention with an education only group versus routine treatment in 48 subjects with schizophrenia. The education group was a two-session educational programme giving information about schizophrenia and how to manage it in the home environment to patients and relatives. The behavioural interventions were both of 9 months duration and similar content. Families initially received the education programme followed by stress management, goal setting, and training in procedures to achieve these goals. Both behavioural interventions were didactic in that families were taught skills to manage schizophrenia. Patients were allocated to interventions according to whether their relatives expressed high emotion. Results showed that medication adherence was achieved by 68% of all patients with no significant difference between groups.

Cognitive behavioural therapy

Lecompte and Pelc (1996) tested a cognitive behavioural programme targeted at changing adherence patterns through the use of five therapeutic strategies: engagement, psycho-education, identifying prodromal symptoms, developing coping strategies, and behavioural strategies for reinforcing adherence behaviour and correcting false beliefs about medication. The primary outcome measure was the duration of hospitalization, which the authors argued was a useful indirect measure of adherence. Patients receiving the cognitive behavioural intervention spent significantly less time in hospital in the year after the intervention compared with the year before the intervention but no difference was found in the control group. This improvement cannot be certainly attributed to adherence.

In bipolar disorder, Cochran (1984) described the effect of a modified cognitive behavioural therapy intervention aimed at altering cognitions and behaviours that interfere with adherence with lithium in individuals recently prescribed this mood stabilizer. The intervention consisted of one hour a week for 6 weeks and was based on Beck et al.'s (1979) model. Results showed that patients in the intervention group were significantly more adherent and significantly less likely to be hospitalized than those in the standard care group immediately post-CBT and at 6-month follow-up. This study suggests a potentially cost-effective intervention but was of small size ($N = 28$) and required replication. A pilot study of cognitive concordance therapy in 10 outpatients with bipolar disorder who were non-adherent with lithium also showed improvement in adherence following a six-session intervention (Scott & Tacchi 2002). The intervention utilized a health belief model to allow clinician and patient to reach a collaborative understanding of the disorder, its treatment, and each others' aims and goals. Specific behavioural cognitive interventions were then employed to effect changes in adherence behaviour. The intervention was also highly acceptable to patients treated by junior doctors who were trained in this approach (Boilson et al. 2004).

In Lam et al.'s (2003) randomized controlled trail of 103 individuals with bipolar disorder allocated to routine care alone or routine care with a flexible schedule of

12 to 18 individual sessions of CBT, the CBT group had significantly greater adherence on self-report measures at 6 months but non-significant differences in serum levels of mood stabilizers. However, a large-scale effectiveness trial involving patients with more frequent and severe bipolar episodes did not find any benefit on adherence in those receiving CBT (Scott et al. 2006).

Motivational interviewing

Motivational interviewing is an intervention that was described by Miller and Rollnick (1991) to help people identify the costs and benefits related to their personal goals as well as the advantages and disadvantages of services that help people achieve these goals. Motivational interviewing has been applied to a broad range of problems in chronic illness management and substance misuse. Rollnick and Miller (1995) defined it as a directive, client-centred counselling style for eliciting behavioural change by helping clients to explore and resolve ambivalence. It includes behavioural analysis but does not try to force the person into accepting the evidence of advantages of a new behaviour but considers the value of letting a person carefully discover the advantages and disadvantages of their behaviour for themselves. It has been suggested that for this intervention to be successful in improving medication adherence in schizophrenia modifications have to be made to combat the presence of negative symptoms (Corrigan et al. 2001).

Hayward et al. (1995) used an intervention of medication self-management based on motivational interviewing. The patients received three 30-minute sessions either of medication and self-management or of non-directive discussion on any issue except medication. The pilot work showed trends in favour of the intervention group with regard to adherence but these were not statistically significant. This work led to the development of compliance therapy described by Kemp et al. (1996). Compliance therapy utilizes motivational interviewing and cognitive behavioural approaches and is described in detail in the treatment manual (Kemp et al. 1997). The key techniques are those of reflective listening, regular summarizing, inductive questioning, exploring ambivalence, developing discrepancies between present behaviour and broader goals, and using normalizing rationales. In an RCT by Kemp et al. (1998), 74 patients with psychosis were allocated to 4 to 6 sessions of compliance therapy versus 4 to 6 sessions of supportive counselling. Results showed a significant effect upon adherence in the intervention group as compared with the control group immediately post-treatment and at 18-month follow-up. O'Donnell et al. (2003) failed to replicate Kemp's findings but did show that attitudes to treatment at baseline predicted adherence at one year suggesting early identification of attitudes towards medication may be useful in clinical practice. A recent large pan-European trial by Gray et al. (2006) also failed to find a significant additional benefit from a similar intervention.

Multi-model approaches

Kelly and Scott (1990) described a study where patients were assigned to one of three intervention groups or a control group receiving standard treatment alone. The first intervention group included the development of an individual compliance plan that focused on assessing the patient's current level of adherence, devised an appropriate behavioural approach for improving it, and encouraged a positive and supportive environment. This intervention was carried out in the patient's home. The second intervention was carried out at a clinic and was aimed at improving patient provider communication designed to teach the patient to become an active health care consumer. The third intervention was the two interventions combined. Results showed significant difference in adherence between the active treatment groups and the control group.

Azrin and Teichner (1998) examined a behavioural intervention delivered to individual patients or to patients and their family and compared this with a control group receiving an information pack describing psychotropic medications. The two intervention groups were taught detailed behavioural guidelines for each step of the medication taking sequence and in the family group, families collaborated with the patients in implementing these behavioural strategies. The intervention groups showed significantly greater adherence than the comparison group but the active treatment groups were not significantly different from each other.

Cognitive adaptation training (CAT) is a manual-driven intervention employing a series of compensatory strategies based on neuropsychological, behavioural, and occupational therapy principles. Training includes a comprehensive behavioural assessment to quantify the level of apathy and disinhibited behaviour and neuropsychological assessment to examine the level of executive functioning, attention, and memory. Velligan et al. (2008) studied 95 patients with schizophrenia who were randomly assigned to CAT focused on many aspects of community adaptation, CAT focused on medication and appointment keeping and treatment as usual. Treatment lasted for 9 months and patients were followed up for 6 months after the withdrawal of home visits. Medication was a primary outcome of this study as measured by unannounced pill counts. Results showed that both CAT interventions improved medication adherence and these effects remained even after visits were withdrawn. The full CAT intervention improved functional outcome relative to the other two treatment groups but this difference reduced after the withdrawal of home visits.

Service responses In the United Kingdom and several other countries community-based care models, involving several specialist teams, have been developed to meet the needs of those with severe mental disorders. Most models include assertive outreach programmes, and improving medication adherence is a recognized target for these services. Marshall and Lockwood (2002) have stated that the key components of such interventions are the provision of a strong and supportive social network, close monitoring of clinical status including the medication regime, provision of stable housing, and other supported services. Zygmunt et al. (2002) noted that 4 of the 10 community-based studies reviewed reported the intervention was associated with significantly greater medication adherence. Stein and Test (1980) described a conceptual model of community treatment titled 'Training in Community Living' and compared this with short-term hospitalization plus aftercare. At 8- and 12-month follow-up adherence with antipsychotic medication in the experimental group was significantly improved compared with the control group. Following the intervention, patients returned to a traditional community programme and these benefits were lost.

Bush et al. (1990) compared assertive community treatment versus standard case management and showed improvement in medication adherence at 24 months as did Ford et al. (1995) who compared intensive case management with standard case management. Some studies of enhanced care management have failed to show such improvements e.g. Bond et al. (1988) who compared assertive community treatment with standard case management. Modrcin et al. (1988) compared 'strengths case management' versus standard case management and showed no difference in adherence between the two groups at 4 months.

A naturalistic survey by Grunebaum et al. (2001) of adults with schizophrenia living in supportive housing facilities in New York City showed that direct supervision of medication was associated with better adherence. A structured interview was used to assess medication adherence, degree of medication supervision, opinions about medication, and regime complexity. A study by Fenton et al. (1997) showed that supervision of medication by family members or friends was associated with better adherence but persons living in supportive housing are often without significant others to supervision their treatment. Ziguras et al. (2001) extended the notion of significant others to mental health professionals noting the beneficial effect on medication adherence of matching the cultural background of the patient and their case manager.

Summary of interventions to improve medication adherence

The evidence from the studies reviewed shows that purely didactic psycho-educational interventions are the least effective for improving medication adherence (Merinder 2000). In those with impaired capacity direct supervision may be helpful, but in those who can and do make choices, the interventions that employ educational and behavioural strategies are more likely to be successful. Individual and group approaches utilizing these strategies produce significant improvements in medication adherence, with or without changes in knowledge about the disorder. The quality of the educational programme and therapy delivered to patients is a strong predictor of gains in knowledge and adherence.

Successful interventions that improve both knowledge and adherence are often highly focused on a particular model (e.g. compliance therapy). The different forms of behavioural and cognitive therapies that were most successful at improving adherence were those that (i) targeted the therapeutic relationship, (ii) had a method of exploring the patient's model of their disorder including their beliefs and expectations and (iii) employed concrete problem-solving techniques (Tacchi & Scott 2005).

Interventions can be subdivided according to the format such as individual, group, or family interventions or service approaches. The most significant finding when studies are assessed in this way is that family interventions are less effective than other formats unless this incorporates significant behavioural elements. Intriguingly, group psycho-education interventions may be more effective than individual approaches, especially in bipolar disorders where patients appear to learn from the experiences of their peer group. Multi-modal approaches are generally helpful across a range of problem areas but it is difficult to distil the active ingredients that may specifically improve adherence. Interventions utilizing combined psycho-education, cognitive and behavioural

Box 9.4 Summary of interventions to enhance medication adherence in schizophrenia (Scott 2004)

Intervention (number of studies)	Improved knowledge	Improved adherence	Improved outcomes
Didactic psychoeducation (N = 7)	85%	14%	14%
Psychoeducation plus behavioural interventions (N = 11)	83%	75%	45%
Behavioural and cognitive behavioural interventions (N = 5)	100%	80%	60%
Multi-modal interventions (N = 12)	75%	75%	50%
Service-based responses (N = 10)	Not known	40%	50%

strategies, and homework strategies are more effective in increasing adherence. There is little research specifically targeting improved adherence to LAIs. In most studies those on LAIs are often not distinguished from those on oral medications. Box 9.4 shows a summary of interventions addressing adherence in schizophrenia. Box 9.5 identifies types of interventions that are reported in the literature on schizophrenia and BAD that may be useful strategies for improving adherence.

Clinical techniques to improve adherence

The stringent entry criteria for efficacy research studies are such that they would exclude 80% of patients seen in clinical practice. The trial results, therefore, are difficult

Box 9.5 Interventions used in effective approaches to adherence in schizophrenia and bipolar disorder

1. Exploration of patients model of disorder with attention to cultural beliefs and context
2. Education regarding disorder and its treatment, provided in verbal, written, didactic video, interactive formats
3. Attention to therapeutic alliance, avoiding confrontation
4. Enhancing motivation by linking adherence to personal goals
5. Behavioural and concrete problem-solving strategies: using reminders, cues and reinforcements, regular medication routines, self-monitoring
6. Identification of attitudes and beliefs about treatment, particularly those that reduce use of coping behaviours such as adherence
7. Simple cognitive interventions to modify maladaptive ideas

to relate to the patients we actually see. To effectively enhance adherence, clinicians also need to make informed choices about the strategies that may help their patients stick with the prescribed treatment regime. Once choice has been made, the following simple techniques are worth utilizing no matter what type of mediation has been decided upon.

Education

We have shown that education alone is a necessary part of treatment but is not sufficient to promote adherence. The principle in providing education or imparting knowledge to the patient is to ask and not tell. It is useful to start with the patient's own knowledge about his or her illness and medication e.g. using the five-area model i.e. establishing identity (what is it?), cause (what caused it?), timeline (how long will it last, will it recur?), consequences, and cure/control (can I solve the problem or can someone else cure it?). This will provide an essential baseline from which further discussion can take place and be put into context.

When thinking about a particular medication it is useful to ask what the patient already knows about this or whether they know someone else who has taken such medication. Subsequently specific questions can be asked and gaps in knowledge or misconceptions corrected. Such an approach is usually far more effective in engaging a patient and improving knowledge than the clinician giving a didactic presentation. Questions can be encouraged and specific information can be given in simple everyday language but should be limited to a few major points per discussion. Education should be repeated and reinforced by recapping and giving summaries and using written material or other supplements. Regular checking with the patient by asking questions will also reinforce education.

It is also important to distinguish between a patient's general knowledge (they usually know that 80% patients with bipolar disorder will experience a relapse in the next 5 years) and their application of that knowledge to themselves (when asked, most patients with bipolar disorder state they will not be one of the people who has a relapse). This is a critical issue for clinicians to be aware of. General information leaflets or pronouncements on research that state that bad outcomes will 'happen to them' do not have the same impact on patients as when patients have identified this information for themselves and can discover in what ways they or may not fit into the high risk of relapse group etc.

Behavioural interventions

Unintentional non-adherence (such as forgetting) is likely to respond to a behavioural approach. In practice all forms of non-adherence will be improved by some behavioural intervention. Simplifying the treatment regime is thought to improve adherence (Goodwin & Jamison 1990). It has been shown that if a patient chooses the type of medication to suit him or her, this will increase the chances of adherence (Lingham & Scott 2002). Providing a list of written instructions with regard to medication on a wallet-sized card is helpful to patients. For some patients the use of a medi pack or dosette box can be useful although too few clinicians actually realize that patients may

Box 9.6 Behavioural techniques that can be used in the clinical practice to promote adherence

1. Give written instructions about medication regime
2. Use prompts to remind patient when to take medication e.g. notes stuck in prominent places, text message alerts
3. Pair tablet taking with routine activities e.g. brushing teeth
4. Rehearse each step of adherence with the regime, particularly when anticipating exposure to high risk situations where non-adherence is likely
5. Engage families, significant others or support workers in the process
6. Keep a diary of medication taken
7. Simplify the medication regime
8. Match the prescription to the patient's lifestyle

not find these simple. It must be established that the patient knows how to use these and that arrangements are in place for this to be regularly prescribed and updated. Prompts such as text message alerts or notes in prominent places can improve adherence (Scott 2001). Pairing tablet taking with routine activities such as brushing the teeth can be useful although care needs to be taken to ensure that medication is not left where children might find it. Matching the prescription to the patient's lifestyle and activities e.g. taking into account when medication can be taken for night-shift workers is important as are rehearsing high-risk situations e.g. rehearsing how medication will be taken when the patient is away from home, a scenario that is often associated with non-adherence. The benefits of each strategy can be monitored through keeping a simple medication diary that can be reviewed with the clinician to monitor progress on the effectiveness of the intervention (Box 9.6). Indeed, as with other interventions (reducing alcohol intake, maintaining a diet plan), self-monitoring of adherence is a beneficial intervention in its own right and a quick and simple communication tool if clinicians and patients are being open in discussing adherence problems. Sometimes it is helpful to recruit family members or prompting when relationships are good and the patient sees this as supportive rather than undermining.

Cognitive techniques

Cognitive techniques are useful when non-adherence is intentional. Recent research highlights that patient beliefs that impair adherence can be broadly classified as concerns versus necessity (Clatworthy et al. 2009). The clinician should therefore start by exploring the patient's concerns about medication—are these specific to this medication? Are they stigmatized by others who disapprove of psychotropics, or does the patient not believe there is a role for medication believing that 'will power' should be the cure for their problem? It is worth taking time to hear all the concerns and recognizing that none is trivial to patients; if the clinician can help reduce concerns through providing accurate information or solve problems or simply sympathize, the patient will be more likely to try to adhere (Clatworthy et al. 2009). Next it is important to help the patient re-assess the necessity of medication in their treatment. To do this, the patient should be provided with a realistic appraisal of the disorder and his or her prognosis in whatever format seems appropriate and understandable. This can be done by the patient themselves e.g. by using the Internet or by providing information, or both.

The next step is to explore the pattern of non-adherence and identify specific situations where there is high risk of omitting prescribed medication. Any negative thoughts with regard to medication are noted and these can be explored with the clinician who can guide the patient to examine his or her own cognitions. An example would be does the patient omit medication before a meeting, worrying it will make him or her drowsy or because he or she thinks that everyone will know he or she is taking tablets (and therefore an inadequate person)? Alternative explanations and rating of the degree of belief and thoughts need to be generated; however, this must be by the patient not the doctor—you are trying to establish the patients' reaction not second guess them (especially as this will be influenced by the doctor's personal beliefs).

Behavioural 'experiments' can be used to test out negative thoughts and also provide further evidence-based information (rather than assumptions) on which to base discussions to generate alternative views e.g. what about taking a tablet before the meeting and recording what actually happens? The particular stage of recovery that the patient is in will influence their beliefs and the discussion. Patients who are well and symptom free may have different beliefs and attitudes to a patient who has recently relapsed and can equate relapse with stopping medication. It is important to remember this as medication adherence is not all or none and is not constant—it varies between individuals and within an individual; it is usually partial (rather than completely all or nothing); and it often cycles depending on the patients' perception of how necessary medication is to help them function at that moment in time or how much they wish to avoid future negative consequences.

Conclusions

Patient choice is at the centre of maximizing effectiveness of treatment in its broadest form. The political and clinical agenda behind the 'patient choice' movement has merged seamlessly with the recovery model. A health belief model that promotes patient choice and integrates with the 'personal treatment goals' philosophy such as the 'cognitive representation of illness model' is a useful asset as it promotes a dialogue between clinicians and patients that reflects all of the concepts encompassed by the recovery model. Research models on effective interventions to promote adherence in psychosis and severe mood disorders are less consistent that might be anticipated but it is possible to extract some practical approaches that can be used to effect positive patient choice and enhance adherence in day to day practice.

Although LAIs have been available for many decades, the early use of these 'depots' stigmatized this treatment for two generations of prescribers. Trainee psychiatrists and other clinicians were too often left with the impression that LAIs were actually the alternative to choice! Listening to the views of participants of our adherence workshops we found that there was too often an assumption that injectable antipsychotics were solely for use with uncooperative non-adherent patients who frequently disengaged from services—it was almost seen as the ultimate punishment for patients who did not respond to the care and treatment provided.

In contemporary clinical practice, the practical application of choice and personal recovery models has also led to the recognition that patients also deserve the option of using LAIs. These medications may well be convenient and preferable to some patients. Also reserving LAIs for the non-adherent patient is misplaced optimism; even the availability of SGA rather than FGA-LAIs will not prevent adherence problems in those patients where the clinician is struggling to establish a working therapeutic alliance or there is no shared understanding of how to tackle the patients' problems.

Finally, it is noteworthy that although clinically we are again viewing the use of LAIs as a choice patients may make (despite some prescribers retaining mixed views of such treatments), there is now a need for further studies on who most often chooses or benefits from LAIs. Importantly, there is a need for clinical trials to assess the effectiveness of interventions to enhance adherence with antipsychotic medication, whether this be oral or an LAI in those with both schizophrenia and bipolar disorder.

References

Atkinson JM, Coia DA, Gilmour WH, Harper JP. (1996). The impact of education groups for people with schizophrenia on social functioning and quality of life. *Br J Psychiatry,*168(2), 199–204.

Azrin NH, Teichner G. (1998). Evaluation of an instructional program for improving medication compliance for chronically mentally ill outpatients. *Behavioural Res Ther*, **36**, 849–61.

Bauml J, Kissling W, Pitschel W.G. (1996). Psychoedukative Gruppen Fur schizophrenie Patienten: Einfluss auf Wissensstand und Compliance. *Nervenheilkunde,*15, 145–50.

Beck AT, Rush AJ, Shaw BF, Emery G. (1979). *Cognitive Therapy of Depression*. New York: Guilford Press.

Boczkowski JA, Zeichner A, DeSanto N. (1985). Neuroleptic compliance among chronic schizophrenic outpatients: an intervention outcome report. *J Consult Clin Psychol*, **53**(5), 666–71.

Boilson M, Murdoch J, Hull A, Hamilton R, Scott J. (2004). A brief adherence therapy: training issues and patient satisfaction. *Ir J Mede*, **21**, 91–4.

Bond GR, Miller LD, Krumwied RD, Ward RS. (1988). Assertive case management in three CMHCs: a controlled study. *Hosp Community Psychiaty*, **39**(4), 411–18.

Brown CS, Wright RG, Christensen DB. (1987). Association between type of medication instruction and patients' knowledge, side effects, and compliance. *Hosp Community Psychiatry*, **38**(1), 55–60.

Bush CT, Langford MW, Rosen P, Gott W. (1990). Operation outreach: intensive case management for severely psychiatrically disabled adults. *Hosp Community Psychiatry*, **41**(6), 647–9.

Clarkin J, Carpenter D, Hull J, Wilner P, Glick I. (1998). Effects of psycho-educational intervention for married patients with bipolar disorders and their spouses. *Psychiatr Serv,*49(4), 531–3.

Clatworthy J, Bowskill R, Parham R, Rank T, Scott J, Horne R. (2009) Understanding medication non-adherence in bipolar disorders using a necessity-concerns framework. *J Affect Disord*, **116**(1–2), 51–5.

Cochran S, (1984). Preventing medication non -compliance in the out-patient treatment of bipolar affective disorder.. *J Consult Clin Psycho*,**52**(5), 873–8.

Colom F, Vieta E, Martinez-Aran A, Reinares M, Goikolea JM, Benabarre A, et al. (2003). A randomized trial on the efficacy of group psychoeducation in the prophylaxis of recurrences in bipolar patients whose disease is in remission. *Arch Gen Psychiatry*,**60**(4), 402–7.

Colom F, Vieta E, Sanchez-Moreno J, Martinez-Aran A, Reinares M, Goikolea JM, et al. (2005) Stabilizing the stabilizer: group psychoeducation enhances the stability of serum lithium levels. *Bipolar Disorders*, **7**, 32–6.

Corrigan PW, McCracken SG, Holmes EP. (2001). Motivational interviews as goal assessment for persons with psychiatric disability. *Community Ment Health J*,**37**(2), 113–22.

Cramer JA, Rosenheck R. (1999). Enhancing medication compliance for people with serious mental illness. *J Nerv Ment Dis*, **187**, 53–5.

Department of Health (2009). *NHS Constitution: A Consultation on New Patient Rights*. London: Department of Health.

DiMatteo MR. (1979). A social-psychological analysis of physician patient rapport: toward a science of the art of medicine. *J Soc Issues*,**35**, 12–33.

Dolder CR, Lacro JP, Leckband S, Jeste D.(2003). Interventions to improve antipsychotic medication adherence: review of recent literature. *J Clinl Psychopharmacol*, **23**(4), 389–99.

Eckman TA, Liberman RP, Phipps CC, Blair KE. (1990). Teaching medication management skills to schizophrenic patients. *J Clin Psychopharmacoly*, **10**(1), 33–8.

Falloon MD, Boyd JL, McGill CW, Williamson M, Razani J, Moss HB, et al. (1985). Family management in the prevention of morbidity of schizophrenia. *Arch Gen Psychiatry*, **42**(9), 887–96.

Fenton WS, Biller CR, Heinssen RK. (1997). Determinants of medication compliance in schizophrenia: empirical and clinical findings. *Schizophr Bull*, **23**, 637–51.

Ford R, Beadsmore A, Ryan P, Repper J, Craig T, Mujen M. (1995). Providing the safety net: case management for people with serious mental illness. *J Ment Health*, **1**, 91–7.

Goodwin FK, Jamison KR. (1990). *Manic-depressive Illness*. New York: Oxford University Press.

Goulet J, Lalonde P, Lavoe G, Jodoin F. (1993). The impact of a neuroleptic education program on young adults with psychosis. *Can J Psychiatry*, **38**(8), 571–3.

Gray R, Leese M, Bindman J, Becker T, Burti L, David A, et al. (2006) Adherence therapy for people with schizophrenia. European multicentre randomised controlled trial. *Br J Psychiatry*, **189**, 508–14.

Gray R, Spilling R, Burgess D, Newey T. (2009). Antipsychotic long-acting injections in clinical practice: medication management and patient choice. *Brit J Psychiatry*, **195**, 51–6.

Grunebaum MF, Weiden Peter J, Olfson M. (2001). Medication supervision and adherence of persons with psychotropic disorders in residential treatment settings: a pilot study. *J Clin Psychiatry*, **62**, 5.

Harvey NS, Peet M. (1991). Lithium maintenance: 2. Effects of personality and attitude on health information acquisition and compliance. *Brit J Psychiatry*, **158**, 200–4.

Hayward P, Chan N, Kemp R, Cavanaugh JL Jr, Davis JM, Lewis DA. (1995). Predicting the revolving door phenomenon among patients with schizophrenia, schizoaffective, and affective disorders. *Am J Psychiatry*, **152**(6), 856–61.

Hill S, Laugharne R. (2006). *Patient choice survey in general adult psychiatry. Psychiatry on line.* http//www.priory.com/psych/cornwall.pdf (accessed 23 May 2010).

Hogarty GE, Andeson CM, Reiss DJ, Kornblith SJ, Greenwald DP, Ulrich RF, et al (1991). Family psychoeducation, social skills training, and maintenance chemotherapy in the aftercare treatment of schizophrenia. *Arch Gen Psychiatry*, **48**(4), 340–7.

Hope, T. (2002). Evidence-based patient choice and psychiatry. *Evid Based Ment Health*, **5**(4), 100–1.

Horne R, Weinman J. (1995). *The Beliefs about Medication Questionnaire: A New Measure for Assessing Lay Beliefs about Medicines.* London: BPS.

Kelly GR, Scott JE. (1990). Medication compliance and health education among outpatients with chronic mental disorders. *Med Care*, **28**, 1181–97.

Kemp R, Hayward P, David A. (1987). *Compliance Therapy Manual.* London: The Maudsley.

Kemp R, Hayward P, Grantley A, Everitt B, David A. (1996). Compliance therapy in psychotic patients, randomised controlled trial. *BMJ*, **312**(7027), 1302.

Kemp R, Kirov G, Everitt B, David A. (1998). Randomised controlled trial of compliance therapy. *Br J Psychiatry*, **172**, 413–9.

Kikkert MJ, Schene AH, Koeter MWJ, Robson D, Born A, Helm H, et al. (2006). Medication adherence in schizophrenia: exploring patients', carers' and professionals' views. *Schizophr Bull*, **32**(4), 786–94.

Lam DH, Watkinser, Hayward P, Bright J, Wright K, Kerr N, et al (2003). A randomised controlled study of cognitive therapy for relapse prevention for bipolar affective disorder. *Archf Gen Psychiatry*, **60**(2), 145–52.

Lecompte D, Pelc I. (1996). A cognitive-behavioural program to improve compliance with medication in patients with schizophrenia. *International J Ment Health*, **25**, 51–6.

Lehman AF, Goldman HH, Dixon LB, Churchill R. (2004). *Evidence-based Mental Health Treatments and Services: Examples to Inform Public Policy.* New York: Milbank Memorial Fund.

Leventhal H, Diefenbach M, Leventhal EA. (1992). Illness cognition: using common sense to understand treatment adherence and affect cognition interactions. *Cognit Ther Res*, **16**(2), 143–63.

Lingam R, Scott J. (2002). Treatment non-adherence in affective disorders. *Acta Psychiatr Scand*, **105**, 164–72.

MacPherson R, Jerrom B, Hughes A. (1996). A controlled study of education about drug treatment in schizophrenia. *Br J Psychiatry*, **168**, 709–17.

Marshall M, Lockwood A. (2002). Assertive community treatment for people with severe mental disorders. *Cochrane Database Syst Rev*, (2), CD001089.

Mendonca PJ, Brehm SS. (1983) Effects of choice on behavioral treatment of overweight children. *J Soc Clin Psychol*, **1**(4), 343–58.

Merinder LB, Viuff AG, Laugesen H, Clemmensen K, Misfelt S, Espensen B. (1999). Patient and relative education in community psychiatry; a randomised controlled trial regarding its effectiveness. *Soc Psychiatry Psychiatr Epidemiol*, **34**(6), 287–94.

Merinder LB. (2000). Education in schizophrenia: a review. *Acta Psychiatr Scand,*, **102**(2), 98–106.

Merinder LB. (2002). Patient education in schizophrenia: a review. *Acta Psychiatr Scand*, **102**(2), 98–106.

Miller WR, Rollnick S. (1991). *Motivational Interviewing, Preparing People to Change Addictive Behaviour*. New York: Guilford Press.

Modrcin M, Rapp CA, Poertner J. (1998). The evaluation of case management services with the chronically mentally ill. *Eval Program Plann*, **11**, 307–14.

National Institute for Health and Clinical Excellence. (2009). Schizophrenia: core interventions. In, *The Treatment and Management of Schizophrenia in Primary and Secondary Care* (Update): National Clinical Practice Guideline Number 82.

O'Donnell C, Donohoe G, Sharkey L, Owens N, Migone M, Harries R, et al. (2003). Compliance therapy, a randomised controlled trial in schizophrenia. *BMJ*, **327**, 834.

Patel MX, de Zoysa N, David AS., (2008). A cross-sectional study of patients' perspectives on adherence to antipsychotic medication, LAI versus oral, *J Clin Psychiatry*, **69**(10), 1548–56.

Patel MX, Haddad PM, Chaudhry IB, McLoughlin S, Husain N, David AS. (2009). Psychiatrists' use, knowledge and attitudes to first and second generation antipsychotic long-acting injections, comparisons over five years. *Journal of Psychopharmacology*, in press. (published online ahead of print 28 May 2009, doi, 10.1177/0269881109104882).

Patel MX, Nikolaou V, David AS. (2003) Psychiatrists' attitudes to maintenance medication for patients with schizophrenia. *Psychol Med*, **33**, 83–9.

Pekkala E, Merinder L (2002). Psychoeducation for schizophrenia. *Cochrane Database Syst Rev*, (2), CD002831.

Rankin, J. (2005). *A Good Choice for Mental Health; Working Paper Three*. London: Institute for Public Policy Research.

Razali SM, Hasanah CL, Khan A, Subramaniam M. (2000). Psychosocial interventions for schizophrenia. *J MentHealth*, **9**, 283–9.

Razali MS, Yahua H. (1995). Compliance with treatment in schizophrenia: a drug intervention program in a developing country. *Acta Psychiatr Scand*, **91**, 331–5.

Rennie TW, Bothamley GH, Engova D, Bates IP. (2007). Patient choice promotes adherence in preventive treatment for latent tuberculosis. *Eur Respir J*,**30**(4), 728–35.

Rollnick S, Miller WR. (1995). What is motivational interviewing? *Behav & CognPsychother*, **23**, 325–34.

Royal College of Psychiatrists. (2009). *Good Practice Report* (Third Edition). Dorchester: Dorset Press.

Samele C, Lawton-Smith S, Warner L, Mariathasan J. (2007) Patient choice in psychiatry. *Br J Psychiatry*, **191**, 1–2.

Scott J. (1999). Cognitive and behavioural approaches to medication adherence. *Adv Pychiatr Treatment*, **5**, 338–47.

Scott J. (2001). *Overcoming Mood Swings*. New York: Constable Robinson.

Scott J. (2004). Patient treatment issues and the successful combining of pharmacotherapy with psychoeducation. *Intl J Neuropsychopharmacol*, **7**, S96–7.

Scott J, Colom F. (2005). Psychological treatments for bipolar disorders. *Psychiatr Clin North Am*, **28**, 371–84.

Scott J, Paykel E, Morriss R, Bentall R, Kinderman P, Johnston T, et al. (2006) A randomised controlled trial of CBT versus usual treatment in severe and recurrent bipolar disorders. *Br J Psychiatry*, **188**, 313–20.

Scott J, Tacch MJ. (2002). A pilot study of concordance therapy for individuals with bipolar disorder who are non-adherent with lithium prophylaxis. *Bipolar Disorders*, **4**, 286–93.

Seltzer A, Roncar I, Garfinkel P. (1980). Effect of patient education on medication compliance. *Can J Psychiatry*, **25**, 638–45.

Shakir AS, Volkmar FR, Bacon S, Pfefferbaum A. (1979). Group psychotherapy as an adjunct to lithium maintenance *Am Journal Psychiatry*, **136**(4A), 455–6.

Smith J, Birchwood M, Haddrell A. (1992). Informing people with schizophrenia about their illness: the effect of residual symptoms. *J Ment Health*, **1**(1), 61–70.

Stein LI, Test MA. (1980). Alternative to mental hospital treatment, I: conceptual model, treatment program, and clinical evaluation. *Arch Gen Psychiatry*, **37**, 392–7.

Streicker SK, Amdur M, Dincin J. (1986). Educating patients about psychiatric medications: failure to enhance compliance. *Psychosoc Rehabil J*, **4**, 15–28.

Tacchi MJ, Scott J. (2005). *Improving Adherence in Schizophrenia and Bipolar Disorders*. Chichester, England: John Wiley.

Tarrier N, Barrowclough C, Vaughan C, Bamrah JS, Porceddu K, Watts S, et al. (1988). The community management of schizophrenia. A controlled trial of a behavioural intervention with families to reduce relapse. *Br. J. Psychiatry*, **153**, 532–42.

Telles C, Karno M, Mintz J, Paz G, Arias M, Tucker D, et al. (1995). Immigrant families coping with schizophrenia. *Br J Psychiatry*, **167**, 473–9.

Tiihonen J, Wahlbeck K, Lönnqvist J, Klaukka T, Ioannidis JP, Volavka J, et al. (2006). Effectiveness of antipsychotic treatments in a nationwide cohort of patients in community care after first hospitalisation due to schizophrenia and schizoaffective disorder, observational follow-up study. *BMJ*, **333**(7561): 224.

Van Gent C, Zwart F. (1991). Psycho-education of partners of bipolar-manic patients. *J Affective Disorders*, **21**, 15–18.

Velligan DI, Diamond PM, Mintz J, Maples N, Li X, Zeber J, et al. (2008). The use of individually tailored environmental supports to improve medication adherence and outcomes in schizophrenia. *Schizophr Bull*, **34**(3), 483–93.

Velligan D, Weiden P, Sajativic M, Scott J, Carpenter D, Ross R, et al. (2009). The expert consensus on medication adherence in schizophrenia and bipolar disorders. *J Clin Psych*, **70** (Suppl 4), 1–46.

Walburn J, Gray R, Gournay K, Quraishi S, David AS. (2001) Systematic review of patient and nurse attitudes to lai antipsychotic medication. *Br J Psychiatry*, **179**, 300–7.

Warner R. (2010). Does the scientific evidence support the recovery model? *The Psychiatrist*, **34**, 3–5.

Xiong W, Phillips MR, Hu X, Wang R, Dai Q, Kleinman J, et al. (1994). A family-based intervention for schizophrenic patients in China: a randomised controlled trial. *Br J Psychiatry*, **165**, 239–47.

Ziguras SJ, Klimidis S, Lambert TJ, Jackson AC. (2001). Determinants of anti-psychotic medication compliance in a multicultural population. *Community Ment Health J*, **37**(3), 273–83.

Zygmunt A, Olfson M, Boyer CA, David M. (2002). Interventions to improve medication adherence in schizophrenia. *Am J Psychiatry*, **159**(10), 1653–64.

Chapter 10

Prescribing patterns and determinants of use of antipsychotic long-acting injections: an international perspective

Tim Lambert

Correspondence: tim.lambert@sydney.edu.au

Introduction

As has been discussed in Chapter 1, medication adherence in psychotic patients is important because of the link to relapse, and the consequences of this for the progress of the illness and for the nature of the patient's treatment regime (Fenton et al. 1997; Haywood et al. 1995; Weiden & Glazer 1997). Concern for adherence with antipsychotic medications is not new. Knudsen (1985), in his review of depot issues, noted that as early as the 1960s it was known that approximately 50% of outpatients and up to 25% of inpatients did not take their medicine as prescribed. It was also understood at that time that the most important cause of re-hospitalization of schizophrenic patients was non-adherence (Christensen 1974; Hare & Willcox 1967; Knudsen 1985; Willcox et al. 1965). The rates of adherence to oral antipsychotics have not substantially improved over the decades, even with the advent of the oral SGAs (Dolder et al. 2002; Oehl et al. 2000).

Complicating the issue is the global trend towards a substantial reduction in psychiatric beds, falling from 4 per 1000 in 1960 to 1.3 per 1000 in 1996 in the United States. In Australia the reduction has been even more pronounced with a fall from 3.1 to 0.3 per 1000 over the corresponding period (Currier 2000). In both countries, and in many others in which available psychiatric beds have fallen, there has been a move from institutional care to community-based models of care. Whereas this promotes care in the least restrictive environment and may enhance a patient's quality of life (Newton et al. 2000), it does place greater reliance on the patient, their family, and other sources of non-direct care to promote adherence with physical and psychosocial treatments. It is likely that this trend places further pressure on the ability of persons with persistent psychosis to maintain their adherence to oral antipsychotic treatment.

Owing to their ability to deal effectively with oral antipsychotic non-adherence, LAIs have been described as a pivotal development in antipsychotic treatments as well as an important facet of deinstitutionalization and the maintenance of community psychiatry (Daniel 1968; Gerlach 1995; Hale 1993; Haring et al. 1981; Simpson 1984). Figure 10.1 shows the evolution of antipsychotic use and the target domains of therapy from the 1950s to the present. It is clear that after the introduction of each 'generation' of antipsychotics (first generation, or 'typicals' and second generation, or 'atypicals') there is a lag of less than a decade before LAI forms of the medications are introduced, presumably to help address the issue of non-adherence and relapse (Simpson 1984).

In this chapter we will review the rates of LAI prescription across the world, where possible note some of the trends in use over time, and discuss reasons that might account for the differences in prescription rates.

LAI prescription rates

Logically, if we consider that (i) the point prevalence of schizophrenia appears to be approximately in the range of 0.4% to 0.7% in most countries (Saha et al. 2005), (ii) antipsychotics are universally considered the bedrock of treatment for persistent psychosis, and (iii) the rate of clinically relevant non-adherence is likely to be of the order of one to two in three patients in most parts of the world, then we might logically expect that the rates of use of LAIs to be non-trivial and be approximately equal in a global sense. However, despite the use of LAIs in clinical practice since the 1960s, 'figures on the use of depots are sparse' (Adams et al. 2001, p. 290), and it is difficult to find readily available figures of prescription patterns that can be easily compared across regions. For descriptive purposes, rates of LAI use that have been able to be abstracted from the literature are presented for four regions: (i) Europe and the Middle East, (ii) North America (iii) Australasia and, (iv) rest of world (ROW) (see Tables 10.1–10.4).

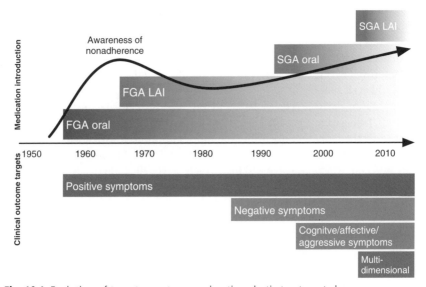

Fig. 10.1 Evolution of target symptoms and antipsychotic treatment classes.

Table 10.1 Use of LAIs in Europe and Middle East

Study	Study year	Country	Setting	LAI %
Johnson and Wright (1990)	1970	UK	O	High
Haring et al. (1981)	Late 1970s	Germany	U	33
Edwards and Kumar (1984)	1980s	UK	I	26
		UK	I	46
Muscettola et al. (1991)	1984	Italy	I, O	7.6[a]
Johnson and Wright (1990)	1987	UK	O	>37[a]
Meise et al. (1994)	1989	Austria	M	50
Lindström et al. (1996)	1991	Sweden	U	46.2
Kiivet et al. (1995)	1992	Spain	I	13
		Sweden	I	21
		Estonia	I	21
Tavcar et al. (2000)	1994	Slovenia	O	74
Barnes and Curson (1994)	To 1994	UK	LR/U	27–39
		Scandinavia	LR/U	≤ 60
Paton et al. (2003)	2003	UK	I	29
Foster et al. (1996)	1994	UK	O	29
Tognoni et al. (1999)	1994–1997	Italy	O	31.7[b]
Knapp et al. (2002)	1990s	UK (London)	M	33
		UK	M	50
Hanssens et al. (2006)	2006??	Belgium	O	21.5
Kovacs (2005)	2005	Hungary		26
Magliano et al. (2004)	1998	Italy		25
Bitter et al. (2003)	1999	Budapest,	I	26.9
		Hungary		42.0
Barnes et al. (2009)	2005–2007	UK	O	36
			F	28
			I	35
Heresco-Levy et al. (1989)	1985	Israel	O	45
	1987	Israel	O	58

LAI % = proportion of patients in sample receiving LAI.
U = unknown, presumed system-wide (M); O = outpatient/community; I = inpatient; F = forensic;
    LR = literature review.
[a] Not described; figures are estimated from data in paper.
[b] Average of participating centres.

Table 10.2 Use of LAIs in United States and Canada

Study	Year	Setting	LAI %
Price et al. (1985)	Early 1980s	O, CMHC	20
Remington et al. (1993)	Early 1990s	M	50
Citrome et al. (1996)	1994	I, VA	28(12–39
Rothbard et al. (2003)	1991	O, Medicaid	20
	1996		15
Valenstein et al. (2001)	1991–95	? O, VA	18(2–28
Rosenheck et al. (2000)	1994–96	O, VA	11.8
		O, non-VA	29.7
		I, VA	15.7
		I, non-VA	16.5
Remington et al. (2001)	1997 (Canada)	O, UNI O/P	23
		O, GEN O/P	15
		O, PH O/P	43
Bitter et al. (2003)	1999	I	1.2
Covell et al. (2002)	1998	O, non-VA	28
Barnes and Curson (1994)	<1994	Review	5–20

U = unknown, presumed system-wide (M); O = outpatient/community; I = inpatient; VA = veteran's affairs; CMHC = community mental health centres; non-VA = other non-VA setting, na = not available; UNI = university hospital, PH= psychiatric hospital, GEN = general hospital psych unit.
LAI % = proportion of patients in sample receiving LAI.

Europe and Middle East

Outside of inpatient settings, the general trend in Europe is supportive of antipsychotic LAIs being used in between one-quarter and one-half of non-hospitalized patients. In the 1980s, Israel was a robust user of LAIs with rates of use of up to 58%, perhaps reflecting the community focused care. The reported rates for inpatient use appear somewhat less but there are no studies that serially follow a cohort of patients from inpatient to outpatients and monitor changes in depot prescriptions. Thus the rates cannot be compared directly. Given the trend in the care of those with persistent psychosis is towards general community clinic care, the outpatient figures are the most relevant with respect to comparisons.

As Table 10.1 indicates, for many European regions, there are little data over time. In the United Kingdom there is some suggestion that in the 1970s the rates were 'high' (Johnson & Wright 1990) and by the 1990s had fallen to about one-third of prescriptions, a figure that appears to be somewhat stable into the 2000s (Barnes et al. 2009). There is some indication that in Italy rates declined over the 1990s to about 25%, a trend that is also reflected in countries such Australia and New Zealand (see below).

Table 10.3 Use of LAIs in Australia and New Zealand

Study	Year	Setting	LAI %
Lambert (1989–1991)[a]	1989-91	I, PH	61[b]
Galletly (1992)	1992	I, PH	61
Lambert (1994)[a]	1994	I, PH	72
Galletly and Tsourtos (1997)	1997	O, PH	48
Ziguras et al. (1999)[a]	1997	O, CP	42
Jablensky et al. (1999) (Low prevalence study)	1997–98	All	34.7[b]
		I	24.8
		O	29.2
Jablensky et al. (2000)	1998	All	25.6[c]
Keks et al. (1999)	1998	CP	33.2
Callaly and Trauer (2000)	1999	CP	28.3[b]
Humberstone et al. (2004)	2000	O	22.3
Mond et al. (2003)	2001	All; HIC	16.7
Lambert (2005)	1998	CP	47.6
	2000		33
	2002		28

O = outpatient; I = inpatient; TH = teaching hospital; PH = psychiatric hospital; CP = community psychiatric setting; HIC = Health Insurance Commission.
[a] Unpublished hospital-based audits undertaken by author.
[b] Rate for schizophrenia only.
[c] Any psychosis.
LAI % = proportion of patients in sample receiving LAI.

United States and Canada

The use of LAIs in the United States and Canada is shown in Table 10.2. It has been considered by some commentators that antipsychotic LAIs are underutilized in the United States, especially when compared to Europe and Australasia, with rates estimated to be from 4% to 15% (Barnes & Curson 1994; Remington & Adams 1995; Glazer 2007). However, the wide variety of service models in the United States, the fragmentation of services following deinstitutionalization, and the predominance of studies performed in the Veteran's Affairs (VA) systems suggest that this may be a simplification of a more regionally diverse and complex pattern.

A number of observations can be gleaned from the North American data. Rates of use of LAIs in non-hospital populations are lower than in Europe; those treated in community-based services may receive LAI prescriptions more frequently than those in hospital-based outpatient services, especially those associated with the VA system

Table 10.4 Use of LAIs in the rest of the world (Asia, South America etc)

Study	Study year	Country	Setting	LAI %
Chong et al. (2000)	1999	Singapore	I	66
Tan CH et al. (2008) See the breakdown in Sim et al. (2004)		East Asia	I	≤15.3
Xiang et al (2008)		Hong Kong	O	36.1
		Beijing		10
Bitter et al. (2003)	1999	Shanghai, China	I	0.0
		Hong Kong	I	26.0
		Tokyo	I	17.7
Ungvari et al. (1996)	1994	Hong Kong	I	46.8
Ungvari et al. (1997)	1996	Hong Kong	I	48.0
Kanazawa et al. (2008)	2008	Japan	U	1.5

U= unknown; O = outpatient/community; I = inpatient; LAI % = proportion of patients in sample receiving LAI.

or attached to psychiatric hospitals (Covell et al. 2002; Rosenheck et al. 2000). Little can be said concerning the trends over time, although US commentators have described a replacement of FGA-oral and FGA-LAI medications by SGAs (Rothbard et al. 2003), a picture that may also be present in Canada.

The impression that LAI use is 'low' in the United States might be further illuminated by examining the LAI prescription rates in specifically identified populations of non-adherent patients. In a survey of US psychiatrists, for patients who had demonstrated non-adherence, only 17.6% were prescribed LAIs (West et al. 2008). In a 3-year study of non-adherent patients only 12.4% were initiated on LAIs (Ascher-Svanum et al. 2009). Thus, US psychiatrists knowing that their patients are non-adherent are still reticent to prescribe LAIs. There may be 'culture-bound' forces that drive such prescribing disparities i.e. in the United States, LAI use may be viewed as a 'punitive' rather than an adherence tool (Glazer 2007).

Another problem of cross-sectional surveys, both in the United States and elsewhere, is that we are unable to get an impression of the persistence of LAI prescriptions (discussed below). For example, in the US-SCAP study, 26% of patients received an FGA-LAI at least once in the course of the 6-year study (Shi et al. 2007). This would undoubtedly translate into lower-point prevalence rates of LAI use.

Australasia

Despite the concerted move to a community-based care model in Australia and New Zealand, there is, as elsewhere, a paucity of studies that have reported on the prescription rate of LAI antipsychotics. The studies that were identified as well as further unpublished data are shown in Table 10.3. A number of reports have examined the use of antipsychotics in community or outpatient settings in the 1990s and from which estimates of LAI use could be obtained (Callaly & Trauer 2000; Galletly & Tsourtos 1997; Keks et al. 1999; Morgan et al. 2002; Wheeler et al. 2008; Ziguras et al. 1999). There are two studies that have examined serial trends over time (Lambert 2005; Wheeler et al. 2008).

For Australian non-hospitalized patients during the mid- to late 1990s the use of LAIs medication ranged between 28% and 48% of patients. By the early 2000s, well after the introduction of oral SGAs as the principal form of antipsychotic management (Mond et al. 2003), percentage rates for LAI prescribing in Australia had fallen to the high twenties (at least as can be determined from rates determined for those treated in the public sector in Victoria (Lambert 2005)), and in New Zealand, to the lower twenties (again from public sector prescribing audits, using the same protocol as in the Victorian study (Humberstone et al. 2004; Wheeler et al. 2008)). The time trends for antipsychotic use in Victoria between 1998 and 2002 are shown in Figure 10.2.

The Victorian data were obtained in a period where the last of the long-stay hospital beds closed (2000) to make way for an essentially community-based model of care (see Meadows & Singh 2001). These public-setting data show that FGA-orals are almost completely supplanted by SGA-orals. The high rates of LAI use found in the 1970s (see Table 10.3) fell progressively and appeared to be stabilizing around 29% of prescriptions for those with schizophrenia. This figure was not found to be significantly different from the rate of absolute non-adherence of 33% proposed for those with schizophrenia (Lambert 2005; Oehl et al. 2000).

To date, no formal studies have been carried out with respect to prescribing trends in the era of SGA-LAIs (i.e. risperidone LAI, which has been available in Australia since 2005 and olanzapine LAI, which became available in 2009).

The rest of the world

In this group of regions, there is wide disparity. Commonly held wisdom posits that overall rates of LAI use in China, Korea, and Japan are less than 2% (supported by

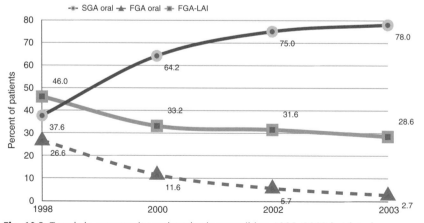

Fig. 10.2 Trends in community antipsychotic prescribing 1998–2003 in Victoria, Australia.

Kanazawa et al. 2008, Japan) and Bitter et al. (2003; China); yet studies that have examined particular services find higher rates, as shown in Table 10.4. More recent studies across East Asia estimate the *mean* rate of LAI use to be 15.3% in inpatient populations (Sim et al. 2004). Community-based LAI treatment data are sparse in comparison to hospitalized patient statistics. Hong Kong's non-hospital usage rate of 33% is much higher than in mainland China; this may reflect the very different health delivery systems for those with psychiatric illness that are found in the two regions. The outpatient rates for LAI use in southern Thailand of approximately 15% are consistent with the inpatient findings in the REAP study (Sim et al. 2004). All in all it is likely that there is wide variation in use (especially in inpatient settings) but there is a dearth of data for prescription rates in the community. Estimates from the above tables would suggest that the average LAI prescription rates may be on par with North America but less than in Australia and parts of Europe. At the time of writing it is not possible to describe temporal trends in community prescribing of LAIs.

Overview of influences on LAI prescription rates

Variations in the use of depots across and within countries, suggest the existence of factors that influence prescription rates in addition to levels of non-adherence alone. Identification of these factors would assist in informing us concerning the optimal the use of these agents (Curson et al. 1985; Remington & Adams 1995) and in recognizing the barriers to better implementing these agents. Indeed 'Only sparse information is available on the clinical and functional characteristics of patients treated with first-generation depot antipsychotics' (Shi et al. 2007 p.483), and the existing disparities in use suggest 'research questions for which we have inadequate data' (Essock 2002).

A number of factors have been proposed that may influence choice of a medicine in general: the rank order to market since class introduction; price; ease of use; prescribers' idiosyncratic beliefs and attitudes (perhaps based on a small number of personal experiences); marketing by pharmaceutical companies; the local prescribing culture; staff attitudes, training, and experience; the influence of the pharmacist (where available); perceived greater efficacy of one drug over another or perceived decrements in toxicity; whether a drug is seen as a 'breakthrough' medication; and other mechanisms beyond the effectiveness of the medication, including elements of the patient's sociodemographic background (Citrome et al. 1996; Domino et al. 2003; Essock 2002). However, it should be noted that a substantial proportion of the influence on prescribing remains unexplained (Domino et al. 2003).

In the following sections we shall consider influences on LAI use under the general headings of (i) the patient, (ii) the model of care, and (iii) the nature of the antipsychotic medication (see Figure 10. 3).

The patient

A number of patient-related associations have been made with the likelihood of receiving an LAI rather than an oral prescription.

Accommodation The patients' living situation and condition may influence prescriptions of LAIs, with those living in less well-supervised housing being more likely to receive LAIs (Tavcar et al. 2000).

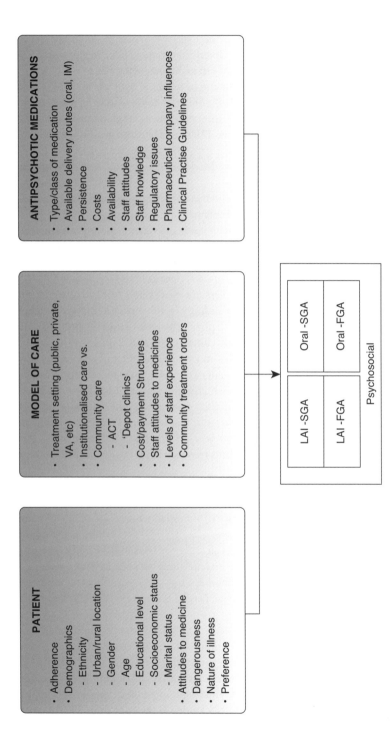

Fig. 10.3 Influences on the decision to prescribe treatment in schizophrenia.

Gender Gender has been variously reported as being unrelated to LAI use (Covell et al. 2002; Lindström et al. 1996) and higher in males (Arnold et al. 2004; Mark et al. 2003; Price et al. 1985; Shi et al. 2007). Given that male gender is a predictor of non-adherence, arguably the higher LAI rates in males may reflect this.

Age In terms of age, LAI use has been found to be higher in older persons (Magliano et al. 2004), younger persons (Price et al. 1985; Shi et al. 2007), and to be unrelated to age (Covell et al. 2002). On the whole, significant differences, when found, may not be particularly clinically significant as mean age differences between groups are often on the order of only 2 years.

Educational level LAI use has been linked to lower educational levels (Magliano et al. 2004; Shi et al. 2007).

Illness characteristics Those with more enduring negative symptoms may be targeted for this therapy as they have 'passive acceptance' of LAIs, although negative symptom states may make LAI adherence through clinic attendance more problematical (Macpherson et al. 1998; Tattan & Creed 2001). In the US-SCAP study, those receiving FGA-LAIs were more likely to have higher levels of psychopathology (PANSS total, PANSS positive, hostility and excitement factors, and disorganization) (Shi et al. 2007).

Psychiatric and forensic history LAI users are more likely to have more recent hospitalizations (Shi et al. 2007), to demonstrating a 'revolving door' history, perhaps as a proxy for severity of illness admixed with poor adherence (Tavcar et al. 2000), and have higher likelihood of arrests and forensic contacts (Shi et al. 2007). In terms of the temporal relationship between key variables and commencement of an LAI, Ascher-Svanum et al. (2009) showed that certain events were more likely to 'recently' precede initiation of an LAI compared to patients who did not start an LAI. These included recent hospitalization, recent arrest, recent illicit drug use, recent switching, or augmentation of oral antipsychotics, and recent treatment with oral FGAs. Depending on the variable 'recent' was defined as within 30 days to 6 months of starting the LAI. It is reasonable to suggest that these 'trigger' events may lead in part to the decision to start an LAI.

Substance use disorders Substance use problems are more likely in LAI-treated than orally treated patients (Shi et al. 2007). This is not an unexpected association given that substance misuse is highly predictive of non-adherence, for which LAIs are a common solution.

Patient preferences The patient's own preference for LAIs may be a key determinant of use. Patient support for their LAIs is somewhere between 39% and 89% (see Anderson et al. 1989; Desai 1999; Eastwood & Pugh 1997; Goldbeck et al. 1999; Hoencamp et al. 1995; Larsen & Gerlach 1996; Pereira & Pinto 1997; Singh et al. 1995; Warren 1995; Wistedt 1995).

Static cross-sectional estimations of satisfaction with LAIs may be confounded by a time dimension to attitude formation, with those who are stable on LAI medications providing higher rates of satisfaction than those who are newly switched to LAIs (Desai 1999). Periera and Pinto (1997) addressed the issue of patients' preference for taking depots relative to other medications and found those on depots are less happy with their medications than those on oral medications. At the same time, 59% of those on depots were happy to remain on depots and 89% were happy to remain on depots if they were given the choice of taking an oral medication also. Ninety-four per cent of those on orals were happy to remain on these medications. Similar rankings were produced from the Australian low-prevalence study (Castle et al. 2002; Jablensky et al. 2000). Needless to say, if a patient is vocal with regard to their preference, this may have a strong influence on the treatment team's decision to place the patient on a particular form of medicine.

Interpretation of these findings is not straightforward, especially when one considers that those on LAIs are often likely to have complicated clinical histories, including the poorest adherence history, which may itself be a consequence of negative attitudes to medicines in general. The patient preferences are further complicated by the attitudes towards the medication of those caring for the patient (see Chapter 8), which may run counter to those held by the patient. Some clinicians view LAIs (relatively) adversely and may believe that patients have the same attitude. Patients, left to their own devices, may be more accepting, for reasons that differ from what mental health staff might consider important (Finn et al. 1990; Kennedy et al. 2004; Svedberg et al. 2003; Van Dongen 1997).

Ethnicity With respect to ethnicity and antipsychotic prescribing in the United States, the United Kingdom, and New Zealand, non-Caucasian ethnic groups have significantly increased risks of receiving LAIs. In particular, this relates to those from dark-skinned ethnic minorities (Arnold et al. 2004; Kuno & Rothbard 2002; Wheeler et al. 2008). For non-black migrant populations e.g. Europeans in the United Kingdom and Australia, ethnic influences on medication management have not previously been found to be significant (Ziguras et al. 1999).

These ethnic differences may be accounted for in many ways although it appears that there may be a link between ethnicity and adherence with non-Caucasian patients having reduced adherence (Lawson 1996; Opolka et al. 2003).

In a more general framework, evidence exists for disparities in the health care of those of ethnic minority backgrounds. The US Surgeon-General's 2001 report on 'Race, Culture, and Ethnicity and Mental Health' demonstrated that there were clear disparities in access and treatment for ethnic minorities that resulted in them receiving inadequate or improper treatment (US Department of Health and Human Services 2001). In the US population, this seems to be most clear for those African-American and Afro-Caribbean background compared to Caucasians and other ethnic minorities (Mark et al. 2003). In Britain a similar situation may exist for Afro-Caribbean patients whose outcomes are in general poorer than for the predominant Caucasian population (Bhugra et al. 1997). The issue of ethnicity and prescribing has attracted much interest and in view of this it is considered in detail in the next section.

Ethnic differences and LAI prescribing rates

Table 10.5 summarizes literature on the influence of ethnicity on LAI usage and indicates a number of main trends appearing in the treatment profiles of different ethnic populations. In the United States, ethnic disparities in the prescription of LAIs have been described for more than 20 years. African-American inpatients have elevated risks of receiving LAIs compared to Caucasians. Although less is known of this group, Hispanic inpatients have odds ratios of the order of 1.5 compared to Caucasians.

Table 10.5 Ethnicity and depot antipsychotic use

Ethnic group	Year	Country	Setting	Data source	Use	Findings	Comments	Reference(s)
African-American	1985	US	C	RFA	More	OR 2.2	Young male black most likely; 37.1% vs. 14.9%	(Price et al. 1985)
African-American	1994	US	I	ADB	More	OR 1.99a	36% vs. 22%; $p < .05$	(Citrome et al. 1996)
Hispanic	1994	US	I	ADB	More	OR 1.52a	30% vs. 22%; $p < .05$	(Citrome et al. 1996)
African-Americans	1996	US	M	PORT	More	OR 2.91	40% vs. 18%	(Kreyenbuhl et al., 2003)
African-Americans	1991–95	US	O	P	More	OR 1.5	Controlled for adherence estimates	(Valenstein et al. 2001)
African-American	1995	US	O	ADB	More	OR 2.1a	26% vs. 14%; similar across 3 service settings	(Kuno and Rothbard, 2002)
Caribbeans	1985	UK	C	RFA+CI	More	$p < .01$	Bivariate analysis; young males in particular	(Glover and Malcolm, 1988)
Caribbeans	1991	UK	O	RTA	More		First episode cohort	(Chen et al., 1991)
Non-caucasian	1996–98	US	C	RFA	More	OR 2.12	Computed from OR for Caucasians (.47, $p = .005$).	(Covell et al., 2002)
East Asian	1997	UK	C	RFA+CI	More	$p < .01$	Bivariate analysis; mainly females of all ages	(Glover and Malcolm, 1988)
NESB	1997	AUS	C	RFA+CI	Equal	OR 1.42	33.9% vs. 50%	(Ziguras et al., 1999)
African-Americans	1999	US	O	RFA	More	OR 2.0	20% vs. 10%	(Woods et al., 2003)

African-Americans	1999–2001	US	M	P (SCAP)	More	$p < .05$	36% vs. 19% males; 27 vs. 15% females	(Mark et al., 2003)
African-Americans	1997–2003	US	M	P (SCAP)	More	OR 1.53		(Shi et al. 2007)
Maori	2000	NZ	C	RFA	More	OR 2.07		
Pacific Islander					More	OR 1.71		(Wheeler et al. 2008)
Asian					Equal	OR 0.95		

Where possible data represents schizophrenia, or non-affective psychotic disorders. NESB = non-English-speaking background; *Country*: US = USA, UK = Britain, AUS = Australia; *Setting*: I = inpatient, O = outpatients, C = community, PORT = Patient Outcomes Research Team, M = mixed, U =not known; *Source*: P = prospective study, RFA = retrospective file audit, ADB = administrative database, CI =clinician interview. *Findings*: OR =odds ratios. Significant wherever use is 'more' or 'less'.
[a] Crude OR calculated from reported raw rates/frequencies.
[b] From the dataset of Ziguras et al. (1999).

In outpatient/community settings the relative risk of receiving LAIs is between 1.3 and 1.6 times higher for African-Americans. In the United Kingdom, Afro-Caribbean patients and those of East-Asian background are also significantly more likely to receive LAIs. In the United Kingdom, inner-city morbidity patterns reflect a preponderance of Afro-Caribbean patients presenting in a disturbed state—the same group also appears to have higher rates of compulsory admission (Owens et al. 1991).

In a small study in the United Kingdom, Glover and Malcolm (1988) found that in community-treated patients, young males of African-Caribbean (West-Indian) background, more so than West-Indian women of all ages and older Asian women, were all more likely to receive LAI medications. The finding that 'extreme non-compliance' is predicted by ethnicity and gender might help explain the higher use of LAIs in the Afro-Caribbean male population; findings that may be helpful in understanding the high use of LAIs in African-Americans in other settings (Sellwood & Tarrier 1994).

In New Zealand both Maori and Pacific Islanders (dark-skinned ethnic groups) were found to have higher rates of LAI use compared to whites and Asian groups (Wheeler et al. 2008). It is noteworthy that these differences were not static. In a repeat study 4 years after the original, the ethnic differences in LAI prescription rates had disappeared.

Using data from an unpublished study of antipsychotic prescribing in Victoria, Australia (Lambert & Singh, unpublished data), when considering ethnicity dichotomously, differences between groups is significant in the late 1990s but equilibrates a number of years later (see Table 10.6). In this study, comprising many community urban and rural mental health centres, the largest of the centres with the highest proportion of ethnically diverse patients, showed no differences between ethnic groups in terms of LAI prescribing at any time point. What differences were found were in rural and smaller communities. Notably, the ethnically diverse populations did not comprise patients of Aboriginal or Torres Straits backgrounds (i.e. dark skinned) and so generally were Europid or Asian. This finding is consistent with that of a previous study in the same population, which indicated LAI use was equivocal between those of NESB and ES groups (Ziguras et al. 1999). The trend towards equal prescription rates between white and non-white populations over time (Table 10.6) parallels that seen in New Zealand. Unfortunately, there are no readily available data showing temporal trends in ethnically diverse populations in other countries.

In some of these studies attempts have been made to variously control for confounders such as age, gender, substance misuse, education, socio-economic class, and diagnosis. Even allowing for the influence of these covariates, ethnicity remains an independent predictor of LAI use. For example, in one study clinician-rated estimates of adherence were specifically controlled for (Valenstein et al. 2001). Despite this, African-American patients were a little less than 1.5 times more likely to be prescribed LAIs compared to Caucasians.

Ethnicity and SGAs

In a manner complementary to the findings above, the same populations that receive higher rates of LAIs receive significantly lower rates of SGA orals (Daumit et al. 2003; Mark et al. 2002; Opolka et al. 2003, 2004). The disparity in ethnic groups with respect

Table 10.6 Antipsychotic use by ethnicity and year

	Country of birth	N (%)		
		1998	2000	2002
LAIs	Non-ESB	137 (51.3)	88 (40.2)[b]	134 (34.2)
	ESB	188 (45.2)	239 (31.2)	377 (31.9)
	Any ethnicity	325 (47.6)	327 (33.2)	511 (32.5)
	All Vic patients (%)[a]	46.0	33.2	31.6
SGAs	Non-ESB	72 (27)[c]	133 (60.7)	282 (71.9)
	ESB	157 (37.7)	497 (65)	889 (75.3)
	Any ethnicity	229 (33.5)	630 (64)	1171 (74.5)
FGAs	Non-ESB	81 (30.3)	24 (11)	18 (4.6)
	ESB	110 (26.4)	90 (11.8)	75 (6.4)
	Any ethnicity	191 (28)	114 (11.6)	93 (5.9)

Data are from community-treated patients with schizophrenia in Western Melbourne, Victoria, Australia (unpublished data, Lambert & Singh 2005).
ESB = English-speaking background; NESB = non-English speaking background.
[a] Includes schizophrenia patients where ethnicity data is missing.
Odds ratios for ES vs. NESB patients:
[b] OR 0.696, 95% CI 0.496–0.923, p =.014.
[c] OR 1.642, 95% CI 1.174–2.295, p =.004
Percentages reflect proportions (point prevalence) of patients with schizophrenia receiving prescriptions for the antipsychotic class/type.

to SGA use has been suggested to be on account of an ethnic-specific time lag of some years between the introduction of a new agent and its implementation in usual practice. There remains the possibility that different groups will 'catch up' (Copeland et al. 2003; Daumit et al. 2003; Kreyenbuhl et al. 2003; Woods et al. 2003). The implication is that as SGA use equilibrates between ethnic groups, there will be a corresponding equilibration in the prescription of LAIs. For New Zealand Maori and Pacific Islanders this appears to have some validity (Wheeler et al. 2008).

Fully exploring the reasons for such ethnic differences in antipsychotic prescribing is beyond the scope of this chapter. However, a number of issues may be germane. As suggested by Glazer (2007), LAI use in certain countries or regions may be linked to prescriber perceptions relating to 'dangerousness' and go hand in hand with other methods of social control for this such as involuntary treatment. In multicultural societies certain ethnic minorities may stigmatize mental issues more than the host culture, a fact that is blamed for the reluctant and late presentation of many minority patients to psychiatric services. This in turn may affect the type of services required and/or provided, which can lead to interpretations by treating agencies such that a different set of rules applies to this group of patients, affording a part rationalization of different treatments given. Counter to this is the proposal of a specific culture of 'organizational racism', which is said to exist within psychiatry (quoted in Callan & Littlewood 1998). Impaired service delivery to black and ethnic minority patients may be linked to society's broader perceptions of minorities and their status (Lipsedge 1993). For example, treatments for Afro-Caribbean patients are geared towards pharmacotherapy rather than psychotherapy when compared to Caucasian patients. Furthermore, the use of involuntary admissions is twice as high in Afro-Caribbeans when compared to Caucasians and European migrants to Britain (Harrison et al. 1988) and remains so when controlling for age, gender, diagnosis, risk of violence, socio-economic status, and level of social support (Singh et al. 1998).

Blacks (Afro-Caribbeans, Africans, Somalis) are also over-represented in secure psychiatric facilities in the United Kingdom. The proportion of blacks in medium secure units in London has been found to be three times their population rate. As no differences from Caucasians on previous history, offending, and other variables that might predict use of this type of service have been found, the reason for this over-representation is not readily apparent (Lelliott et al. 2001). Perceived 'potential for dangerousness' has been suggested to underlie some of the more coercive approaches. For example, those assessed as being at risk of committing violence are more likely to receive involuntary detention (Singh et al. 1998). The issue of racial bias, perhaps expressed as racial perceptions rather than actual cultural differences, should be considered when examining disparities of care, including LAI treatments (Callan & Littlewood 1998, p. 3.; Snowden 2003,). Bias, should it exist, ultimately impairs the therapeutic alliance resulting in lack of trust and alienation (Misdrahi et al. 2009). That in turn is a major predictor of poor adherence, which in turn leads to the likelihood of increased LAI antipsychotic use.

It is possible that the issue of communication and ethnic relatedness is an important one. Ziguras et al. (1999, p. 884) examined the matching of case manager's ethnic background to that of their clients. In terms of access to SGAs versus LAI antipsychotics, matching for a case manager of the same background had no effect on access to SGAs but did make it less likely that a patient would receive LAI medication. In a later report, matching the case manager's ethnic background to that of the patient was a significant predictor of increased adherence when controlling specifically for the level of patient cooperativeness (Ziguras et al. 2003). This finding is consistent with US studies of ethnic matching (Flaskerud 1986; Flaskerud & Liu 1991) and would help explain reduced LAI prescribing in ethnically matched therapist–patient dyads.

In summary, there appears to be a consistent trend towards greater use of LAIs in patients of dark-skinned ethnic backgrounds compared to whites and Asians. Although there are some indications that the black population might be less adherent than white, which would justify the greater use of LAIs, that there may be independent factors such as perceived 'dangerousness' in the absence of solid evidence, suggests that it is not only the United States but other countries as well that may use LAIs for punitive reasons (Glazer 2007). Future research should address whether these findings that were largely published in the 1990s remain in the current era.

Model of care

As indicated in Figure 10.3 the second part of the framework for considering LAIs use looks at the Model of Care. The principal components first include the treatment setting. These vary widely and include public community mental health clinic settings, hospital outpatient departments, special services such as Veteran's Affairs in the United States, private medical systems, inpatient care, long-term institutional care, forensic systems, non-specialist care such as general practitioners (for a contrast between state and local versus federal service providers in the United States, see Rosenheck et al. 2000).

Second, the cost or payment structures may have a profound influence on the availability of certain treatments. Such structures include public insurance (Medicaid, Medicare in the United States; the NHS in the United Kingdom; Medicare in Australia), HMOs, and other private insurance variations.

Third is the provision of specialized treatment services such as assertive community teams (ACT), depot clinics, homelessness teams, and the other programmes that specifically address issues of the difficult to treat group of patients with SMI.

Fourth, the organizational culture itself may be overt or covert and be driven by specific staff attitudes, levels of experience, skills, and training. This may lead to idiosyncratic ways of doing business that reveal a specific medical micro-culture, replete with attitudes, behaviours, and rules that are particular to the micro-culture (Hughes et al. 2007; Hull et al. 2001).

Finally, and most important, is the role of community treatment orders (CTOs also known as outpatient commitment orders) in service models that are largely community focused.

In this section, we will deal briefly with the issues relating to the medical microculture and then focus on CTOs, as 'the relationship between receiving an LAI and being subject to a CTO is significant, and reflects the consideration given to enhancing adherence in a community mental health setting' (Lambert et al. 2009).

Treatment setting (micro-medical culture)

In the first part of this chapter we saw that in the broadest sense there may be cultural forces that drive LAI prescribing disparities e.g. the low rates in the United States of 10% to 15% versus higher rates elsewhere—and that behind these rates may lie different attitudes to the LAI tool i.e. in the United States is a 'punitive' tool (Glazer 2007), perhaps linked to concerns over dangerousness. When one examines prescribing at a more local level, it is clear that although there may be recognizable aggregate trends that pertain to countries or regions, there are wide variations, even within formal systems of care or cities. For example, those treated in VA settings, in contrast to those without medical insurance or who have other types of insurance, are less likely to receive LAIs (Citrome et al. 1996; Shi et al. 2007). However, even within a particular system of care such as the VA system there has been a great variation in depot rates, suggesting the ultimately dominant effects of local or even hospital prescribing culture (Citrome et al. 1996; Domino et al. 2003; Xiang et al. 2008; Valenstein et al. 2001). This may indicate that the attitudes of the health care providers, and perhaps the medical profession in particular, as discussed in detail in Chapter 8, may have very profound effects on the use of classes of medicine, not only LAIs but with other 'difficult' medications such as clozapine (Conley et al. 2005).

The authors (Bitter et al. 2003) of a multi-country comparative inpatient LAI prescribing study concluded, 'The results indicate that prescription patterns in different centres do not follow any specific guidelines for the treatment of schizophrenia. The results also confirm previous findings that prescribing practices for schizophrenia vary greatly among centres and countries.'

Community treatment orders

'The community treatment order (CTO) is used to address medication non-adherence by provision of involuntary treatment but in a less restrictive environment than that afforded by in-patient care' (Lambert et al. 2009 p.s57). The use of CTOs has been proposed as a specific service-related influence on the implementation of LAI treatments and, at least in Australia where CTOs have been is use since the 1980s, there appears a distinct relationship between their use and the use of LAI antipsychotics (Callaly & Trauer 2000; Lambert et al. 2009; Vaughan et al. 2000). In fact, it has been proposed that a CTO's principal function is in persuading patients to accept LAI antipsychotics (Hardman 1993; Ridley 1993; Swartz et al. 2001; Vaughan et al. 2000), or to help reduce the high defaulting rate of LAI patients in standard care (McLaren & Cookson 1989).

In brief, there exists a literature that supports the link between LAI use and some form of legal sanction. However, the association has largely been suggestive rather than empirically based (McLaren & Cookson 1989; Swartz et al. 2001; Vaughan et al. 2000; Weil 1996).

CTOs should be understood in the clinical context from where their use arises. As part of the process of deinstitutionalization, the locus of care has moved from institutions to the community. For the non-adherent and treatment reluctant patients, especially those identified as displaying the 'revolving door syndrome' (Weiden & Glazer 1997), the CTO provides a mechanism extending the state's power for involuntary treatment beyond the hospital and allows for their continuing treatment in a less restrictive environment (Fernandez & Nygard 1990; McIvor 1998; Power 1999).

CTOs or comparable arrangements are used in parts of the United States, Canada, Israel, New Zealand, Australia, and the United Kingdom (CTO legislation was initiated in November 2008 in England and Wales, see Patel et al. 2010). CTOs differ in their form and function somewhat between jurisdictions. In Victoria, Australia e.g. CTOs are defined as 'orders under the Mental Health Act which enable involuntary patients to live in the community while they receive treatment for their mental illness' (Department of Human Services 2004 p.2). By placing patients under such orders it is hoped that they will 'spend less time in hospital, gain more insight into their condition and be able to make effective use of community resources, even after the order [was] terminated' (McIvor 1998, p. 224).

Despite the proposition that their effect is likely to work through 'persuading the persuadable' to engage in treatment (Bar El et al. 1998; Dedman 1990; Pinfold et al. 2001; Swartz et al. 2001), there are reports of improved outcomes for those treated in the community with CTOs compared to patients not discharged on CTOs (Power 1998; Vaughan et al. 2000). However, the improvements seen with CTOs may simply reflect better, more integrated services being made available to the CTO patient, perhaps in concert with LAI delivery, and more research is required to determine the active therapeutic components of a CTO (McIvor 1998; Swartz et al. 2001).

In the United States for a patient subject to a sustained period on a CTO, it appears that the attendant increase in service intensity that accompanies the order is the effective component of improvement in outcomes rather than the legal order per se. Thus it has been argued that, for patients prescribed an LAI within the US context, adherence is enhanced independently of the main effect of longer-term CTO involvement (Swartz et al. 2001). It is feasible that the legal process first grants access to treating the patient with a LAI and second, provides sufficient time to establish a regular injection routine. The latter may in turn allow difficult to treat patients a better chance of establishing some control over their illness and with it a measure of improved insight which in itself *may* enhance further adherence (Cuffel et al. 1996; Garavan et al. 1998; Kemp et al. 1998).

In Israel the success of the CTO was considered to be owing to its promotion of the use of LAIs in unwilling patients (Weil 1996). It is noteworthy that this report 'detailed statistics related to uncooperative patients . . . [that] reveal that a significant proportion of such patients become cooperative once the process is activated'. Community-treated patients who willingly attended their outpatient appointments were likely to be taken off their order. This suggests the possibility that the CTO functions to engage the reluctant patient in initiating LAI treatment, and that once it is established, the order becomes less critical in and of itself. This finding would be consistent with that found in the North Carolina studies and is also consistent with the that for those receiving LAIs, re-admission, and LAI adherence in an index year is not predicted by CTO status (Lambert et al. 2007), a finding supported by adherence and CTO status in US studies (Swartz et al. 2001).

In Australia, there is common use of LAIs (see Table 10.3) and an established clinical framework for CTO use. Lambert et al. (2009) and Callaly and Trauer (2000)found that the odds ratio of a CTO being used in LAI-treated patients was about four times that of CTO use in all other antipsychotics. Callaly and Trauer's conclusion regarding this relationship is consonant with what is undoubtedly a commonly held point of view of clinicians in Victoria: 'As might be expected, the proportion of patients who were subject to a community treatment order was higher for those prescribed LAI antipsychotics than for those who were prescribed oral antipsychotics. This confirms that LAI antipsychotics tend to be prescribed where there is a clinical perception that the patient is at high risk of non-compliance' (Callaly & Trauer 2000, p. 223). Some authors have linked the potential effectiveness of CTOs (e.g. in reducing hospitalization) more directly to their ability to promote the use of LAIs under the order (Vaughan et al. 2000; Weil 1996).

Vaughan et al.'s (2000) study provided a picture that was consistent with the notion that better outcomes are linked to the ability of CTOs to ensure that patients are (i) treated with LAIs and (ii) that this then enables other psychosocial treatments to be more frequently applied. As noted above, CTO effectiveness may lie in the ability, and inclination, of a mental health service to provide a range and depth of adequate services once the patient is engaged through the mechanism of the CTO (Swartz et al. 1999; Vaughan et al. 2000).

In terms of the framework model proposed in Figure 10.2, the need for LAI medication follows from issues of poor adherence (the patient), interacting with constraints within the case management system (the Model of Care). It would be expected that if there were any degree of drug refusal, or ambiguity about adherence, then LAI treatment would be warranted. However, it is possible that, having made the prescribing decision, patients may still refuse to accept treatment. The CTO provides an avenue to persuade reluctant patients in the community to accept mandated treatment and thus represents an essential component of the Service's response to non-adherence. The strong relationship between CTO use and LAI prescriptions is, therefore, one that might be expected to be found in countries/regions that implement any form of CTO.

The antipsychotic

As shown in Figure 10.3, influences on LAI prescription relating to the nature of the antipsychotic include the type or class of medication, the available delivery routes (oral, IM, orodispersible), availability, direct acquisition cost, staff knowledge, and attitudes towards the agent, regulatory issues, pharmaceutical company influences, and clinical Practice Guidelines.

Class of medicine As discussed in Chapter 8, attitudes towards LAIs can be somewhat negative. Patel et al. (2009, 2003) found that although UK psychiatrists thought that the advent of SGA-LAIs would lead to a broader rate of use, following the introduction of risperidone LAI, the rates of use had instead fallen, although attitudes and knowledge had remained stable. As noted earlier in the chapter, it is as yet unclear as to what the introduction of SGA-LAIs has had on the proportions of patients treated with LAIs in general in settings other than the United Kingdom, especially those with lower LAI usage rates.

Delivery route As discussed in Chapter 2, LAIs differ in their requirement for oral supplementation. The FGA-LAIs in general require some degree of oral antipsychotic augmentation in the first weeks owing to their slow increase in plasma levels over the first few months of use. Similarly, the microsphere-based risperidone LAI requires 3 to 6 weeks of oral augmentation at initiation. Some practitioners may consider that in this augmentation phase it is better to have medication of one type across the phases of illness, despite there being little evidence to support this. It is more likely that if a prescriber has experience with an oral form of the medication, then he or she may be more comfortable with the LAI form. Thus these concerns may limit the choice of LAI prescribed.

Persistence Arguably one might expect that the use of LAIs would be associated with greater medication persistence, given that for many patients the medication has been initiated owing to previous poor adherence with oral medications. The literature varies on this point. For example, in California medicaid patients persistence with LAIs is very short, many discontinuing within the first few months of treatment (Olfson et al. 2007). In the US-SCAP study those initiated on LAI treatment had a significantly longer mean time to all-cause medication discontinuation (292 days and 316 days, respectively for fluphenazine and haloperidol decanoates) and were twice as likely to stay on the LAI in comparison with oral form of the medication for one year (Zhu et al. 2008). Another way of examining persistence is to consider what proportion remains on LAIs for 18 months, a period suggested as necessary to show separation from oral medications in terms of outcomes such as relapse rates. In an Australia study the 18-month LAI persistence rate was 65% (Lambert 2007); in the Connecticut public sector, at 18 months the persistence rate was similar at about 65% to 70% (Covell et al. 2002). In both of these studies individual services were audited and data abstracted within the context of 'real-world' prescriptions. Of the SGA-LAIs, in the Spanish arm of the international e-Star observational study the 18-month persistence was about 85% (Olivares et al. 2009), considerably higher than that seen with FGA-LAIs and also higher than seen in other arms of the e-Star study such as Australia (Lambert et al. 2009). The lack of any head-to-head FGA-LAI versus SGA-LAI studies at this point in time does not allow us to conclude whether in general persistence has changed with the advent of the latter class of agents. To put these data into perspective we need to consider how the data compare to the persistence rates seen with oral medication. It is common to find that both clozapine and oral olanzapine have higher rates of persistence in the 18- to 36-month range (Haro et al. 2007; Lambert 2007). In general for oral medications, SGAs have longer persistence than FGAs (Ascher-Svanum et al. 2006) and there exists a general trend for clozapine and olanzapine to separate from other antipsychotics.

Availability Not all countries have a broad spectrum of agents available, with the United States being limited to two FGA-LAIs (fluphenazine and haloperidol) and two SGA-LAIs (risperidone and paliperidone; perhaps with olanzapine to follow), Europe having a wider selection of FGA-LAIs (perphenazine, zuclopenthixol, flupentixol, pipothiazine, fluphenazine, haloperidol, and others; Adams et al. 2001) and a number of SGA-LAIs, and Asia having in general a reduced range in any one country but overall access to a broader range than in the United States. The disparate availability depends, at least in part, on the influence of pharmaceutical company drives towards country registration and marketing which is in many cases quite country-specific. In Australia e.g. marketing for FGA-LAIs is virtually non-existent, perhaps because they are low-cost items that retain a solid share of prescriptions (Table 10.6).

Direct costs The actual cost of medications also differs widely between countries and this may in part be determined by different reimbursement practices (Danzon & Furukawa 2008; Lexchin & Mintzes 2008). The cost to the individual patient is key here—in a country with a universal health insurance scheme such as Australia, the individual in a community health setting may pay either nothing or the minimum co-payment of a few dollars, whether it be for inexpensive FGA-LAIs or expensive SGA-LAIs. In countries without such protection for patients, the same medications may cost many hundreds of dollars per month and thus for the chronically ill patient without family financial support or an active job, be beyond their means to pay.

Attitudes of mental health staff and patients to LAIs LAIs may be underused in part due to their having an 'image problem', with some mental health professionals and patients holding negative attitudes towards their use (Adams et al. 2001; Lambert et al. 2003; Patel & David 2005). A basic maxim concerning attitudes is that knowledge affects attitudes, which in turn affect behaviour. For a greater understanding of this area, see Chapter 8.

CPGs and evidence-based medicine Most clinical practice guidelines (CPGs) that are issued by professional bodies, governmental departments as well as groups of experts suggest that LAIs should be used in cases of known poor adherence, where there is a clear revolving door syndrome in evidence, or when there is evidence of a particularly difficult course (e.g. see Kane et al. 1998). Despite high rates of non-adherence (see Chapter 1) we have seen that LAI use can be quite low, despite CPG advice. Here, as in many branches of medicine, it is not uncommon for CPGs to be ignored or used variably (Cabana et al. 1999). Some of the common reasons posited for this include problems with awareness, familiarity, ability to overcome the inertia of previous practice, and absence of external barriers to perform recommendations (Cabana et al. 1999).

There is evidence that in health maintenance organization (HMO) sectors, the organizational culture can be modified towards one more in keeping with the evidence base (Kahan et al. 2009). However, imposing an external locus of control through punitive regulation has not been shown to modify poor prescribing (at least in the elderly) (Kahan et al. 2009; Hughes et al. 2007) and it may be that identified barriers in one particular setting—and the requisite solutions—are not generalizable to other settings (Cabana et al. 1999). Furthermore, in many studies of barriers to implementation of guidelines single barriers are identified as targets for intervention, rather than appreciating that within any one micro-medical culture, multiple barriers may be simultaneously operative.

Methodological issues in LAI use research

One of the principal problems in comparing usage rates, and therefore the determinants or association of LAI prescriptions, lies in the nature of where the data are obtained from. Countrywide statistics from a clearly defined population of patients or an epidemiological sample are required to better test the notion that there are cultural forces at work. At present we only have rates from one or a few centres, and these centres may well be unrepresentative of others of the same ilk, or those in completely different systems of care. Often even basic descriptors of the service and its setting are hard to identify, such as whether they are inpatients or outpatients; whether they were drawn from persons with schizophrenia versus non-schizophrenia, and so on. The unknown nature of the service may have a specific bearing on rates of use. For example, the UK community sample described by Barnes et al. (2009; see Table 10.1) is for assertive outreach teams. This may inflate community prescription rates as typically patients in such teams are among the most difficult to manage using standard community/outpatient methods and as such are candidates for LAIs and clozapine (Craig & Pathare 1997).

Furthermore, reports of prescription rates lag some years between data acquisition and reporting—in that time there may be secular trends that alter prescribing (introduction of new agents, other barriers arising, changes in organizational culture, new prescribing guidelines and edicts, and so on). By the time prescription surveys (the few that there are) come into press, they may well be out of date.

Conclusion

Antipsychotic LAIs continue to have a place in therapy. Although they are prescribed in a significant minority of patients with schizophrenia managed by both general community teams and in inpatient settings, their usage rates vary widely between and within countries and cultures. Whether their use is 'enough' or even satisfactory depends on whether adequate numbers of non-adherent patients are being identified first and then treated with LAIs where appropriate. In this chapter we have reviewed the various factors that may influence prescribing rates and considered them within a framework of influences comprising the patient, the model of care, and the nature of the antipsychotics.

Despite our somewhat fragmented knowledge of the associations with LAI use, there remains a significant deficit in our understanding of the consideration for LAI use that occurs at the micro-level of the individual prescriber and/or his or her micro-medical culture. Future research may well benefit from exploring how these issues facilitate or impede the use of these medications in a population with well-established non-adherence, and to promote ways in which the strong evidence base for the role of LAIs in relapse prevention can be better communicated and implemented. The recent establishment of an international educational programme on relapse prevention (CERP) represents a first step in this direction (Lambert et al 2010).

References

Adams, CE, Fenton MK, Quraishi S, David AS. (2001). Systematic meta-review of depot antipsychotic drugs for people with schizophrenia. *Br J Psychiatry*, **179**, 290–9.

Anderson, D, Leadbetter A, Williams B. (1989). In defence of the depot clinic. The consumers opinion. *Psychiatr Bull*, **13**, 177–9.

Arnold, LM, Strakowski SM, Schwiers ML, Amicone J, Fleck DE, Corey KB, et al. (2004). Sex, ethnicity, and antipsychotic medication use in patients with psychosis. *Schizophr Res*, **66**(2–3), 169–75.

Ascher-Svanum, H, Peng X, Faries D, Montgomery W, Haddad PM. (2009). Treatment patterns and clinical characteristics prior to initiating depot typical antipsychotics for nonadherent schizophrenia patients. *BMC Psychiatry*, **9**, 46.

Ascher-Svanum H, Zhu B, Faries D, Landbloom R, Swartz M, Swanson J. (2006). Time to discontinuation of atypical versus typical antipsychotics in the naturalistic treatment of schizophrenia. *BMC Psychiatry*, **6**, 8.

Bar El, YC, Durst R, Rabinowitz J, Kalian M, Teitelbaum A, Shlafman M. (1998). Implementation of order of compulsory ambulatory treatment in Jerusalem. *Int J Law Psych*, **21**, 65–71.

Barnes TRE, Curson DA. (1994). Long-term depot antipsychotics: a risk-benefit assessment, *Drug Safety*, **10**, 464–79.

Barnes TRE, Shingleton-Smith A, Paton C. (2009). Antipsychotic long-acting injections: prescribing practice in the UK. *Br J Psychiatry*, **195**, S37–S42.

Bhugra D, Leff J, Mallett R, Der G, Corridan B, Rudge S. (1997). Incidence and outcome of schizophrenia in whites, African-Caribbeans and Asians in London. *Psychol Med*, **27**(4), 791–8.

Bitter I, Chou JC, Ungvari GS, Tang WK, Xiang Z, Iwanami A, et al. (2003). Prescribing for inpatients with schizophrenia: an international multi-center comparative study. *Pharmacopsychiatry*, **36**(4), 143–9.

Cabana MD, Rand CS, Powe NR, Wu AW, Wilson MH, Abboud PA, et al. (1999). Why dont physicians follow clinical practice guidelines? A framework for improvement. *JAMA*, **282**(15), 1458–65.

Callaly T, Trauer T. (2000). Patterns of use of antipsychotic medication in a regional community mental health service. *Australas Psychiatry*, **8**(3), 220–4.

Callan A, Littlewood R. (1998). Patient satisfaction: ethnic origin or explanatory model? *Int J Soc Psychiatry*, **44**(1), 1–11.

Castle D, Morgan V, Jablensky A. (2002). Antipsychotic use in Australia: the patients perspective. *Aust N Z J Psychiatry*, **36**(5), 633–41.

Chen EY, Harrison G, Standen PJ. (1991). Management of first episode psychotic illness in Afro-Caribbean patients. *Br J Psychiatry*, **158**, 517–22.

Chong SA, Sachdev P, Mahendran R, Chua H-C. (2000). Neuroleptic and anticholinergic drug use in Chinese patients with schizophrenia resident in a state psychiatric hospital in Singapore. *Australas Psychiatry*, **34**(6), 988–91.

Christensen, JK. (1974). A 5-year follow-up study of male schizophrenics: evaluation of factors influencing success and failure in the community. *Acta Psychiatr Scand*, **50**, 60–72.

Citrome L, Levine J, Allingham B. (1996). Utilization of depot neuroleptic medication in psychiatric inpatients. *Psychopharmacol Bull*, **32**(3), 321–6.

Conley RR, Kelly DL, Lambert TJ, Love RC. (2005). Comparison of clozapine use in Maryland and in Victoria, Australia. *Psychiatr Serv*, **56**(3), 320–3.

Copeland LA, Zeber JE, Valenstein, M, Blow FC. (2003). Racial disparity in the use of atypical antipsychotic medications among veterans. *Am J Psychiatry*, **160**(10), 1817–22.

Covell, NH, Jackson CT, Evans AC, Essock SM. (2002). Antipsychotic prescribing practices in Connecticut's public mental health system: rates of changing medications and prescribing styles. *Schizophr Bull*, **28**(1), 17–29.

Craig T, Pathare S. (1997). Assertive community treatment for the severely mentally ill in West Lambeth. *Adv Psychiatr Treatment*, **3**, 111–18.

Cuffel BJ, Alford J, Fischer EP, Owen RR. (1996). Awareness of illness in schizophrenia and outpatient treatment adherence. *J Nerv Ment Dis*, **184**(11), 653–9.

Currier GW. (2000). Psychiatric bed reductions and mortality among persons with mental disorders. *Psychiatr Serv*, **51**(7), 851.

Curson DA, Barnes TR, Bamber RW, Platt SD, Hirsch SR, Duffy JC. (1985). Long-term depot maintenance of chronic schizophrenic out-patients: the seven year follow-up of the Medical Research Council fluphenazine/placebo trial. II. The incidence of compliance problems, side-effects, neurotic symptoms and depression. *Br J Psychiatry*, **146**, 469–74.

Daniel GR. (1968). Social and economic effects of long acting phenothiazines. *Br J Soc Psychiatry*, **2**, 167–9.

Danzon PM, Furukawa MF. (2008). International prices and availability of pharmaceuticals in 2005. *Health Aff ((Millwood)*, **27**(1), 221–33.

Daumit GL, Crum RM, Guallar E, Powe NR, Primm AB, Steinwachs DM, et al. (2003). Outpatient prescriptions for atypical antipsychotics for African Americans, Hispanics, and whites in the United States. *Arch Gen Psychiatry*, **60**(2), 121–8.

Dedman P. (1990). Community treatment orders in Victoria, Australia. *Psychiatr Bull*, **14**, 462–4.

Department of Human Services. (2004). *Involuntary Patients. About Your Rights* (May 2005 edition). Melbourne: Mental Health Branch, Victorian Government Dept of Human Services.

Desai N. (1999). Switching from depot antipsychotics to risperidone: results of a study of chronic schizophrenia. *Adv Ther*, **16**, 78–88.

Dolder CR Lacro JP, Dunn LB, Jeste DV. (2002), Antipsychotic medication adherence: is there a difference between typical and atypical agents? *Am J Psychiatry*, **159**(1), 103–8.

Domino ME, Frank RG, Rosenheck R. (2003). The diffusion of new antipsychotic medications and formulary policy. *Schizophr Bull*, **29**(1), 95–104.

Eastwood N, Pugh R. (1997). Long-term medication in depot clinics and patients rights: an issue for assertive outreach. *Psychiatr Bull*, **21**, 273–5.

Edwards S, Kumar V. (1984). A survey of prescribing of psychotropic drugs in a Birmingham psychiatric hospital. *Br J Psychiatry*, **145**, 502–7.

Essock SM. (2002). Editors introduction: antipsychotic prescribing practices. *Schizophr Bull*, **28**(1), 1–4.

Fenton WS, Blyler CR, Heinssen RK. (1997). Determinants of medication compliance in schizophrenia: empirical and clinical findings. *Schizophr Bull*, **23**(4), 637–51.

Fernandez GA, Nygard S. (1990). Impact of involuntary outpatient commitment on the revolving-door syndrome in North Carolina. *Hosp Community Psychiatry*, **41**(9), 1001–4.

Finn SE, Bailey JM, Schultz RT, Faber R. (1990). Subjective utility ratings of neuroleptics in treating schizophrenia. *Psychol Med*, **35**, 843–8.

Flaskerud, JH. (1986). The effects of culture-compatible intervention on the utilization of mental health services by minority clients. *Community Ment Health J*, **22**(2), 127–41.

Flaskerud JH, Liu PY. (1991). Effects of an Asian client-therapist language, ethnicity and gender match on utilization and outcome of therapy. *Community Ment Health J*, **27**(1), 31–42.

Foster K, Meltzer H, Gill B, Hinds K. (1996). *OPCS Surveys of Psychiatric Morbidity in Great Britain. Report 8: Adults with Psychotic Disorder Living in the Community.* London: HMSO.

Galletly CA. (1992). Antipsychotic drug doses in a schizophrenia inpatient unit. *Aust N Z J Psychiatry*, **26**(4), 574–6.

Galletly CA, Tsourtos G. (1997). Antipsychotic drug doses and adjunctive drugs in the outpatient treatment of schizophrenia. *Ann Clin Psychiatry*, **9**(2), 77–80.

Garavan J, Browne S, Gervin M, Lane A, Larkin C, O'Callaghan E. (1998). Compliance with neuroleptic medication in outpatients with schizophrenia; relationship to subjective response to neuroleptics; attitudes to medication and insight. *Compr Psychiatry*, **39**(4), 215–9.

Gerlach J. (1995). Depot neuroleptics in relapse prevention: advantages and disadvantages. *Int Clin Psychopharmacol*, **9**(Suppl 5), 17–20.

Glazer WM. (2007). Who receives long-acting antipsychotic medications? *Psychiatr Serv*, **58**(4), 437.

Glover G, Malcolm G. (1988). The prevalence of depot neuroleptic treatment among West Indians and Asians in the London borough of Newham. *Soc Psychiatry Psychiatr Epidemiol*, **23**(4), 281–4.

Goldbeck R, Tomlinson S, Bouch J. (1999). Patients knowledge and views of their depot neuroleptic medication, *Schizophr Bull*, **23**, 426–33.

Hale T. (1993). Will the new antipsychotics improve the treatment of schizophrenia? *BMJ*, **307**(6907), 749–50.

Hanssens L, De Hert M, Wampers M, Reginster JY, Peuskens J. (2006). Pharmacological treatment of ambulatory schizophrenic patients in Belgium. *Clin Pract Epidemol Ment Health*, **2**, 11.

Hardman AE. (1993). Community treatment order in Australia. *Br J Psychiatry*, **162**, 710.

Hare EH, Willcox DR. (1967). Do psychiatric in-patients take their pills? *Br J Psychiatry*, **113**, 1435–39.

Haring C, Tegeler J, Lehmann E, Ptock W. (1981). Social aspects of therapy with depot neuroleptics in the Federal Republic of Germany. *Acta Psychiatrica Belgica*, **81**(2), 189–202.

Haro JM, Suarez D, Novick D, Brown J, Usall J, Naber D; SOHO Study Group. (2007). Three-year antipsychotic effectiveness in the outpatient care of schizophrenia: observational versus randomized studies results. *Eur Neuropsychopharmacol*, 17(4), 235–44.

Harrison G, Holton A, Neilson D, Owens D, Boot D, Cooper J. (1988). Severe mental disorder in Afro-Caribbean patients: some social. demographic and service factors. *Psychol Med*, 19(3), 683–96.

Haywood TW, Kravitz HM, Grossman LS, Cavanaugh JL Jr, Davis JM, Lewis DA. (1995). Predicting the 'revolving door' phenomenon among patients with schizophrenic, schizoaffective, and affective disorders. *Am J Psychiatry*, 152(6), 856–61.

Heresco-Levy U, Greenberg D, Wittman L, Dasberg H, Lerer B. (1989). Prescribing patterns of neuroactive drugs in 98 schizophrenic patients. *Isr J Psychiatry Relat Sci*, 26(3), 157–63.

Hoencamp E, Knegtering H, Hooy JJS, van der Molen AEGM. (1995). Patient requests and attitude towards neuroleptics. *Nord J Psychiatry*, 49(Suppl 35), 47–55.

Hughes CM, Lapane K, Watson MC, Davies HT. (2007). Does organisational culture influence prescribing in care homes for older people? A new direction for research. *Drugs Aging*, 24(2), 81–93.

Hull SA Cornwell J, Harvey C, Eldridge S, Bare PO. (2001). Prescribing rates for psychotropic medication amongst East London general practices: low rates where Asian populations are greatest. *Fam Pract*, 18(2), 167–73.

Humberstone V, Wheeler A, Lambert T. (2004). An audit of outpatient antipsychotic usage in the three health sectors of Auckland, New Zealand. *Aust N Z J Psychiatry*, 38(4), 240–5.

Jablensky A, McGrath J, Herrman H, Castle D, Gureje O, Carr V, et al. (1999). National survey of mental health and wellbeing. Report 4. In *People Living with Psychotic Illness: An Australian Study 1997–98. An Overview*. Canberra: Commonwealth Department of Health and Aged Care.

Jablensky, A, McGrath J, Herrman H, Castle D, Gureje O, Evans M, et al. (2000). Psychotic disorders in urban areas: an overview of the study on low prevalence disorders. *Aust N Z J Psychiatry*, 34(2), 221–36.

Johnson DAW, Wright NF. (1990). Drug prescribing for schizophrenic out-patients on depot injections. Repeat surveys over 18 years. *Br J Psychiatry*, 156, 827–34.

Kahan NR, Kahan E, Waitman DA, Kitai E, Chintz DP. (2009). The tools of an evidence-based culture: implementing clinical-practice guidelines in an Israeli HMO. *Acad Med*, 84(9), 1217–25.

Kanazawa, T, Tsutsumi A, Nishimoto Y, Yoneda H. (2008). The questionnaire of the usage of depot injection in Japan. *Eur Neuropsychopharmacol*, 18, S418–19.

Kane JM, Aguglia E, Altamura AC, Ayuso Gutierrez JL, Brunello N, Fleischhacker WW, et al. (1998). Guidelines for depot antipsychotic treatment in schizophrenia, *Eur Neuropsychopharmacol*, 8(1), 55–66.

Keks NA, Altson K, Hope J, Krapivensky N, Culhane C, Tanaghow A, et al. (1999). Use of antipsychosis and adjunctive medications by an inner urban community psychiatric service. *Aust N Z J Psychiatry*, 33(6), 896–901.

Kemp R, Kirov G, Everitt B, Hayward P, David A. (1998). Randomised controlled trial of compliance therapy. 18-month follow-up. *Br J Psychiatry*, 172, 413–19.

Kennedy FC, Seth R, Sinclair S, Levey S, Bentall RP. (2004). Patients appraisals of neuroleptic medication: the measurement and predictive utility of attitudes. *Int J Psychiatry Clin Pract*, 9(1), 21–7.

Kiivet R, Llerena A, Dahl ML, Rootslane L, Sánchez Vega J, Eklundh T, et al. (1995). Patterns of drug Treatment of schizophrenic patients in Estonia, Spain and Sweden. *Br J Clin Pharmacol*, 40(5), 467–76.

Knapp M, Ilson S, David A. (2002). Depot antipsychotic preparations in schizophrenia: the state of the economic evidence. *Int Clin Psychopharmacol*, **17**(3), 135–40.

Knudsen P. (1985). Chemotherapy with neuroleptics. Clinical and pharmacokinetic aspects with a particular view to depot preparations. *Acta Psychiatr Scand Suppl*, **322**, 51–75.

Kovacs G. (2005). [Prescription of psychotropic drugs for schizophrenic outpatients in Hungary]. *Neuropsychopharmacol Hung*, **7**(1), 4–10.

Kreyenbuhl J, Zito JM, Buchanan RW, Soeken KL, Lehman AF. (2003). Racial disparity in the pharmacological management of schizophrenia. *Schizophr Bull*, **29**(2), 183–93.

Kuno E, Rothbard AB. (2002). Racial disparities in antipsychotic prescription patterns for patients with schizophrenia. *Am J Psychiatry*, **159**(4), 567–72.

Lambert T. (2007). *Introduction: Ten Years of Olanzapine in Australia*. Auckland: Adis International Press.

Lambert T, Brennan A, Castle D, Kelly DL, Conley RR. (2003). Perception of depot antipsychotics by mental health professionals. *J Psychiatr Pract*, **9**(3), 252–60.

Lambert T, de Castella A, Kulkarni J, Ong AN, Singh B. (2007). One year estimate of depot antipsychotic adherence and readmission in Australian community mental health settings [abstract]. *Schizophr Bull*, **33**, 485.

Lambert T, Singh B, Patel M. (2009). Community treatment orders and antipsychotic long-acting injections. *Br J Psychiatry*, **195**, S57–S62.

Lambert TJR. (2005). The use of depot antipsychotics in community psychiatry, PhD dissertation. University of Melbourne.

Lambert T, Kane J, Kissling W, Parella E. (2010). CERP – Centres of Excellence in Relapse Prevention. An international educational programme to enhance relapse prevention in schizophrenia [abstract]. *Schizophr Res*, **117**(2-3), 295.

Larsen EB, Gerlach J. (1996). Subjective experience of treatment, side-effects, mental state and quality of life in chronic schizophrenic out-patients treated with neuroleptics. *Acta Psychiatr Scand*, **93**, 381–8.

Lawson WB. (1996). The art and science of the psychopharmacotherapy of African Americans. *Mt Sinai J Med*, **63**(5–6), 301–5.

Lelliott P, Audini B, Duffett R. (2001). Survey of patients from an inner-London health authority in medium secure psychiatric care. *Br J Psychiatry*, **178**(1), 62–6.

Lexchin J, Mintzes B. (2008). Medicine reimbursement recommendations in Canada, Australia, and Scotland. *Am J Manag Care*, **14**(9), 581–8.

Lindström E, Widerlöv B, von Knorring L. (1996). Antipsychotic drug: a study of the prescription pattern in a total sample of patients with a schizophrenic syndrome in one catchment area in the county of Uppland, Sweden, in 1991. *Int Clin Psychopharmacol*, **11**, 241–6.

Lipsedge M. (1993). Mental health access: access to care for black and ethnic minority people. In A Hopkins, V Bahl (eds), *Access to Health Care for People from Black and Ethnic Minorities*. London: Royal College of Physicians, pp. 169–82.

Macpherson R, Alexander M, Jerrom W. (1998). Medication refusal among patients treated in a community mental health rehabilitation service. *Psychiatr Bull*, **22**(12), 744–8.

Magliano L, Fiorillo A, Guarneri M, Marasco C, De Rosa C, Malangone C, et al. (2004). Prescription of psychotropic drugs to patients with schizophrenia: an Italian national survey. *Eur J Clin Pharmacol*, **60**(7), 513–22.

Mark TL, Dirani R, Slade E, Russo PA. (2002). Access to new medications to treat schizophrenia. *J Behav Health Serv Res*, **29**, 15–29.

Mark TL, Palmer LA, Russo PA, Vasey J. (2003). Examination of treatment pattern differences by race. *Ment Health Serv Res*, **5**(4), 241–50.

McIvor R. (1998). The community treatment order: clinical and ethical issues. *Aust N Z J Psychiatry*, **32**(2), 223–8.

McLaren S, Cookson J. (1989). Community treatment orders for mental illness. *Lancet*, **2**(8677), 1457.

Meadows G, Singh B (eds.). (2001). *Mental Health in Australia: Collaborative Community Practice*. Melbourne: Oxford University Press.

Meise U, Kurz M, Fleischhacker WW. (1994). Antipsychotic maintenance treatment of schizophrenia patients: is there a consensus? *Schizophr Bull*, **20**(1), 215–25.

Misdrahi D, Verdoux H, Lançon C, Bayle F. (2009). The 4-point ordinal alliance self-report: a self-report questionnaire for assessing therapeutic relationships in routine mental health. *Compr Psychiatry*, **50**(2), 181–5.

Mond J, Morice R, Owen C, Korten A. (2003). Use of antipsychotic medications in Australia between July 1995 and December 2001. *Aust N Z J Psychiatry*, **37**(1), 55–61.

Morgan V, Castle D, Jablensky A. (2002). The use of psychopharmacological and other treatments by persons with psychosis. *National Survey of Mental Health and Wellbeing. Bulletin 4*. Canberra: Commonwealth Department of Health and Aged Care.

Muscettola G, Bollini P, Pampallona S. (1991). Patterns of neuroleptic drug use in Italian mental health services. *DICP, Ann Pharmacother*, **25**, 296–301.

Newton L, Rosen A, Tennant C, Hobbs C, Lapsley HM, Tribe K. (2000). Deinstitutionalisation for long-term mental illness: an ethnographic study. *Aust N Z J Psychiatry*, **34**(3), 484–90.

Oehl M, Hummer M, Fleischhacker WW. (2000). Compliance with antipsychotic treatment. *Acta Psychiatr Scand, Suppl*, **102**(407), 83–6.

Olfson M, Marcus SC, Ascher-Svanum H. (2007). Treatment of schizophrenia with long-acting fluphenazine, haloperidol, or risperidone. *Schizophr Bull*, **33**(6), 1379–87.

Olivares JM, Rodriguez-Morales A, Diels J, Povey M, Jacobs A, Zhao Z, et al.; e-STAR Spanish Study Group. (2009). Long-term outcomes in patients with schizophrenia treated with risperidone long-acting injection or oral antipsychotics in Spain: results from the electronic Schizophrenia Treatment Adherence Registry (e-STAR). *Eur Psychiatry*, **24**(5), 287–96.

Opolka JL, Rascati KL, Brown CM, Gibson PJ. (2003). Role of ethnicity in predicting antipsychotic medication adherence. *Ann Pharmacother*, **37**(5), 625–30.

Opolka JL, Rascati KL, Brown CM, Gibson PJ. (2004). Ethnicity and prescription patterns for haloperidol, risperidone, and olanzapine [see comment]. *Psychiatr Serv*, **55**(2), 151–6.

Owens, D, Harrison G, Boot D. (1991). Ethnic factors in voluntary and compulsory admissions. *Psychol Med*, **21**(1), 185–96.

Patel M, David A. (2005). Why arent depot antipsychotics prescribed more often and what can be done about it? *Adv Psychiatr Treatment*, **11**, 203–13.

Patel MX, Haddad PM, Chaudhry IB, McLoughlin S, Husain N, David AS. (2009). Psychiatrists use, knowledge and attitudes to first- and second-generation antipsychotic long-acting injections: comparisons over 5 years. *J Psychopharmacol*, doi:10.1177/0269881109104882.

Patel MX, Nikolaou V, David AS. (2003). Psychiatrists attitudes to maintenance medication for patients with schizophrenia. *Psychol Med*, **33**(1), 83–9.

Patel MX, Matonhodze J, Gilleen J, Boydell J, Taylor D, Szmukler G, et al. (2010). Community treatment orders, ethnicity, conditions and psychotropic medication: The first six months. *Eur Neuropsychopharmacol*, **20**(Suppl 1), S74–5.

Paton C, Lelliott P, Harrington M, Okocha C, Sensky T, Duffett R. (2003). Patterns of antipsychotic and anticholinergic prescribing for hospital inpatients. *J Psychopharmacol*, **17**(2), 223–9.

Pereira S, Pinto R. (1997). A survey of the attitudes of chronic psychiatric patients living in the community toward their medication. *Acta Psychiatr Scand*, **95**(6), 464–8.

Pinfold V, Bindman J, Thornicroft G, Franklin D, Hatfield B. (2001). Persuading the persuadable: evaluating compulsory treatment in England using supervised discharge orders. *Soc Psychiatry Psychiatr Epidemiol*, **36** (5), 260–6.

Power P. (1998). Outpatient commitment—is it effective? Doctor of Medicine Thesis, University of Melbourne, Australia.

Power P. (1999). Community treatment orders: the Australian experience. *J Forensic Psychiatry*, **10**, 9–15.

Price N, Glazer W, Morgenstern H. (1985). Demographic predictors of the use of injectable versus oral antipsychotic medications in outpatients. *Am J Psychiatry*, **142**, 1491–2.

Remington G, Adams M. (1995). Depot neuroleptic therapy: clinical considerations. *Can J Psychiatry*, **40**(Suppl 1), S5–S11.

Remington G, Shammi CM, Sethna R, Lawrence R. (2001). Antipsychotic dosing patterns for schizophrenia in three treatment settings. *Psychiatric Services*, **52**(1), 96–8.

Remington GJ, Prendergast P, Bezchlibnyk-Butler KZ. (1993). Dosaging patterns in schizophrenia with depot, oral and combined neuroleptic therapy. *Can J Psychiatry*, **38**(3), 159–61.

Ridley G. (1993). Community treatment orders. *Br J Psychiatry*, **163**, 417.

Rosenheck RA, Desai R, Steinwachs D, Lehman A. (2000). Benchmarking treatment of schizophrenia: a comparison of service delivery by the national government and by state and local providers. *J Nerv Ment Dis*, **188**(4), 209–16.

Rothbard AB, Kuno E, Foley K. (2003). Trends in the rate and type of antipsychotic medications prescribed to persons with schizophrenia. *Schizophr Bull*, **29**(3), 531–40.

Saha S, Chant D, Welham J, McGrath J. (2005). A systematic review of the prevalence of schizophrenia. *PLoS Med*, **2**(5), e141.

Sellwood W, Tarrier N. (1994). Demographic factors associated with extreme non-compliance in schizophrenia. *Soc Psychiatry Psychiatr Epidemiol*, **29**(4), 172–7.

Shi L, Ascher-Svanum H, Zhu B, Faries D, Montgomery W, Marder SR. (2007). Characteristics and use patterns of patients taking first-generation depot antipsychotics or oral antipsychotics for schizophrenia. *Psychiatr Serv*, **58**(4), 482–8.

Sim K, Su A, Ungvari GS, Fujii S, Yang SY, Chong MY, et al. (2004). Depot antipsychotic use in schizophrenia: an East Asian perspective. *Hum Psychopharmacol*, **19**(2), 103–9.

Simpson G. (1984). A brief history of depot neuroleptics. *J Clin Psychiatry*, **45**(5 Pt 2), 3–4.

Singh SP, Croudace T, Beck A, Harrison G. (1998). Perceived ethnicity and the risk of compulsory admission. *Soc Psychiatry Psychiatr Epidemiol*, **33**(1), 39–44.

Singh V, Hughes G, Goh SE. (1995). Depot clinic: consumers' viewpoint. *Psychiatr Bull*, **19**, 728–30.

Snowden, LR . (2003). 'Bias in Mental Health Assessment and Intervention: Theory and Evidence'. *Am J of Public Health*, **93**, (2) 239–43.

Svedberg B, Backenroth-Ohsako G, Lutzen K. (2003). On the path to recovery: patients' experiences of treatment with long-acting injections of antipsychotic medication. *Int J Ment Health Nurs*, **12**(2), 110–18.

Swartz, MS, Swanson JW, Wagner HR, Burns BJ, Hiday VA, Borum R. (1999). Can involuntary outpatient commitment reduce hospital recidivism?: Findings from a randomized trial with severely mentally ill individuals. *Am J Psychiatry*, **156**(12), 1968–75.

Swartz MS, Swanson JW, Wagner HR, Burns BJ, Hiday VA. (2001). Effects of involuntary outpatient commitment and depot antipsychotics on treatment adherence in persons with severe mental illness. *J Nerv Ment Dis*, **189**(9), 583–92.

Tan CH, Shinfuku N, Sim K. (2008). Psychotropic prescription practices in East Asia: looking back and peering ahead. *Curr Opin Psychiatry*, **21**(6), 645–50.

Tattan TM, Creed FH. (2001). Negative symptoms of schizophrenia and compliance with medication. *Schizophr Bull*, **27**(1), 149–55.

Tavcar R, Dernovsek MZ, Zvan V. (2000). Choosing antipsychotic maintenance therapy—a naturalistic study. *Pharmacopsychiatry*, **33**(2), 66–71.

Tognoni G and Italian Collaborative Study Group on the Outcome of Severe Mental Disorders. (1999). Pharmacoepidemiology of psychotropic drugs in patients with severe mental disorder in Italy. *Eur J Clin Pharmacol*, **55**, 685–90.

Ungvari GS, Chow LY, Chiu HF, Ng FS, Leung T. (1997). Modifying psychotropic drug prescriptions patterns: a follow-up survey. *Psychiatry Clin Neurosci*, **51**, 309–14.

Ungvari GS, Pang AH, Chiu HF, Wong CK, Lum FC. (1996). Psychotropic drug prescription in rehabilitation. A survey in Hong Kong. *Soc Psychiatry Psychiatr Epidemiol*, **31**, 288–91.

US Department of Health and Human Services. (2001). *Mental Health: Culture, Race, and Ethnicity—A Supplement to Mental Health: A Report of the Surgeon General*. Rockville, MD: U.S. Department of Health and Human Services, Substance Abuse and Mental Health Services Administration, Center for Mental Health Services.

Valenstein M, Copeland LA, Owen R, Blow FC, Visnic S. (2001). Adherence assessments and the use of depot antipsychotics in patients with schizophrenia. *J Clin Psychiatry*, **62**(7), 545–51.

Van Dongen CJ. (1997). Is the treatment worse than the cure? Attitudes toward medications among persons with severe mental illness. *J Psychosoc Nurs Ment Health Serv*, **35**(3), 21–5.

Vaughan K, McConaghy N, Wolf C, Myhr C, Black T. (2000). Community treatment orders: relationship to clinical care, medication compliance, behavioural disturbance and readmission. *Aust N Z J Psychiatry*, **34**(5), 801–8.

Warren B. (1995). Developing practice through clinical audit. *J Clin Effectiveness*, **3**, 151–4.

Weiden P, Glazer W. (1997). Assessment and treatment selection for 'revolving door' inpatients with schizophrenia. *Psychiatr Q*, **68**(4), 377–92.

Weil F. (1996). The broadened framework of compulsory interventions in the new Israeli law. Their practical consequences. *Med Law*, **15**(2), 233–9.

West JC, Marcus SC, Wilk J, Countis LM, Regier DA, Olfson M. (2008). Use of depot antipsychotic medications for medication nonadherence in schizophrenia. *Schizophr Bull*, **34**(5), 995–1001.

Wheeler A, Humberstone V, Robinson E. (2008). Ethnic comparisons of antipsychotic use in schizophrenia. *Aust N Z J Psychiatry*, **42**(10), 863–73.

Willcox DR, Gillan R, Hare EH. (1965). Do psychiatric out-patients take their drugs? *BMJ*, **5465**, 790–2.

Wistedt B. (1995). How does the psychiatric patient feel about depot treatment, compulsion or help? *Nord J Psychiatry*, **49**(Suppl 35), 41–6.

Woods SW, Sullivan MC, Neuse EC, Diaz E, Baker CB, Madonick SH, et al. (2003). Best practices: racial and ethnic effects on antipsychotic prescribing practices in a community mental health center. *Psychiatr Serv*, **54**(2), 177–9.

Xiang YT, Weng YZ, Leung CM, Tang WK, Ungvari GS. (2008). Clinical and social correlates with the use of depot antipsychotic drugs in outpatients with schizophrenia in China. *Int J Clin Pharmacol Ther*, **46**(5), 245–51.

Zhu B, Ascher-Svanum H, Shi L, Faries D, Montgomery W, Marder SR. (2008). Time to discontinuation of depot and oral first-generation antipsychotics in the usual care of schizophrenia. *Psychiatr Serv*, **59**(3), 315–7.

Ziguras S, Lambert TJ, McKenzie DP, Pennella J. (1999). The influence of clients ethnicity on psychotropic medication management in community mental health services. *Aust N Z J Psychiatry*, **33**(6), 882–8.

Ziguras S, Klimidis S, Lewis J, Stuart G. (2003). Ethnic matching of clients and clinicians and use of mental health services by ethnic minority clients. *Psychiatr Serv*, **54**(4), 535–41.

Chapter 11

The role of antipsychotic long-acting injections in current practice

Peter Haddad, Tim Lambert, and John Lauriello

Correspondence: peter.haddad@gmw.nhs.uk

Introduction

In this chapter we consider the role of antipsychotic long-acting injections (LAIs) in current practice. We start by highlighting the high prevalence of non-adherence with antipsychotics and its consequences in schizophrenia. This is crucial as it is the foundation on which the use of LAIs rests. We examine the benefits of LAIs as well as their disadvantages. Next we review the position of LAIs in schizophrenia treatment guidelines and address the question of when an LAI should be considered as a treatment option. Finally we examine some key clinical questions that relate to the use of LAIs and make some recommendations for future research. Some of these areas have been examined in previous chapters, and we will refer back to these as appropriate. However this chapter provides an opportunity to bring various elements together and provide a broader picture of the place of LAIs in current practice. For the most part we concentrate on schizophrenia given that published data on the use of LAIs in bipolar disorder are limited. As more data become available the role of LAIs in bipolar disorder and other chronic psychotic disorders will become clearer.

Poor adherence and its consequences

The high prevalence of poor adherence with oral antipsychotics in schizophrenia is the main rationale for using LAIs. Poor adherence is not unique to schizophrenia but is seen in many chronic medical disorders (Cramer & Rosenheck 1998) (see Chapter 1). A systematic review of medication non-adherence in schizophrenia, that included 10 studies, found a mean rate of non-adherence of 41.2% (Lacro et al. 2002). A later study by Valenstein et al. (2006) showed that nearly 40% of patients with schizophrenia had adherence problem in a given year and that the figure rose when a longer period was considered. It is worth reviewing this study in more detail as the findings are important. Antipsychotic adherence was assessed over 4 years in a cohort of approximately 34,000 patients with schizophrenia. Prescribing data were used to calculate the medication possession ratios (MPRs) for individual patients in each year. Patients were divided into three groups: those with consistently good adherence (MPRs > 0.8 in all 4 years), consistently poor adherence (MPRs < 0.8 in all 4 years), or inconsistent adherence. In each year 36% to 37% of patients were poorly adherent. Most patients (61%) had adherence difficulties at some point during the 4-year period showing that adherence is not a stable trait. Approximately 18% had consistently poor adherence, 39% had consistently good adherence, and 43% were inconsistently adherent.

Non-adherence may be intentional or unintentional. The former occurs when a patient deliberately stops or reduces the dose of his or her medication. This may be for various reasons that include a belief that medication is not needed to keep well, or that side-effects of medication outweigh any benefits, or because the patient does not want to rely on medication to keep well. Unintentional non-adherence occurs when doses of medication are missed but this is not deliberate. For example, the patient may forget to take medication, find the medication regimen complicated and difficult to follow, or run out of medication as he or she is late in collecting the next prescription. Adherence lies on a spectrum; at one end a patient stops medication totally, at the other end prescribed medication is taken consistently, and in the middle are patients who miss a varying number of doses, a phenomenon termed partial adherence. Non-adherence is often covert i.e. it is not known to the health professionals involved with the patient. This may be because the patient chooses not to disclose their true adherence, is not aware of it, or because the clinical team fail to inquire about it. Studies that compare electronic monitoring versus subjective reports of antipsychotic adherence in outpatients with schizophrenia show that clinicians, and patients, are poor at identifying non-adherence (Byerly et al. 2005; Velligan et al. 2007).

Poor adherence in schizophrenia can lead to relapse or, in patients who have not achieved remission, persistent symptoms, and both can have serious repercussions. These include costs to the patient as well as increased demands on services, especially as relapse frequently leads to hospitalization (Figure 11.1). Some evidence suggests that treatment responsiveness reduces with each relapse so that an increasing proportion of patients become refractory to treatment (Wiersma et al 1998). Whether this is a consequence of relapse or reflects the fact that patients with a more severe disease process have more frequent relapses is unclear. The social consequences of a relapse, for example the end of a relationship or the loss of a job, can have a serious effect on the patient's quality of life and self-esteem. If poor adherence is not recognized it can lead to inappropriate treatment decisions including the assumption that a patient is treatment resistant or requires a trial of a higher dose of the current antipsychotic. In practice there can be a bi-directional relationship between non-adherence and some of its 'outcomes' e.g. substance misuse and relapse can result from poor adherence but can also contribute to it. Often causality acts in both directions simultaneously so that a vicious circle is set up. For example, partial adherence can lead to relapse which in turn causes adherence to become poorer and so on.

Ascher-Svanum et al. (2006) reported on the relationship between adherence with antipsychotic medication and outcome in schizophrenia using data from a 3-year, prospective, observational study conducted in the United States. Patients were divided

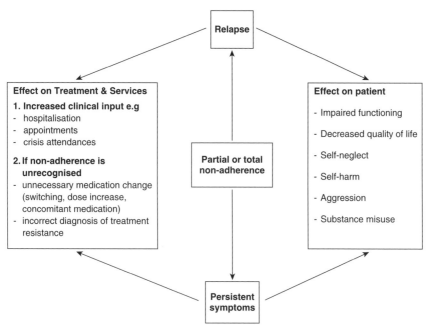

Fig. 11.1 Clinical consequences of non-adherence with antipsychotic medication.

into those who were adherent and non-adherent based on patient-reported adherence plus the medication possession ratio (percent of days with a prescription for any antipsychotic). Non-adherence was associated with a significantly increased risk of a range of adverse outcomes that included psychiatric hospitalization, use of emergency psychiatric services, arrests, violence, victimizations, poorer mental functioning, poorer quality of life, substance misuse, and alcohol-related problems. Non-adherence in the first year of the study predicted significantly poorer outcomes in the following 2 years.

Similar results were reported by Novick et al. (2010) using data from a 3-year, prospective, observational, European study of patients with schizophrenia (Schizophrenia Outpatients Health Outcomes [SOHO] study). Outpatients entered the study when they started or changed antipsychotics and were assessed at 6-month intervals thereafter. At each assessment, patients were divided into those who were adherent or non-adherent based on physician ratings. Regression models, correcting for baseline variables, investigated the associations between adherence and future outcome measures. Data for 6731 patients were analysed. Non-adherence was significantly associated with an increased risk of relapse, hospitalization, and suicide attempts and a decreased likelihood of achieving remission.

Many other studies have demonstrated that stopping antipsychotic medication or non-adherence is associated with a poorer outcome in schizophrenia. A 5-year prospective study of patients with a first psychotic episode showed that stopping medication increased the risk of relapse fivefold compared to those who continued medication

(Robinson et al. 1999). An analysis based on prescription refills showed that patients who missed 30 days or more of antipsychotic medication had a fourfold greater risk of deliberate self-harm than those without treatment gaps (Herings & Erkens 2003). Two studies using medication refill data showed that missing medication for 10 consecutive days was associated with a 1.5- to 2-fold increase in the risk of hospitalization (Law et al. 2008; Weiden et al. 2004). In one study the risk of rehospitalization increased as the length of time without medication increased (Weiden et al. 2004).

People with schizophrenia pose far more risk to themselves, in terms of deliberate self-harm and suicide, than risk to others. Nevertheless, a small number of people with schizophrenia commit violent offences, including homicide, when psychotic and poor adherence is associated with an increased risk of violence to others (Alia-Klein et al. 2007). In the United Kingdom, the National Confidential Enquiry into Suicide and Homicide concluded that only 5% of all perpetrators of homicide in England and Wales suffered from schizophrenia (Appleby et al. 2001). Only a small number of these cases, 14 in the 4 years between 1996 and 2000, were deemed preventable by mental health teams involved. Nevertheless, these 'preventable' cases were characterized by a high rate of non-adherence with treatment (54%).

Advantages and disadvantages of LAIs

The main advantage of an LAI is that covert non-adherence is impossible as both the patient and the treating team know exactly what dose of medication has been administered and when. In contrast adherence with oral medication is often unclear. Some patients tell their clinician that they are taking their medication but later, often after a relapse, disclose that they had stopped medication months earlier. Critics may argue that a patient who adheres poorly with oral medication will adhere poorly with an LAI too. This is undoubtedly true for some patients. Nevertheless several observational studies report adherence rates with LAIs that are high and, where there is a comparator group, superior to those seen with oral medication (Heyscue et al. 1998; Lambert et al. 2007; Olivares et al. 2009; Shi et al. 2007; Tiihonen et al. 2006; Zhu et al. 2008).

A large prospective observational study of patients with schizophrenia in the United States (the SCAP study) reported a 91% one-year mean medication possession ratio (MMPR) in those treated with an FGA-LAI (Shi et al. 2007). The MMPR was the number of days covered by the LAI divided by 365 days. A retrospective assessment of all patients prescribed an FGA-LAI over one year in two US centres found that 95% of injections were given on or near the due date (Heyscue et al. 1998). A one-year study in Australia showed a mean LAI adherence rate of 93% (Lambert et al. 2007). The continuation rate with medication can be regarded as an indirect measure of adherence. In Spain the e-STAR study reported a higher mean 2-year continuation rate for risperidone long-acting injection (RLAI) than for oral medication (81.8% vs. 63.4%) (Olivares et al. 2009). Patients in the SCAP study in the United States who were treated with one of two FGA-LAIs had a higher continuation rate than patients treated with the same two antipsychotics in oral form (Zhu et al. 2008). A study of patients with early schizophrenia in Finland found a higher continuation rate for perphenazine LAI compared to oral haloperidol (Tiihonen et al. 2006).

Not all studies find high adherence or continuation rates with LAIs. For example, Taylor et al. (2009) reported a high discontinuation rate for treatment with RLAI in London (84% over 3 years) but this may reflect various confounders. These include the study taking place soon after RLAI was licensed, when clinicians may have been less familiar with dosing and selecting patients who were suitable for treatment. In addition, LAIs tend to be prescribed to patients with complex histories and established poor adherence i.e. there is a prescribing bias that needs to be considered or adjusted for in observational data. Undoubtedly, the persistence of LAI use also depends on the local service delivery model and local micro-medical cultural attitudes to LAIs as discussed in Chapter 10.

In summary some, but not all, studies report relatively high adherence rates with LAIs. There is also a limited evidence base, discussed later in this chapter, for better long-term outcomes in terms of global improvement, relapse, or rehospitalization with LAIs compared to oral medication. Improved adherence with an LAI may reflect the regular contact and a positive relationship with the nurse who administers the LAI and the fact that if a patient misses an LAI it is immediately known about and is likely to be assertively followed up. In contrast, non-adherence with oral medication is often covert and so the clinical team cannot intervene when it occurs. The decision to use an LAI should usually result from shared decision-making, as discussed in Chapter 9, so that the patient understands the rationale for an LAI and is committed to the treatment plan. Without this involvement an LAI is unlikely to be successful in increasing adherence. There is no clear evidence that community treatment orders (CTOs) extend the length of LAI treatment, although many clinicians who use these orders believe this to be the case. Further research is required regarding the role of CTOs and LAI adherence (see Chapter 10).

Although the avoidance of covert non-adherence and improved adherence are the main reasons for using an LAI, these medications have other advantages (Table 11.1). If a person becomes non-adherent with an LAI then plasma antipsychotic levels will fall gradually, and relapse will be delayed compared to that seen after stopping oral medication. This provides a longer 'window of opportunity' in which to try and re-engage the patient. Some patients find an LAI more convenient than having to collect prescriptions and take daily medication. LAIs are also useful in differentiating the contribution of new medications to the patient's regimen. Sometimes psychotropic medication is added to an oral antipsychotic medication to gain better symptom control, when in reality the original antipsychotic is not being taken consistently. Having the primary antipsychotic established through a guaranteed route helps better understand the effects and side-effects of adjunctive medication. The optimal design of a study examining an adjunctive treatment, pharmaceutical or psychosocial, to an antipsychotic regimen should include an LAI. If a patient has a persistent high risk of impulsive overdoses e.g. owing to a personality disorder co-morbid with their schizophrenia, then an LAI may reduce the risk of overdose by minimizing the prescribed oral medication that the patient has access to.

It is often difficult to differentiate treatment refractory schizophrenia (i.e. a person who does not respond to a therapeutic dose of an antipsychotic) from a person who has not responded because they have not taken medication consistently

Table 11.1 Principal advantages and disadvantages of LAIs compared to oral medication

---

Advantages

1. Covert adherence is eliminated; overt non-adherence can be addressed
2. Early warning of non-adherence allowing closer monitoring
3. Adherence often better than with oral medication (assumes that prescribing has resulted from shared decision making and depending on service delivery model)
4. Some evidence of better long term outcomes e.g. lower relapse rates
5. Allows regular contact with administering health professional
6. Long apparent half-life means that missed doses may be less problematic and there may be delayed relapse after ceasing LAI
7. More convenient for some patients
8. Less risk of overdose
9. Allows differentiation of lack of efficacy and poor adherence
10. Bypasses the pharmacokinetic hurdles of absorption and first-pass hepatic elimination
11. Delivers a reasonably constant dose of antipsychotic throughout the injection cycle

Disadvantages

1. Understanding the pharmacokinetics and dosing requires specific LAI knowledge
   -Delayed time until steady state is reached
   -Clinical improvement may be delayed after dose increase
   -Elimination may take some weeks to months
2. Adverse effects may persist after stopping/reducing dose
3. Less scope for dynamic dose titration
4. Injection related adverse effects e.g. pain, nodules.
5. Some patients regard an LAI as indicating a lack of control or autonomy
6. There may be ethical concerns with involuntary use of LAIs under mental health acts, including the use of community treatment orders
7. Need for an organized community system to deliver LAIs
8. LAI storage, reconstitution, and administration may require special precautions, and/or training
9. SGA-LAIs have high acquisition costs

(Addington et al. 2009). An LAI allows differentiation. Various authorities have recommended that a trial of an LAI is considered, particularly where poor adherence with oral medication is suspected, before making a definitive diagnosis of treatment resistant schizophrenia and commencing treatment with clozapine (Conley & Buchanan 1997; Lambert 2006; Moore et al. 2007). For some treatment resistant patients, the LAI can allow the patient enough medication and clinical stability to agree to the logistics of taking clozapine.

The main advantage of LAIs, improved adherence, follows from their long apparent half-life that allows administration at 2- to 5-weekly intervals depending on the medication (see Chapter 2). The corollary is that there is a lag period after increasing the dose of an LAI before steady state plasma levels are reached and this means it is less easy to titrate the dose against a person's symptoms than with oral medication. This problem is particularly marked with RLAI as there is little appreciable drug release from the microspheres for the first 3 weeks after an injection. For the same reasons the resolution of adverse effects can be delayed for weeks or even months after reducing the dose of, or stopping, an LAI (see Chapter 3). The delay before reaching steady state is less of an issue than it may first seem as the main role of LAIs is in maintenance and not acute treatment. Also the time to reach steady state can be reduced by using loading doses, which are routinely recommended when starting paliperidone long-acting injection (PLAI) and olanzapine long-acting injection (OLAI). Finally in many patients on maintenance treatment with an LAI, breakthrough psychotic symptoms can be treated with a short course of the equivalent oral antipsychotic. If a long-term higher maintenance dose of medication is needed the LAI can be increased at the same time that oral supplementation is started and at a later date the oral medication gradually withdrawn. Unfortunately in practice the oral is sometimes not withdrawn leading to complicated issues, relating to polypharmacy, for the patient and treating team.

Pain and local injection site reactions are not usually a major issue with LAIs (see Chapter 3). The occurrence of post-injection syndrome alters the risk:benefit ratio for OLAI compared to other LAIs (see Chapters 3 and 6). In addition, the close monitoring and restrictions that post-injection syndrome places on the use of OLAI are likely to act as a major barrier to its widespread use. Some patients equate an LAI with losing control over their medication-taking. Engaging the patient, as discussed in Chapter 9, may allow the patient to reappraise their views. The person may then regard deciding to have an LAI, after several relapses on oral medication, as taking control of their illness rather than surrendering autonomy.

The effective use of LAIs requires an organized system of nursing staff to monitor and administer the medication, and this is not available in all countries. In countries such as the United Kingdom, Australia, and New Zealand, community mental health teams (CMHTs) are well established. Community psychiatric nurses are key members of CMHTs and are usually responsible for administering LAIs and monitoring the patients receiving this treatment. One reason for the lower use of FGA-LAIs in the United States compared to the United Kingdom is a lack of organized community services, although a number of negative attitudes towards LAIs may also be relevant (see Chapters 8 and 10). SGA-LAIs are relatively expensive and in some countries this may act as a barrier to use. In practice the drug treatment costs of schizophrenia form only a small part of the total treatment costs but unfortunately budgets are usually examined in isolation (e.g. separate budgets for pharmacy, community team, inpatient centre, crisis team, etc), which prevents an overview of treatment costs being taken.

LAIs and schizophrenia treatment guidelines

All major treatment guidelines for schizophrenia recommend that LAIs are considered when adherence with oral medication is either a concern or has been poor (Table 11.2). Some suggest that non-adherence should have led to recurrent relapses before an LAI is offered; these include the guidance from the American Psychiatric Association (Lehman et al. 2004a), the Patient Outcomes Research Team (PORT; Lehman et al. 2004b), the Canadian Psychiatric Association (2005), and the Royal Australian and New Zealand College of Psychiatrists (RANZCP 2005). This seems unduly restrictive. It implies that one waits until 'the damage has been done' before intervening. A physician will not wait until a patient had suffered a stroke before deciding to treat hypertension or hyperlipidaemia! In our opinion, concern about the possibility of poor adherence or poor adherence itself, without waiting for its consequences to manifest, is sufficient for a clinician to consider an LAI and discuss this with a patient. This is broadly consistent with the NICE (2009) schizophrenia guidance that states that an LAI should be considered when preventing covert non-adherence is a clinical priority i.e. the guidance does not specify that non-adherence has to have occurred or led to negative consequences before an LAI is considered.

Table 11.2 Recommendations for the use of antipsychotic LAIs in some recent schizophrenia guidelines

Schizophrenia guideline	Relation to non-adherence and/or relapse. Consider an LAI if:	LAI indicated if patient expresses preference for this treatment
American Psychiatric Association Guidelines (Lehman et al. 2004a)	Partial or full non-adherence leading to recurrent relapses	–
Canadian Clinical Practice Guidelines (Canadian Psychiatric Association 2005)	Non-adherence in multi-episode patients or those with persistent positive symptoms	–
NICE[a] Guidelines (NICE 2009)	Avoidance of covert non-adherence is a priority	yes
Patient Outcomes Research Team (PORT) treatment recommendations (Lehman et al. 2004b)	Frequent relapses on oral medication or a history of problems with poor adherence on oral medication	yes
RANZCP[b] (2005)	Despite psychosocial adherence interventions a patient repeatedly fails to adhere to necessary medication and relapses frequently	yes
Texas Medication Algorithm (Miller et al. 2004)	Inadequate adherence at any stage	–

[a] NICE: National Institute of Clinical Excellence.
[b] RANZCP: Royal Australian and New Zealand College of Psychiatrists.

Although the NICE guidance (2009) supports the use of LAIs in specific situations, LAIs, we feel it unduly emphasizes the avoidance of 'covert' non-adherence. In clinical practice, LAIs are useful in overcoming both overt and covert non-adherence. For example, the patient who forgets to take medication or who has a chaotic lifestyle that interferes with regular taking of medication but discusses this with his clinical team has overt non-adherence. Nevertheless, an LAI may be acceptable to such a patient and improve adherence.

The importance of patient choice is discussed in detail by Tacchi and colleagues in Chapter 9. Patient choice in treatment is a key principle of the health services in many countries, including the UK National Health Service (Department of Health 2004, 2009) and is highlighted in various schizophrenia guidelines (e.g. NICE 2009). Three of the guidelines in Table 11.2 state that patient preference is an appropriate reason to consider an LAI (NICE 2009; PORT; RANZCP 2005). Of course, patients can only exercise choice and express a preference if they have been provided with sufficient information about different medication strategies. Some patients may source this information themselves from friends, self-help groups, leaflets, or the Internet but most will rely on the key health professional they work with to provide this. As discussed by Patel in Chapter 8, a proportion of clinicians have negative views about LAIs, and this may prevent them offering impartial information and so limit patient choice.

A survey of UK psychiatrists showed that a significant proportion believed that FGA-LAIs were stigmatizing (36%), old-fashioned (27%), and coercive (17%; Patel et al. 2009a). One-third believed that patients always preferred oral medication over an LAI (Patel et al. 2009a). In contrast, studies investigating patient attitudes show that, among those currently prescribed an LAI, the majority either prefer an LAI to oral medication or have no preference. (Heres et al. 2007; Patel et al. 2009b; Walburn et al. 2001). A weakness with this data is that patients will tend to favour their current treatment, whether it be an oral medication or an LAI. Given this, the finding that 23% of LAI-naïve patients currently receiving an oral antipsychotic regarded an LAI as an acceptable treatment is illuminating (Heres et al. 2007). There is no doubt that some patients dislike the idea of an LAI. However, the assumption that patients always prefer oral medication, expressed by one-third of psychiatrists in the survey by Patel et al. (2009a), is unduly negative and shows that some psychiatrists are making inappropriate assumptions about their patients' preferences. Many patients are open to considering an LAI and of those established on this treatment most have positive views. The consequences of non-adherence, especially relapse, are so important for the patient's long-term well-being, it is key that treatment teams openly discuss their attitudes to the role of LAIs so that unstated biases do not impact on the treatment choices offered to patients.

When should an LAI be considered?

Traditionally LAIs have often been reserved for revolving door patients i.e. patients who have had multiple relapses owing to non-adherence with oral antipsychotic medication. Some commentators have recommended that LAIs be considered for a wider group of patients. For example, Kane et al. (1998) suggested that LAIs should be considered as an option for all patients who require maintenance treatment for schizophrenia. We broadly agree with this. More specifically there are three main indications to consider an LAI as a maintenance agent, namely when a patient expresses a preference for an LAI, when avoiding poor adherence is a priority, and when prior non-adherence with oral medication has led to relapse. All three indications appear in one or more of the schizophrenia guidelines previously reviewed (see Table 11.2). We will consider these indications in turn.

Patient preference may relate to an LAI being more convenient than taking daily medication or because the patient recognizes the potential benefits of an LAI in terms of improved adherence and a possible lower risk of relapse. Preference can be exercised only if an LAI is routinely considered as an alternative to oral maintenance medication. The second indication to consider an LAI is when avoiding poor adherence is a priority. This may be because a patient's previous history suggests that a relapse may be associated with high risks or because the individual stands to lose a great deal by non-adherence leading to a relapse. Patients with early psychosis fall into the latter group. Often these patients are high functioning, may be in education or have a job, and have not yet accrued the social and cognitive deficits that are seen in many chronic patients and that seem to partly result from repeated relapses. Alternative strategies to enhance or guarantee adherence should be considered alongside an LAI e.g. adherence therapy or the possibility of a relative supervising oral medication. The third indication to consider an LAI is when prior non-adherence with oral medication has led to relapse. In such cases it is essential to try and understand the reasons that underlie the poor adherence and to consider different ways to address this; an LAI is not the only solution to poor adherence or necessarily the right one. For example, if poor adherence is because of adverse effects then the solution may be to try and minimize these e.g. by dose reduction, simplification of the drug regimen, or a switch to a better tolerated oral antipsychotic. Other indications for considering an LAI include those with pharmacokinetic hurdles to achieving adequate antipsychotic levels with oral medication, those in whom oral side effects have presaged likely non-adherence, and in differentiating treatment resistance from non-adherence (Lambert 2006).

Whenever an LAI is considered the clinician needs to discuss the pros and cons of an LAI versus oral medication with the patient. The discussion should address the patient's beliefs about medication, situation, and goals. Clearly many factors require consideration when choosing a maintenance agent, including the effectiveness and tolerability of any currently prescribed oral antipsychotic. Often the decision about what antipsychotic drug to use will be more important than the choice of formulation. In many cases the patient and clinician will decide, appropriately, to use an oral antipsychotic as a maintenance agent. If a specific oral drug has been effective during acute treatment but is not available as an LAI, there will be a strong rationale to continue the current oral drug on a long-term basis. However if a patient and clinician decide that an LAI is an appropriate maintenance treatment at the time of a relapse, then it makes sense to use the equivalent oral drug for acute treatment and switch to the LAI if the oral drug shows effectiveness. Discussing LAIs more widely, even if the decision is not to prescribe one, facilitates the patient or clinician returning to consider an LAI in the future, if problems with adherence become prominent.

It is helpful to also consider when it is not appropriate to use an LAI as a maintenance treatment (Kane & Garcia-Ribera 2009). The most obvious case is when a patient has considered an LAI but decided that he or she does not want this form of treatment. Next are patients who have demonstrated good adherence with oral medication; such patients have little to gain by switching to an LAI. An LAI is not suitable for patients who are intolerant to, or have not shown a therapeutic response to, antipsychotics available as LAIs or patients with a severe needle phobia.

It is important not to avoid the issue that there is a small group of patients who require compulsion to take an LAI. These are generally people with recurrent psychotic disorders who do not want any form of medication, oral or LAI, and in many cases who want no contact with psychiatric services. If the person's illness poses a high level of risk to themselves or others, then the relevant mental health law in most countries will allow treatment to be enforced under a community treatment order (see Chapter 10; also Lambert et al. 2009). In such cases an LAI can be an important part of the treatment plan. The administration of an LAI under a community treatment order provides a clear reason for the patient to meet their psychiatric nurse. This can allow various issues to be discussed and hopefully a therapeutic alliance to be built up. Because adherence with an LAI is 'transparent', meetings with the nurse can be 'free' to focus on non-medication related matters. In contrast in high-risk patients who are prescribed oral medication, consultations may be spent repeatedly assessing adherence, or persuading the patient to take medication, and in some cases daily supervision of medication taking may be required. In difficult cases such as this, the patient and clinician may regard an LAI as the 'lesser of two evils'. Even when an LAI is enforced under a community treatment order, or under the appropriate mental health legislation for inpatients, it is important to try and engage the patient and explain the rationale for the prescribing decision.

Key issues and future research

In this section we consider some key issues related to the use of LAIs. We briefly review the current evidence and discuss how future research would be helpful.

Effectiveness of LAIs versus oral medication

If LAIs improve adherence in schizophrenia it follows that they should improve clinical outcomes and in particular reduce the risk of relapse and/or rehospitalization. In reality the evidence for this from randomized controlled trial is limited and not compelling although observational studies are generally more supportive. The Adams et al. (2001) Cochrane review included a meta-analysis of randomized controlled trials (RCTs) that compared FGA-LAIs and FGA oral medication in the treatment of schizophrenia. It found no difference in relapse rates between oral medication and LAIs, although LAIs increased the likelihood of global improvement (see Chapter 4). The lack of difference in relapse may reflect a design bias; the advantage of LAIs is likely to be most marked in non-adherent patients yet such patients are unlikely to enter a traditional RCT with its multiple exclusion criteria. Furthermore, RCTs of LAIs often include sham injections for those receiving oral medication and an equal visit interval for the oral and LAI arms.

In most busy psychiatric services, patients on oral maintenance medication will receive a lower visit or appointment frequency. As a result the oral comparator arm in many trials is not representative of usual clinical practice. The Adams et al. (2001) relapse data need to be considered alongside a recent open RCT that compared RLAI to oral quetiapine over 2 years in patients with schizophrenia or schizoaffective disorder (Gaebel et al 2010). The Kaplan-Meier estimate of time-to-relapse was significantly longer with RLAI. Relapse occurred in 16.5% of patients treated with RLAI and 31.3% of those treated with quetiapine.

With regard to observational studies, virtually all mirror-image studies show that FGA-LAIs (Davis 1994; Haddad et al. 2009; Chapter 4) and RLAI (e.g. Chang et al. 2009; Fuller et al. 2009; Taylor et al. 2008; Willis et al. 2010; Chapter 5) reduce inpatient days compared to prior treatment although the methodological weaknesses of this design need to be considered (Haddad et al. 2009). Prospective observational studies have produced variable results but selection bias may act against LAIs in this design (see Chapters 4 and 5; Haddad et al. 2009). Two prospective studies that reported better outcomes with LAIs than with oral antipsychotics are those of Tiihonen et al. (2006) and Olivares et al. (2009). Tiihonen et al. (2006) reported on a Finnish cohort followed up for a mean of 3.6 years after a first admission with schizophrenia. Compared to oral haloperidol, perphenazine LAI was associated with a lower relative risk of rehospitalization (68% reduction in fully adjusted relative risk). In contrast, oral perphenazine showed no difference to oral haloperidol in rehospitalization risk suggesting that it was the mode of administration rather than the drug per se that was responsible for the improved outcome with perphenazine LAI. Olivares et al. (2009) reported an analysis of e-STAR data from Spain that compared patients who started RLAI with a group that commenced oral risperidone or olanzapine. The continuation rate at 24 months was greater for RLAI than for the oral antipsychotic group (81.8% RLAI vs. 63.4% for oral antipsychotics, $p < .0001$). Compared to the pre-switch period, patients treated with RLAI showed a significantly greater reduction in the number and days of hospitalizations at 24 months than patients treated with oral antipsychotics.

The results of several ongoing prospective trials of oral versus LAIs are awaited. These include the National Institute of Mental Health PROACTIVE trial (Preventing Relapse in Schizophrenia: Oral Antipsychotics Compared to Injectables—Evaluating Efficacy), which compares RLAI to treatment with available oral atypical antipsychotics. This trial has enrolled more than 300 subjects in eight sites and will follow all subjects for a minimum of 18 months and many up to 30 months.

In summary the evidence from RCTs that LAIs lead to a lower relapse rate than seen with oral medication is weak and limited to one positive RCT (Gaebel et al. 2010) and one neutral meta-analysis (Adams et al. 2001). Most retrospective observational studies, and some prospective studies, report better long-term outcomes for LAIs (e.g. see Chapters 4 and 5; Davis 1994; Haddad et al. 2009; Olivares et al. 2009; Tiihonen et al. 2006). Further RCTs that compare LAIs to oral medication in terms of relapse are needed. Such trials need to be at least 18 months long and should have a pragmatic design to ensure that they recruit patients representative of those who are likely to receive an LAI in clinical practice i.e. those with frequent relapses and adherence problems.

LAIs and early psychosis

Surveys have shown that a sizeable minority of psychiatrists think that LAIs should not be used during the first episode of psychosis (Patel et al. 2009a). Such beliefs are not consistent with what many clinicians practice and what is known about the early course of the illness. Certainly LAIs should be avoided in patients who have *never* received antipsychotics because of the risk of a side-effect persisting should the patient not tolerate the drug. However, once it has been shown that a patient with first episode or early psychosis tolerates a specific antipsychotic then there is no reason why that drug should not be given as an LAI assuming that the patient and clinician make this choice. As first-episode patients have as high a rate of non-adherence as multi-episode patients, and given that many consider there to be a somewhat brief window of opportunity to ameliorate the course of illness by effective intervention, key services do consider LAI use within the first year of treatment (Addington et al. 2009). In further support of this, there have been several encouraging studies of the use of LAIs in early psychosis, as reviewed by Emsley and colleagues in Chapter 7. A long-term RCT of an LAI versus oral medication is required in this patient group.

Safety and adverse effects

There are few randomized trials that compare different LAIs. Studies that have compared different FGA-LAIs show no significant differences in efficacy or side-effect profiles with the possible exception of zuclopenthixol decanoate, which may be associated with fewer relapses, though this finding may reflect publication bias (Adams et al. 2001). Only one RCT has compared an FGA-LAI to an SGA-LAI (Rubio et al. 2006) and this showed less extrapyramidal symptoms with RLAI compared to zuclopenthixol decanoate. Extrapolating from data on oral antipsychotics it is unlikely that different LAIs will differ significantly in symptom efficacy in schizophrenia but one would expect marked differences in the risk of adverse effects, including extrapyramidal symptoms, weight gain, and metabolic abnormalities (Haddad & Sharma 2007; Leucht et al. 2009; Lieberman et al. 2005). It would be helpful to have head-to-head comparison studies of different LAIs to confirm this.

With the exception of the post-injection syndrome, injection-related adverse events do not appear problematic for most patients (see Chapter 3). Nevertheless there are individuals who find LAIs painful and those who develop local injection-site complications including tenderness, lumps, and nodules. A head-to-head comparison of two LAIs would help determine whether the risk of injection-site complications differs between agents. Further work is also needed to determine whether the incidence and severity of injection-site problems differ at the deltoid and gluteal sites.

Post-injection syndrome is a potentially serious adverse effect seen with OLAI (see Chapter 6). Virtually all current data on this syndrome have emerged from registration studies. The manufacturer is planning to conduct a multi-national phase IV prospective observational study of approximately 5000 patients treated with OLAI. This will assess the incidence and severity of post-injection syndrome in real world clinical practice and determine whether it differs to that seen during RCTs (Eli Lilly 2009).

Health economics

Potential costs savings are often put forward as an argument to support the use of LAIs. This is based on the fact that poor adherence with antipsychotics (Knapp et al. 2004; Sun et al. 2007) and relapse (Almond et al. 2004) are well-recognized cost-drivers in schizophrenia. If an LAI reduces relapse and hospitalization costs, compared to oral treatment, then it may be cost-effective even though its acquisition and administration costs will be higher than for most oral antipsychotics. However, a systematic review of the economic evidence for LAIs found few studies of relevance or quality (Knapp et al. 2002). The authors concluded that it was not possible to draw conclusions as to the cost-effectiveness of LAIs in the treatment of schizophrenia. Eight years on, this conclusion still holds. Although various studies suggest cost savings with LAIs none can be regarded as a high-quality economic analysis.

Decision modelling studies compare two or more treatments by simulating the clinical management of patients and the services they use and so estimate costs and outcomes of each treatment. Various modelling studies have found that under certain conditions an FGA-LAI (Glazer & Ereshefsky 1996; Hale & Wood 1996) or RLAI (Haycox 2005) is more cost-effective than the comparator, usually a specific oral antipsychotic. Modelling has the advantage of being able to reflect country-specific clinical practice and economic data. Its limitations include reliance on expert opinion, that can introduce bias, and in some cases lack of clarity regarding the methodology and assumptions of the model.

Virtually all mirror-image studies show that FGA-LAIs and RLAI are associated with reduced inpatient care compared to prior treatment (see Chapters 4 and 5 for a review of these studies). However, the methodological weaknesses of mirror-image designs need to be considered. These include regression to the mean, selection bias, and the impact of confounders (Haddad et al. 2009). These points apart, most mirror-image studies do not incorporate any economic analysis and those that do are rudimentary e.g. estimating drug acquisition costs and the cost of inpatient care but ignoring other costs such as outpatient attendances. A recent observational study reported cost savings for RLAI compared to oral antipsychotic treatment but methodological weaknesses include a limited estimate of costs and comparing the current treatment (either oral medication or RLAI) with a retrospective prior-treatment period (Olivares et al. 2008).

A high-quality economic analysis of alternative treatments should be based on data from a prospective study and consider all treatment costs e.g. drug acquisition costs, the cost of inpatient care, out patient and emergency contacts, and any additional overheads e.g. nursing time spent administering an LAI and specialist monitoring in the case of OLAI owing to post-injection syndrome. Treatment costs should be linked to a chosen outcome and ideally a range of outcomes should be considered. Different types of economic evaluation can be conducted depending on the outcome adopted e.g. cost-effectiveness analysis and cost-utility analysis (McKrone 2007). In cost-utility analysis a generic outcome measure is used, the most common of which is the quality-adjusted life year (QALY). This produces a cost-utility ratio for the treatment e.g. the cost per QALY gained. This enables the cost-utility of interventions in diverse disease areas to be compared e.g. cancer, ischaemic heart disease, and schizophrenia.

Such studies are important to those making funding decisions at a broad public policy level. To date there are very few cost-utility analyses in schizophrenia and, with the exception of the some modelling studies (e.g. Laux et al. 2005), none that relate to the use of LAIs.

In summary there are good reasons to suggest that in certain populations an LAI may reduce treatment costs compared to oral antipsychotic treatment and some preliminary data support this. However, a high-quality economic evaluation of an LAI against an oral comparator has not yet been conducted. Given the higher acquisition costs of SGA-LAIs compared to FGA-LAIs, future research should also compare cost-effectiveness in a head-to-head comparison of an FGA-LAI with an SGA-LAI.

Bipolar disorder

Poor adherence with medication is a common problem in bipolar disorder and as in schizophrenia the consequences can be devastating (Sajatovic et al. 2006). There is an emerging evidence base for the use of LAIs as maintenance agents in bipolar disorder, primarily to prevent relapse of mania. Taylor and Shajahan review the relevant studies for FGA-LAIs in Chapter 4. RLAI has recently been licensed for use in bipolar disorder in the United States, and Chue reviews the key trials in Chapter 5. Currently most bipolar treatment guidelines give little attention to LAIs. This reflects the paucity of published RCTs of LAIs in bipolar disorder. In addition, although several FGA-LAIs are licensed for use in schizophrenia and related psychoses, it was only in 2009 that an LAI (RLAI) was specifically licensed for use in bipolar disorder in the United States. Most bipolar guidelines pre-date this and guidelines tend to be reluctant to recommend the unlicensed use of medications. Despite this some bipolar guidelines support the use of an LAI in certain situations. For example, the NICE (2006) bipolar guideline does not recommend the routine use of LAIs but states that it is appropriate to consider an LAI if a patient was successfully treated for mania with an oral antipsychotic but then relapses secondary to non-adherence.

Further research in bipolar disorder is needed. There is, in particular, a need for observational studies to assess the effectiveness, as opposed to efficacy, of LAIs in bipolar disorder as well as studies of bipolar patients' attitudes to receiving their treatment in LAI form. Another key area is whether FGA-LAIs and SGA-LAIs differ in their effect on depressive episodes. Currently there is insufficient information to definitely answer this question. However, some studies suggest that FGA-LAIs may cause depressive relapse in bipolar patients (Bond et al. 2007). In contrast there is strong evidence that quetiapine is effective in treating and preventing relapse of bipolar depression with a weaker evidence base supporting the antidepressant effects of olanzapine (Derry & Moore 2007).

Summary and conclusions

Antipsychotic LAIs have been used for nearly 50 years but the last 8 years have seen the introduction of three SGA-LAIs, which increases the choice for patients and prescribers. This has been accompanied by an increase in the evidence base for LAIs, although in several areas it remains weak. The main rationale for the use of LAIs is the high rate of non-adherence in schizophrenia that leads to a wide range of patient, family, and societal costs. LAIs eliminate covert non-adherence by making adherence transparent. They can improve adherence rates although this requires that their prescribing is the result of a shared decision-making process with the patient and prescriber committed to the treatment. LAIs offer several other benefits that include regular contact with a health professional and greater convenience for some patients. Their main disadvantages are a lack of dose flexibility, a lag period between dose change and steady state plasma levels being achieved, the persistence of adverse effects after reducing or stopping an LAI, the occurrence of injection-related adverse effects and the fact that some patients do not like receiving antipsychotic medication by injection. In some countries service constraints may also limit their use.

Although all treatment guidelines for schizophrenia accept that LAIs have a role, several are unduly restrictive suggesting that LAIs are only offered after non-adherence has led to recurrent relapses. Given the high rate of non-adherence, its serious repercussions, and the importance of patient choice, we advocate a broader approach so that LAIs are considered routinely as a potential option for maintenance treatment in schizophrenia. The decision about the formulation, oral or LAI, and what specific drug is used will involve the patient and prescriber considering many factors apart from the potential benefits of an LAI in terms of convenience and improved adherence. In many cases it will be decided, appropriately, to use oral medication in the maintenance phase. The rationale for using an LAI is strongest in patients where non-adherence has recently occurred or its prevention is a priority. In these cases a more detailed discussion about an LAI should take place with the patient.

There are many areas where further research is needed. These include clarifying how LAIs compare to oral medication in terms of long-term health outcomes and health economics. Currently most data on LAIs relate to their use in schizophrenia but data are emerging on their role in bipolar disorder and further work is need here. In addition comparisons of different LAIs are needed in terms of efficacy, tolerability and safety, and ultimately, their effectiveness in allowing patients with complicated illness profiles to achieve a more solid and reliable recovery trajectory.

References

Adams CE, Fenton MKP, Quraishi S, David AS. (2001). Systematic meta-review of depot antipsychotic drugs for people with schizophrenia. *Br J Psych*,**179**, 290–9.

Addington J, Lambert T, Burnett P. (2009). Complete and incomplete recovery from first-episode psychosis. In HJ Jackson, PD McGorry (eds), *The Recognition and Management of Early Psychosis: A Preventive Approach*. Cambridge: Cambridge University Press, (pp. 201–21).

Alia-Klein N, O'Rourke TM, Goldstein RZ, Malaspina D. (2007). Insight into illness and adherence to psychotropic medications are separately associated with violence severity in a forensic sample. *Aggress Behav*, **33**(1), 86–96.

Almond S, Knapp M, Francois C, Toumi M, Brugha T. (2004). Relapse in schizophrenia: costs, clinical outcomes and quality of life. *Br J Psychiatry*, **184**, 346–51.

Appleby L, Shaw J, Sherratt J, Amos T, Robinson J, McDonnell R, et al. (2001). *Safety First: Report of the National Confidential Inquiry into Suicide and Homicide by People with Mental Illness*. Report for the Department of Health.

Ascher-Svanum H, Faries DE, Zhu B, Ernst FR, Swartz MS, Swanson JW. (2006). Medication adherence and long-term functional outcomes in the treatment of schizophrenia in usual care. *J Clin Psychiatry*, **67**(3), 453–60.

Bond DJ, Pratoomsri W, Yatham LN (2007). Depot antipsychotic medications in bipolar disorder: a review of the literature. *Acta Psychiatr Scand Suppl*, (434), 3–16.

Byerly M, Fisher R, Whatley K, Holland R, Varghese F, Carmody T, Magouirk B, Rush AJ. (2005) A comparison of electronic monitoring vs clinician rating of antipsychotic adherence in outpatients with schizophrenia. *Psychiatry Res*, **133**, 129–33.

Canadian Psychiatric Association. (2005). Clinical practice guidelines. Treatment of schizophrenia. *Can J Psychiatry*, **50**(13 Suppl 1),7S–57S.

Chang HC, Tang CH, Tsai SJ, Yen FC, Su KP. (2009). Long-acting injectable risperidone and hospital readmission: a mirror-image study using a national claim-based database in Taiwan. *J Clin Psychiatry*, **70**, 141.

Conley RR, Buchanan RW (1997) Evaluation of treatment-resistant schizophrenia. *Schizophr Bull*, **23**(4), 663–74.

Cramer JA, Rosenheck R. (1998). Compliance with medication regimens for mental and physical disorders. *Psychiatr Serv*, **49**(2), 196–201.

Davis JM, Matalon L, Watanabe MD, Blake L, Matalon L. (1994). Depot antipsychotic drugs. Place in therapy. *Drugs*, **47**(5), 741–73.

Department of Health. (2004). *The NHS Improvement Plan: Putting People at the Heart of Public Services*. London: Department of Health.

Department of Health. (2009). *NHS Constitution: A Consultation on New Patient Rights*. London: Department of Health.

Derry S, Moore RA. (2007). Atypical antipsychotics in bipolar disorder: systematic review of randomised trials. *BMC Psychiatry*, **7**, 40.

Eli Lilly. (2009). *Zyprexa olanzapine pamoate (OP) depot, Psychopharmacological Drugs Advisory Committee Briefing Document, 3rd January 2008*. http://www.fda.gov/ohrms/dockets/ac/08/briefing/2008-4338b1-03-Lilly.pdf (accessed 14 February 2010).

Fuller M, Shermock K, Russo P, Secic M, Dirani R, Vallow S, et al. (2009). Hospitalisation and resource utilisation in patients with schizophrenia following initiation of risperidone long-acting therapy in the Veterans Affairs Healthcare System. *J Med Econ*, **12**(4), 317–24.

Gaebel W, Schreiner A, Bergmans P, et al. (2010). Relapse Prevention in Schizophrenia and Schizoaffective Disorder with Risperidone Long-Acting Injectable Versus Quetiapine: Results of a Long-Term, Open-Label, Randomized Clinical Trial. Neuropsychopharmacology. In press.

Glazer WM, Ereshefsky L. (1996). A pharmacoeconomic model of outpatient antipsychotic therapy in 'revolving door' schizophrenic patients. *J Clin Psychiatry*, **57**(8), 337–45.

Haddad PM, Sharma SG. (2007). Adverse effects of atypical antipsychotic drugs: differential risk and clinical implications. *CNS Drugs*, **21**(11), 911–36.

Haddad PM, Taylor M, Niaz OS. (2009). First-generation antipsychotic long-acting injections v. oral antipsychotics in schizophrenia: systematic review of randomised controlled trials and observational studies. *Br J Psychiatry*, **195**, S20–8.

Hale AS, Wood C. (1996) Comparison of direct treatment costs for schizophrenia using oral or depot neuroleptics. *Br J Med Econ*, **10**, 37–45.

Haycox A. (2005) Pharmacoeconomics of long-acting risperidone: results and validity of cost-effectiveness models. *Pharmacoeconomics*, **23**(Suppl 1), 3–16.

Heres S, Schmitz FS, Leucht S, Pajonk F-G. (2007) The attitude of patients towards antipsychotic depot treatment. *Int Clin Psychopharmacol*, **22**, 275–82.

Herings RM, Erkens JA. (2003). Increased suicide attempt rate among patients interrupting use of atypical antipsychotics. *Pharmacoepidemiol Drug Saf*, **12**(5), 423–4.

Heyscue BE, Levin GM, Merrick JP. (1998). Compliance with depot antipsychotic medication by patients attending outpatient clinics. *Psychiatr Serv*, **49**(9), 1232–4.

Kane JM, Aguglia E, Altamura AC, Ayuso Gutierrez JL, Brunello N, Fleischhacker WW, et al. (1998). Guidelines for depot antipsychotic treatment in schizophrenia. European Neuropsychopharmacology Consensus Conference in Siena, Italy. *Eur Neuropsychopharmacol*, **8**(1), 55–66.

Kane JM, Garcia-Ribera, C. (2009). Clinical guideline recommendations for antipsychotic long-acting injections. *Br J Psychiatry*, **195**, S63–7.

Knapp M, Ilson S, David A. (2002). Depot antipsychotic preparations in schizophrenia: the state of the economic evidence. *Int Clin Psychopharmacol*, **17**(3), 135–40.

Knapp M, King D, Pugner K, Lapuerta P. (2004). Non-adherence to antipsychotic medication regimens: associations with resource use and costs. *Br J Psychiatry*, **184**, 509–16.

Lacro JP, Dunn LB, Dolder CR, Leckband SG, Jeste DV. (2002). Prevalence of and risk factors for medication nonadherence in patients with schizophrenia: a comprehensive review of recent literature. *J Clin Psychiatry*, **63**(10), 892–909.

Lambert, T. (2006). Selecting patients for long-acting novel antipsychotic therapy. *Australas Psychiatry*, **14**(1), 38–42.

Lambert T, de Castella A, Kulkarni J, Ong AN, Singh B. (2007). One year estimate of depot antipsychotic adherence and readmission in Australian community mental health settings [abstract]. *Schizophr Bull*, **33**, 485.

Lambert T, Singh B, Patel M. (2009). Community treatment orders and antipsychotic long-acting injections. *Br J Psychiatry*, **195**, S57–S62.

Laux G, Heeg B, van Hout BA, Mehnert A. (2005). Costs and effects of long-acting risperidone compared with oral atypical and conventional depot formulations in Germany. *Pharmacoeconomics*, **23**(Suppl 1), 49–61.

Law MR, Soumerai SB, Ross-Degnan D, Adams AS. (2008). A longitudinal study of medication nonadherence and hospitalization risk in schizophrenia. *J Clin Psychiatry*, **69**(1), 47–53.

Lehman AF, Lieberman JA, Dixon LB, McGlashan TH, Miller AL, Perkins DO, Kreyenbuhl J; American Psychiatric Association; Steering Committee on Practice Guidelines. (2004a) Practice guideline for the treatment of patients with schizophrenia, second edition. *Am J Psychiatry*, **161**(Suppl 2),1–56.

Lehman AF, Kreyenbuhl J, Buchanan RW, Dickerson FB, Dixon LB, Goldberg R, et al. (2004b). The Schizophrenia Patient Outcomes Research Team (PORT): updated treatment recommendations 2003. *Schizophr Bull*, **30**(2), 193–217.

Lieberman JA, Stroup TS, McEvoy JP, Swartz MS, Rosenheck RA, Perkins DO, et al.; Clinical Antipsychotic Trials of Intervention Effectiveness (CATIE) Investigators (2005). *N Engl J Med*, **353**(12), 1209–23.

Leucht S, Corves C, Arbter D, Engel RR, Li C, Davis JM. (2009). Second-generation versus first-generation antipsychotic drugs for schizophrenia: a meta-analysis. *Lancet*, **373**(9657), 31–41.

McCrone P. (2007). Health economic measures in schizophrenia research. *Br J Psychiatry*, (Suppl 50), S42–5.

Miller AL, Hall CS, Buchanan RW, Buckley PF, Chiles JA, Conley RR, et al. (2004). The Texas Medication Algorithm Project antipsychotic algorithm for schizophrenia: 2003 update. *J Clin Psychiatry*, **65**(4), 500–8.

Moore TA, Buchanan RW, Buckley PF, Chiles JA, Conley RR, Crismon ML, et al. (2007). The Texas Medication Algorithm Project antipsychotic algorithm for schizophrenia: 2006 update. *J Clin Psychiatry*, **68**(11), 1751–62.

NICE. (2006). Bipolar disorder: the management of bipolar disorder in children, adolescents and adults, in primary and secondary care. NICE clinical guideline 38. London: NICE.

NICE. (2009). Schizophrenia: core interventions in the treatment and management of schizophrenia in primary and secondary care (update) Clinical guideline. Date issued: March 2009; Replaces original guidance from December 2002 NICE. *NICE Clinical Guideline 82*. London: NICE.

Novick D, Haro JM, Suarez D, Perez V, Dittmann RW, Haddad PM. (2010). Predictors and Clinical consequences of non-adherence with antipsychotic medication in the outpatient treatment of schizophrenia. *Psychiatry Res*, **176**(2–3), 109–13.

Olivares JM, Rodriguez-Martinez A, Burón JA, Alonso-Escolano D, Rodriguez-Morales A; e-STAR Study Group. (2008). Cost-effectiveness analysis of switching antipsychotic medication to long-acting injectable risperidone in patients with schizophrenia: a 12- and 24-month follow-up from the e-STAR database in Spain. *Appl Health Econ Health Policy*, **6**(1), 41–53.

Olivares JM, Rodriguez-Morales A, Diels J, Povey M, Jacobs A, Zhao Z, et al.; e-STAR Spanish Study Group. (2009). Long-term outcomes in patients with schizophrenia treated with risperidone long-acting injection or oral antipsychotics in Spain: results from the electronic Schizophrenia Treatment Adherence Registry (e-STAR). *Eur Psychiatry*, **24**(5), 287–96.

Patel MX, Haddad PM, Chaudhry IB, McLoughlin S, Husain N, David AS. (2009a). Psychiatrists' use, knowledge and attitudes to first and second generation antipsychotic long-acting injections: comparisons over five years. *J Psychopharmacol*, in press (published online ahead of print 28 May 2009, doi: 10.1177/0269881109104882).

Patel, MX, deZoysa N, Bernadt M, David AS. (2009b) Depot and oral antipsychotics: Patient preferences and attitudes are not the same thing. *J Psychopharmacol*, **23**, 789–96.

RANZCP. (2005). Royal Australian and New Zealand College of Psychiatrists Clinical Practice Guidelines Team for the Treatment of Schizophrenia and Related Disorders. Royal Australian and New Zealand College of Psychiatrists clinical practice guidelines for the treatment of schizophrenia and related disorders. *Aust N Z J Psychiatry*, **39**(1–2), 1–30.

Robinson D, Woerner MG, Alvir JM, Bilder R, Goldman R, Geisler S, et al. (1999) Predictors of relapse following response from a first episode of schizophrenia or schizoaffective disorder. *Arch Gen Psychiatry*, **56**(3), 241–7.

Rubio G, Martínez I, Ponce G, Jiménez-Arriero MA, López-Muñoz F, Alamo C. (2006). Long-acting injectable risperidone compared with zuclopenthixol in the treatment of schizophrenia with substance abuse comorbidity. *Can J Psychiatry*, **51**(8), 531–9.

Sajatovic M, Valenstein M, Blow FC, Ganoczy D, Ignacio RV. (2006). Treatment adherence with antipsychotic medications in bipolar disorder. *Bipolar Disord*, **8**(3), 232–41.

Shi L, Ascher-Svanum H, Zhu B, Faries D, Montgomery W, Marder SR. (2007). Characteristics and use patterns of patients taking first-generation depot antipsychotics or oral antipsychotics for schizophrenia. *Psychiatr Serv*, **58**(4), 482–8.

Sun SX, Liu GG, Christensen DB, Fu AZ. (2007). Review and analysis of hospitalization costs associated with antipsychotic nonadherence in the treatment of schizophrenia in the United States. *Curr Med Res Opin*, **23**(10), 2305–12.

Taylor DM, Fischetti C, Sparshatt A, Thomas A, Bishara D, Cornelius V. (2009). Risperidone long-acting injection: a prospective 3-year analysis of its use in clinical practice. *J Clin Psychiatry*, **70**(2), 196–200.

Taylor M, Currie A, Lloyd K, Price M, Price K. (2008). Impact of risperidone long acting injection on resource utilization in psychiatric secondary care. *J Psychopharmacol*, **22**(2), 128–3.

Tiihonen J, Wahlbeck K, Lönnqvist J, Klaukka T, Ioannidis JP, Volavka J, et al. (2006). Effectiveness of antipsychotic treatments in a nationwide cohort of patients in community care after first hospitalisation due to schizophrenia and schizoaffective disorder: observational follow-up study. *BMJ*, **333**(7561), 224.

Valenstein M, Ganoczy D, McCarthy JF, Myra Kim H, Lee TA, Blow FC. (2006). Antipsychotic adherence over time among patients receiving treatment for schizophrenia: a retrospective review. *J Clin Psychiatry*, **67**(10), 1542–50.

Velligan DI, Wang M, Diamond P, Glahn DC, Castillo D, Bendle S, et al. (2007). Relationships among subjective and objective measures of adherence to oral antipsychotic medications. *Psychiatr Serv*, **58**(9), 1187–92.

Walburn J, Gray R, Gournay K, Quraishi S, David AS. (2001) A systematic review of patient and nurse attitudes to depot antipsychotic medication. *Br J Psychiatry*, **179**, 300–7.

Weiden PJ, Kozma C, Grogg A, Locklear J. (2004). Partial compliance and risk of rehospitalization among California Medicaid patients with schizophrenia. *Psychiatr Serv*, **55**(8), 886–91."http://www.ncbi.nlm.nih.gov/pubmed?term=%22Wiersma%20D%22%5BAuthor%5D" Wiersma D, HYPERLINK "http://www.ncbi.nlm.nih.gov/pubmed?term=%22Nienhuis%20FJ%22%5BAuthor%5D" Nienhuis FJ, HYPERLINK "http://www.ncbi.nlm.nih.gov/pubmed?term=%22Slooff%20CJ%22%5BAuthor%5D" Slooff CJ, HYPERLINK"http://www.ncbi.nlm.nih gov/pubmed?term=%22Giel%20R%22%5BAuthor%5D" Giel R (1998). Natural course of schizophrenic disorders: a 15-year followup of a Dutch incidence cohort. HYPERLINK."javascript:AL_get(this,%20'jour',%20'Schizophr%20Bull.');" \o "Schizophrenia bulletin. *Schizophr Bull*, **24**(1), 75–85.

Willis M, Svensson M, Löthgren M, Eriksson B, Berntsson A, Persson U. (2010). The impact on schizophrenia-related hospital utilization and costs of switching to long-acting risperidone injections in Sweden. *Eur J Health Econ* Jan 19. [Epub ahead of print].

Zhu B, Ascher-Svanum H, Shi L, Faries D, Montgomery W, Marder SR. (2008). Time to discontinuation of depot and oral first-generation antipsychotics in the usual care of schizophrenia. *Psychiatr Serv*, **59**(3), 315–17.

Index

Note. The following abbreviations are used in the index: FGA, first-generation antipsychotic; LAI, long-acting injection; SGA, second-generation antipsychotic

bipolar disorder (*cont.*)
  FGA-LAIs 80–5, 86–8, 255
  future research 255
  patient education 194, 201
  risperidone LAI 105, 112–13, 255
Brief Adherence Rating Scale 8, 9
Brief Evaluation of Medication Influences Scale 8
bromperidol decanoate 74

Calgary Depression Scale for Schizophrenia (CDSS) 149
Canada
  community treatment orders 226
  prescribing patterns 212–14, 226
Canadian Network for Mood and Anxiety Treatments (CANMAT) 113
Canadian Psychiatric Association 5, 14, 248
CATIE study 87, 106, 140, 178
cautions in LAI use 63–4
children and adolescents 95, 113
China, prescribing patterns 215–16
cigarette smoking 38, 49
class of medicine, as influence on prescribing pattern 228
clinical practice guidelines (CPGs) 229–30
clozapine
  adherence 10, 107
  epilepsy 64
  guidelines for treatment 6
  neuroleptic malignant syndrome 64
  patients' attitudes to 173
  prescribing patterns 229
  and risperidone LAI 117, 119
  treatment resistant schizophrenia 6, 10, 246–7
  withdrawal phenomena 53
coercion 175–6, 179
cognitive impairment, and adherence problems 10, 11
cognitive representation of illness model 188–90
cognitive techniques to improve adherence 202–3
  cognitive adaptation training (CAT) 13, 198
  cognitive behavioural therapy (CBT) 196–7, 199–200
communication in therapeutic relationship 187–8, 190
community care
  adherence 198–9, 209–10
  costs 12
community mental health teams (CMHTs) 247
community psychiatric nurses *see* nurses
community treatment orders (CTOs) 251
  and adherence 226–8, 245
  prescribing patterns 225–8
compliance *see* adherence
compliance therapy 13, 197, 199
concordance 6
contraindications to LAIs 63–4, 251

conventional antipsychotic LAIs *see* first-generation antipsychotic LAIs
coping strategies, cognitive representation of illness model 189
cost-effectiveness analysis 254
cost issues 253–5
  disadvantages of LAIs 247
  FGA- vs SGA-LAIs 86
  hospitalization 87, 117–18, 254
  non-adherence 12–13
  and prescribing patterns 229
  see also under specific antipsychotics
cost-utility analysis 254
crystal-based preparations 23–5, 27
  see also olanzapine LAI; paliperidone LAI
cultural issues
  adherence to medication 195–6, 199
  behavioural family therapy 195–6
  organizational culture, and prescribing patterns 225–6, 230
CUtLASS 87

deliberate self-harm 244
delivery route, as influence on prescribing pattern 228
deltoid injection site 60
  complications 58, 59, 253
  pain 57
  paliperidone LAI 136
  risperidone LAI 105–6
development phases of LAIs based on delivery mechanism 23, 24
disadvantages of LAIs 245–7
discontinuation of antipsychotics 3, 4, 5
  withdrawal phenomena 39, 40, 53–4
dorsogluteal injection site 60
doses, average 29, 30–1
dosette boxes 201–2
dosing equivalence
  FGAs 28–9, 30
  SGAs 26–7, 29–30
  see also under specific antipsychotics
Drug Attitude Inventory (DAI) 8, 170, 172
  risperidone LAI 114–15
duration of untreated psychosis (DUP) 2–3, 147
dyskinesias 39
dysphoria, neuroleptic 10

e-STAR study, risperidone LAI 102, 108, 110, 244, 252
  cost-effectiveness 118–19
  early psychosis 158
  hospitalization 115
early psychosis (EP) 145–6, 148, 158, 252–3
  consequences of relapse and partial response 147
  consideration of LAI use 250
  FGA-LAIs 149–50
  partial adherence and partial response 147